Praise for *Genetic Roulette*

"Unlabeled GMOs in our food works against what I have learned in my 30 years as a family farmer. Agriculture should be sustainable, food should be healthy and safe, and people deserve to know what they're eating."

—United States Senator Jon Tester

"When I worked at Monsanto, I warned both scientists and executives that our GM foods may cause disease, but no one was even willing to listen, let alone investigate the unpredicted side effects. For them, it was all about profit. Now our whole population is threatened by the serious dangers described in *Genetic Roulette*."

—Kirk J. Azevedo, DC

"The ability to introduce alien genes into a genome is an impressive technological manipulation but we remain too ignorant of how the genome works to anticipate all of the consequences, subtle or obvious, immediate or long-term, of those manipulations. This book validates the concerns of biotech critics who warned that our knowledge is too primitive to avoid unexpected and deleterious consequences."

—David Suzuki, geneticist, author of more than 30 books, awarded UNESCO prize for science

"The most comprehensive, well-documented, and highly readable exposé on the serious health dangers of GM foods."

—Samuel S. Epstein, MD, professor emeritus of Environmental Medicine, University of Illinois at Chicago School of Public Health and chairman, Cancer Prevention Coalition

"I used to test for soy allergies all the time, but now that soy is genetically engineered, it is so dangerous that I tell people never to eat it—unless it says organic. *Genetic Roulette* tells you why you must avoid genetically engineered foods to stay healthy."

—John H. Boyles, MD, ear, nose, and throat, and allergy specialist

"*Genetic Roulette* is dynamite. It totally explodes the complacency and apathy that has been allowing genetically engineered foods to creep into our food supply. Scientifically sound, this book is a must for anyone who wants to know the true answer to whether these foods are safe."

— John Robbins, author of *Healthy At 100, The Food Revolution,* and *Diet For A New America*

"Congratulations, Jeffrey Smith, for your courage. Thanks to your tireless investigations, we need wonder no longer why corporations spreading GMOs are so secretive, why they've spent hundreds of millions to keep us from even knowing which foods contain GMOs. They don't want us to examine the shoddy science, the suppressed evidence, and, most of all, the real health risks that GMOs present. Read *Genetic Roulette* not only to protect yourself and your family but to learn through this breath-taking story what all Americans need to do to reclaim our democracy and protect our planet."

— Frances Moore Lappé, author of *Democracy's Edge* and *Diet for a Small Planet*

"No danger to our health is greater than foods containing genetically modified organisms (GMO). Since knowledge is power, I recommend everyone who cares about their health and the health of the ones they love read the groundbreaking new book *Genetic Roulette* by Jeffrey Smith. As a health educator and parent of a young child, I will do everything within my power to keep these dangerous genetically modified foods out of the cupboards and refrigerators and off of the kitchen tables of those I care about. The best way I can do that is to strongly recommend the book."

—Jordan Rubin, founder and chairman, Garden of Life and *New York Times* best-selling author of *The Maker's Diet*

"*Genetic Roulette* is a MUST READ for all parents. Jeffrey's work highlights untested foods that have been introduced onto our children's plates without informed parental consent. The health risks associated with these new foods have the potential to impact every child in America—not just those with food allergies. The best gift that you could give your children is to read *Genetic Roulette*, as the knowledge you will gain is immeasurable and will last a lifetime—your child's."

—Robyn O'Brien, founder of AllergyKids and mother of four

"Jeffrey Smith raises serious questions concerning the production of genetically modified foods. Based on meticulous research, *Genetic Roulette* offers a chilling reminder that the effects of GM foods on human health are largely untested. And, whilst we cannot assume that all such foods are dangerous, nor can we assume that they are all safe, especially in the long term. Yet in the US there is no labeling, so these products sneak into households in many different foods. If you care about your health and that of your children, buy this book, become aware of the potential problems, and take action."

> —Dr. Jane Goodall, DBE, founder of the Jane Goodall Institute and UN Messenger of Peace, www.janegoodall.org

"Jeffrey Smith is the leading world expert in the understanding and communication of the health issues surrounding genetically modified foods. *Genetic Roulette*, which brings in original contributions by eminent scientists worldwide, makes it crystal clear that the American FDA should not be so cavalier about the potential dangers of these procedures."

> —Candace Pert, PhD, author of *Molecules of Emotion* and *Everything You Need to Know to Feel Go(o)d* and former Chief of the Section, National Institutes of Health

"Educators have a responsibility to be informed about the potential risks of genetically engineered foods. I urge school administrators to read *Genetic Roulette* and take preventive action to protect the long-term health of your students."

> —Richard Beall, PhD, director of the Carolina International School

"Jeffrey Smith's *Genetic Roulette* destroys the myth that genetically modified organisms are safe and will give sleepless nights to uncritical supporters of GMOs. It contains a wealth of up-to-date information, fully describing all the negative findings, mishaps, and actual harms caused by genetic engineering, as well as the possible health problems associated with this technology. In contrast to industry propaganda, all information in the book is fully referenced. I would advise all to grab a copy now and read it, regardless of which side they are on in the GMO debate. It is a real treasure and the most important GMO source book for policy makers, scientists, and the public."

> —Arpad Pusztai, PhD and Susan Bardocz, PhD, DSc, both formerly of the Rowett Institute, consultants to the Norwegian Institute of Gene Ecology, and experts on safety assessments on genetically modified foods

"The process by which crops are currently genetically engineered is a mutagenic process. Scientists still have much to learn regarding the ramifications of putting bacterial, viral or any other genes into the foreign context of a plant's DNA. For these and other reasons he describes in his book, Jeffrey Smith believes the products of this mutagenic genetic engineering process should be more thoroughly studied scientifically and more thoroughly regulated—especially by the FDA—before they are ever released into commerce. He's absolutely right."

> —Belinda Martineau, PhD, molecular geneticist, co-developer of the first commercialized genetically engineered food crop and author of *First Fruit: The Creation of the Flavr Savr™ Tomato and the Birth of Biotech Food*

"If a single short message could sum up this remarkably thorough, well-written, brilliantly designed, and deeply disturbing book about biotechnology in our food supply, it would be the quotation on the left side of page 120, "Biology is so much more complex than technology." This volume would never have needed to be written had scientists and corporations and regulators really believed that; none of them would have participated in the risky, ill-informed experiment that treated plant genomes like Lego pieces, and forced the results past its presumptive guardians and into the food supply. Because the experiment is ongoing despite it's riskiness, Jeffrey Smith has collected into a single volume all of the studies (disturbingly few) of the health effects of biotech foods in animals and humans, together with absorbing explanations of why dangerously negative effects may have occurred, some reasons why regulation has been utterly ineffective, and the technical flaws in industry studies that preclude their finding the unexpected (and inevitably expectable) side effects. Read this book, or skim it—a feat the author has enabled with a format that allows for scanning or thorough reading—then remove from your grocery list everything that might contain genetically modified ingredients, write to the people who process the products you've stopped buying, and help end the experiment."

> —Joan Dye Gussow, author of *This Organic Life*, professor emeritus of Nutrition and Education, Columbia University, former member Diet, Nutrition, and Cancer Panel of the National Academy of Sciences, and former member of Food Advisory Committee of the FDA

"When my 12 year old was born, GM foods weren't a part of the American diet. Today, about 30% of our cropland is planted with GMOs. Most Americans are uncomfortable with the idea of eating GM foods and yet eat them every day without knowing. It's time we made a choice! We ought either to satisfy ourselves with solid scientific answers to the concerns clearly laid out in *Genetic Roulette*—or we should change the way we eat. When shoppers in Europe and Japan acted on their convictions, GM foods were largely eliminated from stores."

> —Alan Greene, MD, pediatrician and author of *From First Kicks to First Steps*, www.DrGreene.com, awarded best health website 2005

Genetic Roulette

The Documented Health Risks of Genetically Engineered Foods

■

JEFFREY M. SMITH

Yes!
BOOKS

P.O. BOX 469
FAIRFIELD, IOWA 52556
888-717-7000

Trademark acknowledgements:
StarLink® is a registered trademark of Aventis Crop Science.
Roundup® and Roundup Ready® are registered trademarks of Monsanto Company.
NutraSweet® is a registered trademark of NutraSweet Property Holding, Inc.

Photos page 22, taken by Stanley Ewen, reproduced with permission.
Photo page 48, taken by Irina Ermakova, reproduced with permission.

Cover Illustration: George Foster
Text Formatting: Bluebird Graphics
Printed in the United States on partially recycled paper.
First printing; April, 2007.
10 9 8 7 6 5 4 3 2 1

Library of Congress Catalog-in-Publication Data
Smith, Jeffrey M.
Genetic roulette : the documented health risks of
genetically engineered foods / Jeffrey M. Smith.
p. cm.
Includes bibliographical references and index.
ISBN 978-0-9729665-2-8
1. Genetically modified foods. 2. Genetically
modified foods--Safety measures. 3. Genetically
modified foods--Government policy--United States.
4. Food--Biotechnology--Safety measures.   I. Title.

TP248.65.F66S65 2007   664
                 QBI06-600714

For information or individual orders, contact:
Yes! Books
P.O. Box 469
Fairfield, IA 52556
888-717-7000
www.seedsofdeception.com

Distributed to the book trade by:
Chelsea Green Publishing
P.O. Box 428
White River Junction VT 05001
802-295-6300
www.chelseagreen.com

Suggestions to Readers

This book is designed for three types of readers: the quick scanner, the casual reader who does not need technical data, and those wanting it all. Here are navigation tips so quick scanners and casual readers can skip the technical stuff.

Introductory material: The section leading up to part 1 gives important basics for everyone.

Part 1 (two-page spreads): Quick scanners can stick with the executive summary on the left page only. Casual readers will have to pick and choose among the explanations on the right, since they vary considerably in their level of technical detail.

Connecting the dots: This section integrates information from part 1 and is good for everyone.

Parts 2–4: For quick scanners, the headlines and subheads are sufficient to give you the big picture. Casual readers can get more substance and context by also reading the narrative. The indented excerpts provide examples and elaborations that casual readers may want to skip.

The **Conclusion** are for everyone, as are the lists of GM crops and foods in the **Appendix**.

To make the text easier for the casual reader, scientific jargon and technical details are often put into parentheses.

For updates, corrections, and an open debate on the material presented here, go to www.GeneticRoulette.com. We welcome scholarly responses to all aspects of this book. Please send to submit@GeneticRoulette.com.

Table of Contents

Foreword

This is *the* authentic book on genetic modification that the world has been waiting for. So much has been written about GM—some of it thoughtful and interesting, much of it mischievous or downright deceitful—but none of it systematic, authoritative, and comprehensive. What has long been needed is not more polemic, but the facts, the unvarnished detail that provides the evidence on which people can make up their own minds. This book is it.

For far too long this war between the pro- and anti-GM factions has been fought in a fog. The anti-group (independent scientists, environmentalists, and millions of small farmers) insisted there has been no systematic testing of GM crops or food, so we cannot be sure whether GM products are safe to eat or not. The pro-group (Monsanto, Bayer, Syngenta, and the other agribusiness majors, plus the US and UK governments) claimed that GM food was safe because there was no evidence to suggest otherwise, and there was no need to look for it because GM and non-GM crops were "substantially equivalent." This impasse, this non-dialogue between opposing camps, has now been broken by this book.

For the first time not only are the facts of adverse health problems associated with genetic engineering methodically set out, but the theory, which might account these episodes of mortality and morbidity, is also carefully presented. It has been too little realized that blasting genetically engineered DNA into a plant arbitrarily—like throwing darts into a haystack—disrupts a sequence of genes that has evolved over hundreds of millions of years so as to optimize the functioning of the organism and is bound to destabilize the biochemistry of the plant. We are still learning about the myriad of ways by which this crude insertion process can mutate or permanently turn genes on or off, alter RNA or proteins in plants, produce allergies or toxicities, or even trigger wider unpredictable impacts elsewhere in the genome.

So why isn't all this better known, or at least exhaustively investigated whenever damaging toxic consequences are discovered? This is where the dry revelation of unexpected biochemical reactions turns into an extraordinary exposition of the use of manipulation, concealment, and corruption for the preservation and enhancement of corporate power. Adverse GM reactions are almost never rigorously followed up, abnormal proliferation of cells—which might be a precursor of cancer—is ignored, evidence of horizontal gene transfer into gut bacteria or human DNA—which could cause long-term damage—is studiously ignored, and mortality data on animals fed GM crops is swept aside or suppressed.

How this can still happen, when the potential risks for human health are so great, lies at the heart of this book. It opens up the secret links between, on the one hand, the hugely powerful GM seed companies seeking to grasp the greatest cash bonanza of all time by cornering the world's food supply and, on the other, the governments led by the United States of many of the world's biggest countries and an international network of ministers, key officials and responsive scientists. It is this power nexus, unseen but ubiquitous, that overshadows the entire debate on GM, using every trick in the book, in the teeth of all the evidence, to protect the GM project from collapse. This book is the best exposure yet of these machinations.

The book brings together, for the first time, data culled from hitherto inaccessible sources. Evidence extracted via Freedom of Information Act requests and from a trawl through of previously unexplored industry submissions and government documents throws a new light on the symbiosis between the GM industry and the regulators who are supposed to represent the public interest. The case presented is absolutely a smoking shotgun that should stop in its tracks any dabbling with GM foods, whether by individual families, food companies, or indeed nations.

Genetic Roulette is a fitting sequel to Jeffrey Smith's earlier best seller *Seeds of Deception,* which has become the bible of the GM campaigner. Bibles make a great read, but are sometimes difficult to use as a reference to obtain needed information in a hurry. This book is now designed to fill that gap, and is clearly going to provide a new, powerful, easy-to-handle tool for policy-makers. I believe it will inspire leaders in many different arenas to take action based on the content—indeed it might even jerk the UK government out of their disregard for science, alerting us to the risks of GM.

Jeffrey Smith is one of the great campaigners of our age, a relentless pursuer of the truth, a fearless advocate in the corporate world of secret influence, and a ceaseless promoter of the public interest across the world. He is the modern David against the GM Goliath. This book may well provide the slingshot to change the global course of events this century.

—*Michael Meacher, MP, former UK government environment minister*

Acknowledgments

This book is the result of a worldwide collaboration of the leading experts on the risks of genetically engineered foods. Each section was reviewed by a minimum of three scientists and most were looked at by many more. I want to acknowledge and thank the many scientists who have generously given their time and expertise. Contributions ranged from simple fact checking to dozens of hours reviewing manuscripts or conferring with me about the details of genetic engineering, DNA, and physiology.

I thank the following contributors, as well as many others not listed who helped bring this work to fruition:

Thanks to experimental biologist Arpad Pusztai, PhD, formerly of the Rowett Institute, the top expert in his field of lectin proteins and one of the leading experts on GMO safety assessments; to biochemist and nutritionist Susan Bardocz, PhD, DSc, formerly of the Rowett Institute who has, with Arpad Pusztai, analyzed the full body of safety assessment research on GMOs; to molecular biologist and protein chemist Dave Schubert, PhD, professor at the Salk Institute for Biological Studies, whose scholarly articles have challenged fundamental safety assumptions of GM crops and highlighted gross inconsistencies and errors in the theories behind the technology; to molecular geneticist Michael Antoniou, PhD, of King's College London, who does human gene therapy research and understands intimately the shortcomings and unpredictable dangers of the technology.

Thanks to nutritional biochemist and epidemiologist Judy Carman, PhD, director of the Institute of Health and Environmental Research, who has carefully analyzed many safety assessments for GM crops and identified massive shortcomings and problems that expose the population to significant risk; to geneticist Joe Cummins, PhD, Professor Emeritus of Genetics, University of Western Ontario, the ravenous researcher and prolific critic of GM technology, who regularly points to the gross and subtle errors and inconsistencies behind the science of altering the DNA of food and crops; to molecular geneticist Jack Heinemann, PhD, director of the Centre for Integrated Research on Biosafety, who, with his colleagues, has documented how the lax safety assessment process used in Australia and New Zealand approves crops that are untested for their potential to create severe health problems.

My thanks to biologist Manuela Malatesta, PhD, researcher at the University of Verona, who, with her colleagues, identified significant and worrisome adverse effects of mice fed GM soy; to Sam Epstein, MD, professor emeritus of Environmental and Occupational Medicine at the University of Illinois School of Public Health, and chairman of the Cancer Prevention Coalition, who is a leading expert in the risks of dairy products from cows injected with genetically modified bovine growth hormone; to plant physiologist E. Ann Clark, PhD, at the University of Guelph, who exposes the gaping holes in the GM crop review process of Canada.

To geomorphologist and environmental scientist Brian John, PhD, who is a prolific and tireless dismantler of industry spin and regulatory shortcomings; to Jonathan Matthews, whose outstanding newsletter and archive at www.GMWatch.org has been an invaluable resource for the world; to geneticist Ricarda Steinbrecher, PhD, of Econexus, who has expertly articulated many risks of GM foods and the faulty assumptions used by the biotech industry to claim safety; to William Freese with the Center for Food Safety and formerly research analyst with Friends of the Earth, who has meticulously analyzed submission documents and other obscure works, which expose how industry has rigged research to avoid finding problems and how consumers continue to be placed at risk from faulty scientific arguments by the biotech industry and US regulators; to Jerry Rosman, an Iowa farmer who traced reproductive problems in his livestock to certain GM corn varieties, and who steadfastly presses for a proper scientific investigation.

Thanks to Warren Porter, PhD, of the University of Wisconsin and Caroline Cox, PhD, research director at the Center for Environmental Health, who are experts on the health impacts of pesticides; to agricultural economist Charles Benbrook, PhD, senior researcher at The Organic Center and former executive director of the Board on Agriculture of the US National Academy of Sciences, who has compiled the agronomic evidence on GM crops that contradicts claims of higher yields and reduced pesticides, among others; to biophysicist and geneticist Mae-Wan Ho, PhD, director of the Institute for Science in Society, whose prolific writings on the faulty science behind GMOs is a terrific resource; to Stanley Ewen, PhD, a consultant histopathologist at Grampian University Hospitals Trust, whose pivotal work with Arpad Pusztai revealed fundamental dangers of GM technology, and who continues to identify the health implications of the uncontrollable aspects of GM foods.

To Doug Gurian-Sherman, PhD, at the Union of Concerned Scientists and formerly a reviewer of the safety of genetically engineered crops with the Environmental Protection Agency, and science adviser on GM food safety to the Food and Drug Administration, whose detailed analysis of submittal documents to the FDA demonstrates how the regulatory system is not competent to protect the public from the health risks; to Brian Tokar, Biotechnology Project director at the Institute for Social Ecology and editor of outstanding anthologies on GMOs, who profoundly understands the complex social, political, environmental and scientific implications of this technology.

To Professor Giles-Eric Seralini, PhD, University of Caen, France, president of the Scientific Council of the Committee for Independant Research and Information on Genetic Engineering and member of two French commissions for GMO evaluation, and an expert panel for the European authorities, who has brought to light adverse reactions of animals fed GM crops and how European regulators approved crops based on unscientific and contradictory claims by biotech producers; to Kirk Azevedo, DC, who boldly left Monsanto after discovering that their products may be damaging the health of the population; to Ken Roseboro, publisher of *The Organic and Non-GMO Report*, who tracks the expanding market for non-GMO products, driven by consumer concerns worldwide; to Michael Meacher, MP, former UK minister of the environment, who is one of the most knowledgeable and articulate politicians on the topic of GM foods, and who refuses to be silenced about the risks and the politicization of science.

There are also numerous scientists to whom I am grateful for helping me fact-check reviews of their research or material within their area of expertise, including Irina Ermakova, PhD, a leading scientist at the Institute of Higher Nervous Activity and Neurophysiology of the Russian Academy of Sciences and the vice president of the Russian National Genetic Safety Association; US food law expert Steve Druker, JD, director of the Alliance for Biointegrity; biochemist Robert Mann, PhD, of the University of Auckland; reproductive toxicologist Barry Markaverich, PhD, associate professor of molecular and cellular biology at Baylor College of Medicine; microbiologist Mark Rasmussen, PhD, formerly with the USDA; plant natural products specialist Richard Firn, PhD, of the University of York; animal scientist Federico Infascelli, PhD, professor in Animal Nutrition at the Faculty of Veterinary Medicine of the University of Naples "Federico II"; professor of agricultural biochemistry Harry Gilbert of the University of Newcastle upon Tyne; pediatrician Jim Diamond, MD; plant physiologist Neil Carman, PhD; environmental biologist Michele Marvier, PhD, of Santa Clara University; Kavitha Kuruganti of the Centre for Sustainable Agriculture; veterinarian Dr Ramesh of ANTHRA; virologist Terje Traavik, PhD, director of the Norwegian Institute for Gene Ecology; Rick North, campaigner against rbGH with the Oregon Physicians for Social Responsibility.

Thanks to James Turner, Esq. for his legal advice and support. I extend deep appreciation to the JMG Foundation for their financial support for this book.

I express my love and appreciation for my family, including Nancy Tarascio, Morton Smith, Rick Smith, and Robynn Smith, who tolerated my absentee status over the past two years while I was perpetually "just about to finish" this book, as it expanded in size and scope. I am especially grateful to my wife Andrea, who helped us create a lifestyle supportive of my seven-day-per-week work schedule. Thanks also to the staff at the Institute for Responsible Technology, who are dedicated to exposing the risks of this technology and mobilizing resources to protect public health and the environment.

INTRODUCTION

Deceptions, Assumptions, and Denial—
Exposing the roots of genetically modified crops

When Kirk Azevedo accepted a Monsanto Company recruiter's offer in 1996 to sell genetically modified (GM) crops, it wasn't the pay increase that inspired him. It was the writings of Monsanto CEO Robert Shapiro that were his motivation. Shapiro had painted a picture of feeding the world and cleaning up the environment with his company's new technology. Kirk was fascinated by the idea of swapping genes between species, creating designer organisms that could reduce manufacturing waste, turning "fields into factories and producing anything from lifesaving drugs to insect-resistant plants."[1] When he visited Monsanto's St. Louis headquarters for new employee training, Azevedo shared his enthusiasm for Shapiro's vision during a meeting. When the session ended, a company vice president pulled him aside and set him straight.

"Wait a second," he told Azevedo. "What Robert Shapiro says is one thing. But what we do is something else. We are here to make money. He is the front man who tells a story. We don't even understand what he is saying."

Azevedo was jolted. His image "of helping and healing" the world through GM crops turned out to be a manufactured reality—a lie—crafted to gain public acceptance and to push products. Azevedo realized he was working for "just another profit-oriented company."

Helping the world is only one of several manufactured realities about GM crops, the most fundamental of which is that the foods are safe. The key source for this claim is the United States Food and Drug Administration (FDA). According to their 1992 policy on GM foods, **"The agency is not aware of any information showing that foods derived by these new methods differ from other foods in any meaningful or uniform way."** On the basis of that sentence, the FDA claimed that no safety studies are necessary and that "Ultimately, it is the food producer who is responsible for assuring safety."[2] Biotech companies thus determine on their own if their products are harmless. This policy set the stage for the rapid deployment of the new technology. The seed industry was consolidated, millions of acres were planted, hundreds of millions were fed, consumers and nations objected, laws were passed, crops were contaminated, billions of dollars were lost—and it turns out that sentence was a lie.

The FDA was *fully* aware that GM crops were meaningfully different. That, in fact, was the overwhelming consensus among "the technical experts in the agency." The scientists agreed that genetic engineering leads to "different risks"[3] than traditional breeding and had repeatedly warned their superiors that GM foods might create unpredictable, hard-to-detect side effects. They urged the political appointees who were in charge at the FDA to require long-term safety studies, including human studies, to guard against possible allergies, toxins, new diseases, and nutritional problems.

The scientists' concerns were kept secret in 1992, when FDA policy was put into place. But seven years later, internal records were made public due to a lawsuit and the deception came to

1

light. The agency's newly released 44,000 pages revealed that government scientists' "references to the unintended negative effects … were progressively deleted from drafts of the policy statement (over the protests of agency scientists)."[4] They further revealed that the FDA was under orders from the White House to promote GM crops and that Michael Taylor, Monsanto's former attorney and later its vice president, was brought into the FDA to oversee policy development. With Taylor in charge, the scientists' warnings were ignored and denied.

As a result, consultation with the FDA on GM food safety is a voluntary exercise, in which the agency receives summaries without data and conclusions without foundation. If the company claims that its foods are safe, the FDA has no further questions. Thus, GM varieties that have never been fed to animals in rigorous safety studies and probably *never* fed to humans at all are approved for sale in grocery stores.

In the mid-1990s, the UK government decided to institute what US leaders refused to—rigorous, long-term safety testing. They commissioned scientists to develop an assessment protocol for GM crop approvals that would be used in the UK and eventually by the EU. In 1998, three years into the project, the scientists discovered that potatoes engineered to produce a harmless insecticide caused extensive health damage to rats. The pro-GM government immediately canceled the project, the lead scientist was fired and the research team dismantled. The assessment requirements that were eventually adopted by the EU were a far cry from those that were being developed in the UK. The superficial testing schemes still have yet to meet the demands of the FDA's stifled scientists.

Industry is in charge of safety

Ironically, policy makers around the world gain confidence in the safety of GM crops because they wrongly assume that the US FDA has approved them based on extensive tests, and approvals everywhere rely on the developers to do safety studies on their own crops. Research does not need to be published and most is kept secret under the guise of "confidential business information." Very little data is available for public scrutiny. In 2003, for example, researchers reviewed published, peer-reviewed animal feeding studies that qualified as safety assessments. There were ten. The correlation between the findings and the funding was telling. Five studies "performed more or less in collaboration with private companies" reported no adverse effects. In the three independent studies, "adverse effects were reported." The authors said, "It is remarkable that these effects have all been observed after feeding for only 10–14 days."[5]

Biotech advocates claim that there is plenty of evidence for safety. In December 2004, for example, Christopher Preston did a database search of peer-reviewed animal feeding studies worldwide and came up with 41.[6] Although this is still an incredibly low number of papers by which to judge safety, according to Arpad Pusztai, an expert in feeding studies, Preston's list failed "to distinguish between a scientific study and an animal production exercise." The latter "may be of some value to commercial animal production but have limited scientific value."[7] When the commercial studies were removed from the list, it left only 18 (4 of which are in Russian or Chinese).

In October 2005, Wayne Parrot compiled 60 abstracts entitled, "General Safety and Safety Assessment of Specific Genetically Modified Crops from Scientific Journal Articles."[8] The list was presented to the minister for agriculture and food in the government of western Australia as evidence that sufficient research had been conducted to conclude that GM food was safe. According to an analysis by epidemiologist Judy Carman, "A review of these abstracts found that most were animal production studies. ... In fact, only nine abstracts could be considered to contain measures applicable to human health. The majority of these (six abstracts; 67%) found adverse effects from eating GM crops." Carman pointed out that several other studies with adverse findings had been omitted from the compilation. She concluded, "The list of abstracts therefore does not support claims that GM crops are safe to eat. On the contrary, it provides evidence that GM crops may be harmful to health."[9]

By the beginning of 2007, there were just over 20 peer-reviewed animal feeding safety studies on GM crops. Only a single human feeding trial has been published and there is no post-marketing surveillance on those eating GM foods. Trials funded or conducted by the GM crop producers, however, are consistently substandard. They typically fail to investigate the impacts of GM food on gut function, liver function, kidney function, the immune system, the endocrine system, blood composition, allergic response, effects on the unborn, the potential to cause cancer, or impacts on gut bacteria. In addition, the industry-funded studies have become notorious for using creative ways to avoid finding problems. They feed older animals instead of more sensitive young ones, keep sample sizes too low to achieve the statistical significance needed for proof in scientific studies, dilute the GM component of the feed, overcook samples, compare results with irrelevant controls, choose obsolete insensitive detection methods, limit the duration of feeding trials, and even ignore animal deaths and sickness. They've got "bad science" down to a science.

Genetic engineering creates wide-spread, unpredictable changes

The prevailing worldview behind the development of GM foods was that genes were like Lego blocks, independent pieces that snap into place. This is false. The process of creating a GM crop can produce massive changes in the natural functioning of the plant's DNA. Native genes can be mutated, deleted, permanently turned off or on, and hundreds may change their levels of expression. The inserted gene can become truncated, fragmented, mixed with other genes, inverted or multiplied, and the GM protein it produces may have unintended characteristics with harmful side effects.

To make this clear, we'll use the popular analogy comparing DNA to a book. The four bases that make up the genetic sequence are the letters in the book; the genes are special pages that describe characters called proteins. The common way people explain and promote genetic engineering is to say, "It is just like taking a page out of one book and putting it into another."

In reality, a book would look quite different after it had undergone genetic engineering. The inserted page (gene) may turn out to be multiple identical pages, partial pages, or small bits of text. Sections of the insert are misspelled, deleted, inverted, or scrambled. Next to the inserts, the story is often indecipherable, with random letters, new text, and pages missing. The rest of the book has also changed. There are now typos throughout, sometimes hundreds or thousands of them. Letters are switched, words are scrambled, and sentences are deleted, repeated, or reversed.

Passages from one part of the book, even whole chapters (chromosomes), may be relocated or repeated elsewhere, and bits of text from entirely different books can show up from time to time. Many of the characters in the story (proteins) now act differently. Some minor roles have become prominent, leads have been demoted and some may have switched roles from hero to villain or vice versa. And, if you get bored with this story, take the original book, insert another page—even the same one—and the changes will be completely different. Or stick with the original book and over time, it might actually rearrange the inserted page.

In addition to unintended changes in the DNA, there are health risks from other aspects of GM crops. When a transgene starts to function in the new cell, for example, it may produce proteins that are different than the one intended. The amino acid sequence may be wrong, the protein's shape may be different, and molecular attachments may make the protein harmful. The fact that proteins act differently in new plant environments was made painfully clear to developers of GM peas in Australia. They canceled their 10-year, $2 million project after their GM protein, supposedly identical to the harmless natural version, caused inflammatory responses in mice. Subtle, unpredicted changes in molecular attachments might have similarly triggered deadly allergic reactions in people if the peas were put on the market.

Even if the GM protein is exactly what is intended, there are still problems. For example, corn and cotton varieties are engineered to produce a pesticidal protein called *Bt*-toxin (from *Bacillus thuringiensis*). Because it is used in spray form by farmers, it was claimed to be harmless to humans. That's clearly wrong. People exposed to *Bt*-toxin spray had all sorts of allergic-type symptoms; mice that ingested *Bt* had powerful immune responses and abnormal and excessive cell growth; and *Bt* crops are being blamed for a growing number of human and livestock illnesses.

Another problem is that inserted genes may transfer from food into gut bacteria or internal organs. This possibility had been dismissed earlier based on the assumption that ingested genes are quickly destroyed by the digestive system. Not so. Animal studies demonstrate that ingested DNA can travel throughout the body, even into the fetus via the placenta. Transgenes from GM crops fed to animals have been found in the blood, liver, spleen, and kidneys. The only published human feeding trial on GM food verified that genetic material inserted into GM soy transfers into the DNA of our intestinal bacteria.

Now combine the two risks above and get a third. If the corn gene that creates *Bt*-toxin were to transfer into gut bacteria (like parts of the soy gene have been doing), it might turn our intestinal flora into living pesticide factories. A biotech proponent may argue that this is just speculation since there are no studies to show that *Bt* genes also transfer. But that is the point. There *are* no studies on *Bt* gene transfer to human gut bacteria—*period*. We don't know if this happens because no one is looking. Thus, biotech companies are gambling that this and many other untested dangers won't materialize. And so are regulators. And so are consumers. It's genetic roulette.

If results from the few animal feeding safety studies are any indication, then the odds are stacked against us. Lab animals tested with GM foods had stunted growth, impaired immune systems, bleeding stomachs, abnormal and potentially precancerous cell growth in the intestines, impaired blood cell development, misshapen cell structures in the liver, pancreas, and testicles, altered gene expression and cell metabolism, liver and kidney lesions, partially atrophied livers, inflamed kidneys, less developed brains and testicles, enlarged livers, pancreases, and intestines, reduced digestive enzymes, higher blood sugar, inflamed lung tissue, increased death rates, and higher offspring mortality. About two dozen farmers report that GM corn varieties caused their pigs or cows to become sterile, 71 shepherds say that 25% of their sheep died from grazing on *Bt* cotton plants, and others say that cows, water buffaloes, chickens, and horses also died from eating GM crops. Filipinos in at least five villages fell sick when nearby *Bt* corn was pollinating and hundreds of laborers in India report allergic reactions from handling *Bt* cotton. Soy allergies skyrocketed by 50% in the United Kingdom, soon after genetically engineered soy was introduced; and one human subject out of the few tested showed a skin prick allergic-type reaction to GM soy, but not to natural soy. In the 1980s, a GM food supplement killed about one hundred Americans and caused sickness and disability in another five to ten thousand people.

How do biotech companies deal with adverse reactions to their products? A cursory look at how Monsanto responded to adverse reactions from its toxic chemical PCBs (polychlorinated biphenyls) gives us some insight. In communication with the US Public Health Service, Monsanto claimed their experience "has been singularly free of difficulties." Their internal files[10] obtained from a lawsuit, however, reveal that this was part of a cover-up and denial that lasted decades. Company memos referred to liver disease, skin problems, and even deaths in workers associated with exposure. Monsanto's medical department wanted to prohibit employees from eating at the factory because research showed that PCBs "were quite toxic materials by ingestion or inhalation."[11] The US Navy refused the product because in their safety study, all exposed animals died.

Monsanto was aware that their industrial customers were mixing PCBs into coatings applied inside "potable water supply storage tanks," swimming pools,[12] and grain silos. In the latter case, Monsanto knew that high levels of PCBs ended up in the milk of cows fed the grain.[13] A Monsanto memo also acknowledged that "one million lbs/year" of PCBs were used in highway paints, and "through abrasion and leaching we can assume that nearly all of this ... winds up in the environment."[14] But Monsanto refused to warn consumers or protect the environment because, as an executive made clear in a 1970 memo, "We can't afford to lose one dollar of business."[15] The court fined the company $700 million.

Monsanto has brought this type of reckless denial into the field of GM foods. They have also added to their repertoire extensive bribery,[16] hijacking of regulatory agencies, and threats to reporters and scientists.

Kirk Azevedo experienced firsthand how the company responded to a potentially serious safety hazard in its GM cotton. In 1997, a few months after he was set straight by the Monsanto Vice President at headquarters, a company scientist told him that Roundup Ready cotton plants contained new, unintended proteins that had likely resulted from the gene insertion process. No safety studies had been conducted on the proteins, none were planned, and the cotton plants, which were part of field trials near his home, were being fed to cattle. Azevedo "was afraid at that time that some of these proteins may be toxic." Azevedo asked the PhD in charge of the test plot to destroy the cotton rather than feed it to cattle. He argued that until the protein had been evaluated, the cows' milk or meat could be harmful. The scientist refused.

He approached everyone on his team at Monsanto to raise concenrs about the unknown protein, but no one was interested. "Once they understood my perspective, I was somewhat ostracized," he said. "Once I started questioning things, people wanted to keep their distance from me. I lost cooperation with other team members. Anything that interfered with advancing the commercialization of this technology was going to be pushed aside."

Azevedo believed that Monsanto's irresponsible practices might devastate the health of consumers. "These Monsanto scientists are very knowledgeable about traditional products, like chemicals, herbicides, and pesticides," he said, "but they don't understand the possible harmful outcomes of genetic engineering."

He tried to blow the whistle. "I spoke to many Ag commissioners. I spoke to people at the University of California. I found no one who would ... even get the connection that proteins might be pathogenic, or that there might be untoward effects associated with these foreign proteins that we knew we were producing. They didn't even want to talk about it really. You'd kind of see a blank stare." Azevedo decided to leave Monsanto. He said, "I'm not going to be part of this disaster."[17]

Azevedo had witnessed an example of an assumption-based safety assessment. His colleagues *assumed* that the protein was safe, so they put it into the food supply without testing their assumptions. Similarly, scientists and regulators assumed that genes act as isolated units, produce only one protein, and are destroyed during digestion. They assumed that GM protein will act the same as before in new organisms, that *Bt*-toxin is harmless, and that disruption of the host DNA poses no concern. These and many other assumptions used as the basis of safety claims have been proven wrong. In spite of that, biotech proponents either adamantly repeat their now-obsolete arguments, or declare that it doesn't matter anyway—the crops are still safe.

But the converging lines of evidence in this book suggest, in fact, that GM crops are inherently dangerous and may be responsible for an unfolding health disaster. What is astounding, moreover, is the absence of research following up this mounting evidence and the continued dismissal of serious adverse reactions. It demonstrates a reckless disregard for safety by the biotech industry and by governmental bodies charged with regulating and ensuring the safety of their products.

How genetic engineering works and why it is not an extension of natural breeding

The discovery in the mid-1970s that scientists could transfer genes from the DNA of one species into that of another was heralded as a major scientific breakthrough. Plants, animals, and other organisms could now become equipped with genes they could never acquire naturally and exhibit traits not previously found in their species or even their kingdom.

Scientists have since worked on some interesting combinations. Spider genes were inserted into goat DNA, in hopes that the goat milk would contain spider web protein for use in bullet-proof vests. Cow genes turned pig skin into cowhides. Jellyfish genes lit up pigs' noses in the dark. Arctic fish genes gave tomatoes and strawberries tolerance to frost. Potatoes glowed in the dark when thirsty. Human genes were inserted into corn to produce spermicide. Pharmaceutical companies inserted genes into bacteria, turning them into living factories to produce drugs. And seed companies gave new traits to crops.

GM crops: Two traits in four crops by five companies in six countries

Five companies comprise the GM seed industry, known as Ag biotech. Monsanto is the largest, with their GM seed technology and traits accounting for 88% of the GM acreage planted in 2005. Due to its global shopping spree, it is now the largest seed supplier of both GM and conventional seeds. The other companies are DuPont, Syngenta, Bayer CropScience, and Dow. Together, these five companies own more than 35% of the worldwide seed market[18] as well as 59% of the pesticide market.[19]

There are four major GM food crops currently in commercial production—soybeans, corn, canola, and cotton. All are used to make vegetable oil, and soy and corn derivatives are used in most processed foods. There are also GM zucchini, crookneck squash, papaya, and alfalfa. GM tomatoes and potatoes were introduced but taken off the market. Also, Quest cigarettes contain GM tobacco.

Although Ag biotech promotes its technology as a solution to feed the hungry world, grow crops in the desert and boost nutritional value, the current generation of GM traits is a far cry from that promise. The single dominant GM trait is herbicide tolerance (HT). HT crops are engineered to survive an otherwise toxic dose of weed killer. Companies bundle their HT crops with their brand of herbicide. Roundup Ready crops can withstand Monsanto's Roundup herbicide (whose active ingredient is glyphosate). Liberty Link crops can tolerate Bayer's Liberty herbicide (active ingredient glufosinate ammonium). They are both broad spectrum herbicides—designed to kill all other plant life. When farmers buy HT seeds, they are also required to buy the company's corresponding herbicide.

The glyphosate in Monsanto's Roundup kills plants by inhibiting an enzyme (EPSPS) that is needed for producing key amino acids. Some scientists discovered bacteria in a chemical waste pond near the Roundup factory that survived in spite of the presence of the herbicide. They discovered that the bacteria's version of the enzyme inactivated glyphosate and thereby resisted inhibition. They found the gene that created this enzyme, modified it, and then placed it into the DNA of Roundup Ready crop varieties. Monsanto began commercialization of these crops in 1996 before their patent on glyphosate was due to expire in 2000. These crops, which now force farmers to choose Monsanto's brand of glyphosate, have effectively extended the company's dominance in the herbicide market. In addition, HT crops dramatically increase the use of herbicide,[20] which further contributes to the company's bottom line.

The second popular GM trait is a built-in pesticide. A gene from the soil bacterium *Bacillus thuringiensis*, or *Bt*, is inserted into corn and cotton DNA, where it produces pesticidal toxins in every cell.

About 68% of the crops are engineered to resist an herbicide, about 19% produce their own pesticide and 13% do both. The zucchini, squash, and papaya, which together comprise less than 1% of the GM crop market, are each engineered with modified viral genes designed to resist infection from a single type of plant virus.

There are six countries growing nearly all commercialized GM crops. The United States dominates production at 54%, followed by Argentina (18%), Brazil (11%), Canada (6%), India (4%), and China (3%).[21]

GM is not like natural breeding

Genetic engineering is a lot of things, but it is not sex. Michael Antoniou, a molecular geneticist who does human gene therapy, says genetic modification "technically and conceptually bears no resemblance to natural breeding." In normal sexual reproduction, genomes from both parents contribute thousands of genes to the offspring; these get sorted and expressed in a highly regulated and natural way. Plant breeders have worked with this system for thousands of years by selecting parents with desired characteristics, such as yield or disease resistance, in the hopes that the offspring express both. With genetic engineering, however, a single gene is removed from the DNA of one organism and forcibly inserted into another. This doesn't happen naturally.

A pig can mate with a pig and a tomato can mate with a tomato. But there is no way that a pig can mate with a tomato. Using genetic engineering, however, pig genes can be inserted into a tomato and vice versa. This transfers genes across the natural barriers that have separated species over millions of years of evolution.

Public relations firms of the biotech industry proposed that genetic engineering is just an extension of natural breeding. This idea is designed to promote acceptance, but is not scientifically defensible. Experts at the FDA, for example, repeatedly emphasized that GM technology and its effects are "different than [those] experienced by traditional breeding techniques." FDA microbiologist Louis Pribyl wrote, "The unintended effects cannot be written off so easily by just implying that they too occur in traditional breeding. There is a profound difference between the types of unexpected effects from traditional breeding and genetic engineering."[22] Compliance officer Linda Kahl said that by "trying to force an ultimate conclusion that there is no difference between foods modified by genetic engineering and foods modified by traditional breeding practices," the agency was "trying to fit a square peg into a round hole." She said, "The processes of genetic engineering and traditional breeding are different and according to the technical experts in the agency, they lead to different risks."[23]

In spite of the obvious differences, biologist David Schubert points out that GM advocates use arguments that are "not only scientifically incorrect but exceptionally deceptive. … The biotech industry misuses language to redefine scientific terms in order to make the GE process sound similar to conventional plant breeding."[24] Biochemist Robert Mann says, "One tawdry old argument we have heard since 1974, and can expect to hear again, is the claim that gene transfers occur naturally so GM is only hastening them. This line of talk is a smoke screen designed to obscure the fact that GM usually performs artificial transfers, which are not known to occur in nature."[25]

Another claim is that radiation and chemicals are regularly used on food crops to promote mutations (mutagenesis) and that the random changes that occur in the DNA are similar to those produced by genetic engineering. One GM advocate, for example, cited a manuscript[26] listing all of the registered crops in the world that have a mutagenized parent—2,275 varieties of 175 species. According to Schubert, however, the list included "flowers and many other non-food crops, and the vast majority are not now and never were used commercially."[27] In fact, only one food crop listed in the manuscript, the sunflower, was commercially grown in the United States. Furthermore, the methods are not comparable, but rather used as a smoke screen to divert attention from those elements unique to GM crops.

How to make a GM crop

To make a GM crop, scientists must identify the gene they want to use and analyze its sequence. Since bacteria produce certain amino acids using a different code than in plants, if the source gene is from bacteria, some of the codes will have to be changed.

On one end of the gene, engineers add a promoter sequence to switch it on. The most popular promoter used in GM crops (CaMV 35S) is designed to force the gene to constantly produce a high volume of protein. On the other end, a terminator sequence is attached, which tells the DNA, "The transgene ends here—stop reading." In addition, scientists add a marker gene, typically an antibiotic-resistant marker gene, which helps in a later step described below.

The combination of these sequences, called the gene cassette, is multiplied by the millions. To do this, the cassette is placed into a circular piece of bacterial DNA called a plasmid, which is also equipped to reproduce over and over again in bacteria. Prior to inserting them into plant cells, scientists these days usually remove the extraneous plasmid DNA and use only the gene cassette. Years ago, when most of the currently commercialized GM crops were engineered, the inserted sequences included extraneous DNA from the plasmid, along with the gene cassette.

The plant cells that receive the inserted gene are first grown in the laboratory using a specific nutrient medium. This process is called tissue culture and is highly mutagenic; that is, it creates many genetic changes in the plant cells that cannot be predicted or controlled.

There are two primary methods for performing the gene insertion. One method uses a bacterium (*Agrobacterium tumefaciens*) which, under normal conditions, infects a plant by inserting a specific portion of its own DNA into plant DNA. Once it is functioning in the plant genome, that specific sequence from the bacterium causes the plant to grow tumors. Genetic engineers, however, replace the tumor-creating section of the bacterial DNA with one or more genes. The newly-equipped bacterium "infects" the plant's DNA with those foreign transgenes instead. (The bacterium uses its circular "plasmid" DNA to infect plants.)

The second method of gene insertion uses a gene gun, or particle insertion method. Scientists coat millions of particles of tungsten or gold with gene cassettes and then shoot these into millions of plant cells. Only a few cells out of millions incorporate the foreign gene. Scientists speculate that both methods of gene insertion trigger a wound response in the plant cell, which helps its DNA integrate the foreign gene.

To select cells that have successfully integrated the gene cassette, scientists rely on marker genes. Antibiotic resistant markers, for example, are designed to confer resistance to a particular antibiotic that would otherwise kill the cell. Therefore, that antibiotic is applied to the cells after the gene insertion process. Those that survive are the ones that have the marker gene operating in their DNA. Most cells die.

The surviving cells are again grown using tissue culture, but the changed nutrient medium allows them to develop into plants. Once fully developed, researchers can multiply the desired transgenic line by planting the seeds or by making more clones through tissue culture of the plants' cells.

Each plant grown from separate gene insertions is unique. The location of the transgene in the host DNA and the consequences of that insertion are different with each insertion. That is why all the plants grown from a single insertion are referred to collectively as an "event," indicating that the integration of the transgene cassette is not repeatable or reproducible.

Thus, genetic engineering takes artificial combinations of genes that have never existed together, forcibly inserts them into random locations in the host genome and then clones the results; it is clear that the process differs from natural breeding. According to an article in *Biotechnology and Genetic Engineering Reviews*, "Traditional breeding methods are based upon natural reproductive processes and involve selection at the level of the organism [breeders choose which plants to cross], the precise orchestration of thousands of genes, relatively infrequent mutations, and products that have been selected for safe use over several thousand years. In contrast, GE crop technology abrogates natural reproductive processes, selection occurs at the single cell level [breeders choose which cell to clone], the procedure is highly mutagenic [causing DNA mutations] and routinely breeches genera barriers, and the technique has only been used commercially for 10 years. Furthermore, normal breeding never introduces a cassette of bacterial genes for drug resistance along with strong ... promoters to express foreign proteins at high levels in all parts of the plant."[28]

It's difficult to identify health problems from GM foods, even if widespread

One of the most unscientific and dangerous statements made by biotech proponents is that millions of people in the US have been eating GM food for a decade and no one has gotten sick. On the contrary, GM foods might already be contributing to serious, widespread health problems, but since no one is monitoring for this, it could take decades to identify.

Judy Carman, a former senior epidemiologist for the government of South Australia, describes the difficulties from a public health perspective.[29] "The first problem is to recognize that there is a new health problem in the community. Without full animal testing, we don't even know which diseases to look for in people." If GM crops created a *new* disease, it would not have an established surveillance system. In fact, most *existing* diseases do not have any effective surveillance systems in place, making it hard to identify a change.

Carman points out that, "The HIV/AIDS epidemic went unnoticed for decades, even though it created memorable secondary infections ... and had a focus in young gay men who tended to cluster geographically and see the same doctors. It was largely picked-up by chance ... even though there were by then thousands of HIV/AIDS cases worldwide."

Once a new disease (or increased incidence of an existing disease) is identified, it must be tracked to its cause. Carman says, "Anything that looks like an infectious disease usually results in an investigation by a state or local health authority. Anything else, for example, an increase in cancer, relies on someone, usually an academic, having an interest in the disease and applying in a competitive medical research grant system, for funding to do the investigation." That could take years. If a research effort is funded, "For an existing disease, existing hypotheses would be considered and tested before GM foods, creating a delay in finding the cause," says Carman.

"Then people would need to accurately remember what they had been eating. Most people cannot even remember everything they ate the day before." Moreover, GM foods in many countries, including the United States, are not labeled. Neither consumers nor manufacturers know how much GM content is in the food. "So how can an investigator properly investigate and hence expose the link between the GM food and the illness?" Carman concludes that it "may be almost impossible to prove that a GM food has caused a disease, even if there are thousands of cases."

Some of the difficulties of tracking a GM food's effects were witnessed when StarLink, a GM corn variety unapproved for human consumption, contaminated the US food supply. The concern was that the properties of StarLink's GM protein may trigger allergic reactions. But even with a recall affecting more than three hundred brands and a major disruption of US corn exports, the investigation mounted by the FDA to determine whether the food was allergenic was miserable.

The agency established only a passive monitoring system, contacting and testing only the tiny percentage of affected people who filed formal complaints with them. They never investigated the thousands of health-related consumer calls made to food companies, including those who were rushed to the hospital. The FDA also failed to contact health professionals or allergy groups around the country. It took them nine months to prepare an allergenicity test, but it was so poorly designed, the EPA's expert panel on allergies rejected its conclusions.

The deadly epidemic caused by the GM food supplement L-Tryptophan (see section 1.20) is another demonstration of the difficulty in tracking a problem. Even with five to ten thousand sick and about one hundred dead, the epidemic was almost missed. The reason it was discovered was that the disease was unique, acute, and came on quickly, and it still required some lucky coincidences.

Carman asks, "What would happen if a link were found between a GM food and human ill-health?" She points out that "experience with the tobacco industry indicates that affected industries tend to argue and lobby against evidence for lucrative plant products. This would be compounded by the political considerations and lobbying of many thousands of disaffected farmers whose livelihoods depended on growing the crops. . . . So, even if a GM food is found to cause harm, it may take many years of effort to remove it from the food supply."

"In short, with the level of current safety testing, if GM foods do cause human health problems, it will be very difficult to determine this, even though there may be many cases, and finding the cause and doing something about it may take decades."

Indeed, the European Commission acknowledged, "in the absence of exposure data in respect of chronic conditions that are common, such as allergy and cancer, there simply is no way of ascertaining whether the introduction of GM products has had any other effect on human health. … On the basis of existing research…it is impossible to know whether the introduction of GM food had had any human health effects other than acute toxic reactions."[30]

What is presented in this book

In the absence of large amounts of published data to evaluate the health risks of GM foods, we must draw from varied sources. We include published peer-reviewed journals, unpublished studies, case studies, medical reports, news reports, and eye-witness accounts. We also address theoretical concerns about GM foods based on scientific principles and question the assumptions used as the basis for approvals.

From an epidemiological standpoint, case studies, anecdotal evidence, medical and eye-witness reports, and news stories all have profound significance. They often provide the starting point for an investigation, which may include evaluating and defining patterns of illness, gathering corroborating evidence and analyzing health effects in relation to medical knowledge and scientific theories. This book documents repeating patterns of illness, corroborating evidence, and health reactions consistent with the known potential risks of GM foods.

Terms and concepts used throughout this book

This book is written for both non-scientists and scientists. A few terms that are used throughout the book that are necessary for everyone to understand are described below.

DNA (Deoxyribonucleic acid) is a long molecule found inside the cells of almost all living things. In plants, animals, and humans, it is found inside the **nucleus** of the cell. Most bacteria don't have **nuclei**, but their DNA is associated with the cell membrane.

The information in the DNA is inherited from parents and is made up of a chemical **sequence** containing combinations of four basic units (nucleotides) called **bases**. They are arranged in pairs, called **base pairs** along two opposing strands of DNA. The full code of the DNA for a particular type of organism is called a **genome**. The human genome contains about 3 billion base pairs or a total of 6 billion bases in the double-stranded DNA.

Functional units, which make up only a small percentage of the DNA in plants, animals, and humans, are sequences called **genes**. Genes **code for** proteins. In the human genome, genes comprise only about 3% of the DNA. The other sequences are **non-coding**. The number of genes in a genome varies a great deal. Humans have about 25,000 genes, but the exact number is still being determined.

When a gene is active or **expressing**, its code is reproduced or **transcribed** into separate **RNA** (ribonucleic acid) strands called **transcripts**. The transcripts can then be **translated** into **amino acids** according to a formula; specific combinations of three bases in the RNA determine which amino acids are produced. A connected sequence of amino acids make up **proteins**, including the type of proteins called **enzymes**. The amount of RNA and protein produced by a gene is its **level of gene expression** and the protein produced is the **gene product**.

[Please note that gene expression is not entirely linear, as presented above. Multiple genes often function as units, RNA and proteins can regulate genes, and some RNA can even make DNA.]

The terms **genetically modified (GM)** and **genetically engineered (GE)** are used interchangeably, referring to the use of **genetic engineering**, also known as **recombinant DNA** technology, which inserts genetic sequences into DNA. The method of insertion into plants can be with a **gene gun** or via bacterial infection using **agrobacterium**. The inserted gene is usually from a different species. It produces a **GM protein**. This protein is selected to confer a new **trait** for the **transgenic** organism into which it is placed. In addition to the **inserted gene**, other genetic materials are added to either inform the scientist that the insertion was successfully **integrated** into the **host's** genome or to help the **foreign gene** function properly in the new DNA. The term used to describe all the genetic material that is inserted is called **gene cassette,** or more commonly the **transgene** (although transgene can also refer to just the trait-carrying gene within the cassette.)

Mutations refer to deviations or errors in the genetic sequence that frequently lead to altered or mutated organisms.

GMOs are **genetically modified organisms**, i.e. organisms whose DNA has undergone gene insertion. They are also called **GEOs**, for **genetically engineered organisms**. If a GMO is used for food or to produce GM proteins used in food, the ingested product is called **GM food. Bio-**

technology refers to a broad set of technologies, which include genetic engineering. For convenience, however, we use the term **biotech companies** specifically to refer to agricultural biotechnology companies that develop and promote GM crops and GM food.

HT refers to herbicide tolerance. HT GM crops are given a trait allowing them to inactivate a particular herbicide and survive its application. It is also called **herbicide resistance**.

CaMV 35S is the Cauliflower mosaic virus 35 S promoter used to drive expression of transgenes in GM crops.

Antinutrients are compounds that decrease the nutritional value of food, usually by making a nutrient unavailable or indigestible.

Organizational abbreviations

FAO: United Nations Food and Agricultural Organization

WHO: World Health Organization

CAC: Codex Alimentarius Commission. The Commission, created in 1963 by FAO and WHO, develops food standards, guidelines and related texts

FDA: Food and Drug Administration, the US regulatory body in charge of food safety

EPA: Environmental Protection Agency, the US regulatory body in charge of environmental safety and the safety of pesticides, including the pesticides created by come GM crops

USDA: United States Department of Agriculture, the US body overseeing agriculture policy

FSANZ: Food Standards Australia and New Zealand, the regulatory body that approves GM foods

ANZFA: Australia New Zealand Food Authority, the previous name for FSANZ

ACRE: Advisory Committee on Releases to the Environment, a UK body that makes recommendations for GM crops approvals based on environmental considerations

ACNFP: The Advisory Committee on Novel Foods and Processes, a UK body that makes recommendations for GM crops approvals based on health considerations

EFSA: European Food Safety Authority, the EU-wide body that makes recommendations for GMO approvals to the EU Commission

"Context is crucial. Yet genetic manipulation of food ignores millions of years of evolutionary context, and that could have serious implications in the future. We aren't dealing with an insignificant change to our diets here, we're dealing with a revolutionary technology being used in our food supply—affecting us, future generations, and the ecosystems on which we depend."

—David Suzuki, geneticist

PART 1

The Documented
Health Risks
of Genetically Engineered
Foods

"If the kind of detrimental effects seen in animals fed GM food were observed in a clinical setting, the use of the product would have been halted and further research instigated to determine the cause and find possible solutions. However, what we find repeatedly in the case of GM food is that both governments and industry plough on ahead with the development, endorsement, and marketing [of] GM foods despite the warnings of potential ill health from animal feeding studies, as if nothing has happened. This is to the point where governments and industry even seem to ignore the results of their own research! There is clearly a need more than ever before for independent research into the potential ill effects of GM food including most importantly extensive animal and human feeding trials."[1]

—Michael Antoniou, molecular geneticist, King's College London

SECTION 1:
Evidence of reactions in animals and humans

Part 1 of the book is presented in a "who done it" sequence. Evidence of adverse health problems are described in section 1 followed by the theoretical reasons that might account for those problems, presented in subsequent sections. A common theme among the adverse effects in this section is that no matter where they were from—peer-reviewed journals, submissions to regulators, medical and news reports, or testimonies by those afflicted—they have not been adequately followed up. Rather, attempts to further study the problems are actively thwarted.

1 . 1

GM potatoes damaged rats

This is "a much better-designed study than the industry-sponsored feeding studies I have seen in peer-reviewed literature that deal with Round-Up Ready soybeans or Bt corn."[2]
—Michael Hansen, research biologist, Consumers Union

"To this day, the Lancet *study is the best designed and carefully controlled study of its type. Compared to industry studies, it is leagues apart."*
—Michael Antoniou, molecular geneticist, King's College London

1. Rats were fed potatoes engineered to produce their own insecticide.

2. They developed potentially precancerous cell growth in the digestive tract, inhibited development of their brains, livers, and testicles, partial atrophy of the liver, enlarged pancreases and intestines, and immune system damage.

3. The cause was not the insecticide, but in all likelihood was the process of genetic engineering.

4. GM foods on the market—which were created from the same process—have not been subject to such an extensive testing protocol.

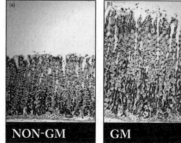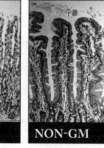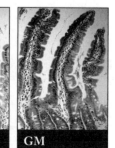

Stomach
The stomach lining of GM-fed rats showed proliferative cell growth.

Intestines
The excessive cell growth was also found in the wall of the small intestines (crypts) in rats fed GM potatoes.

In 1996, the UK government embarked on a plan to require long-term safety tests for all GM foods. A £1.6 million grant was awarded to a team of researchers to develop the testing protocol. Led by Arpad Pusztai of the prestigious Rowett Institute, the team developed a GM potato to use as the first "subject" for their studies. The potatoes were engineered with a gene from the snowdrop plant, which produces an insecticide called the GNA lectin.

Pusztai and his colleagues had conducted extensive research on the GNA lectin for nearly seven years and found it to be harmless to rats. Researchers anticipated that the potato engineered to produce the lectin would similarly be harmless. In fact, the UK government and the Rowett Institute were planning to commercialize the GNA potato and had contracts specifying how the royalties were to be divided.

To test the GM potato, six male rats were assigned to each diet category containing natural potato, natural potato with the lectin added, or GM potato. All three tests were repeated with raw, boiled, and baked potatoes, and rat diets were all supplemented to be complete and balanced. Rats were sacrificed at 10 or 110 days. This protocol had been approved in advance by the office that awarded the grant and similar designs had been used in more than 50 studies conducted at the institute. A 2003 article in *Nutrition and Health* described it as "remarkable in that the experimental conditions were varied and several ways were found by which to demonstrate possible health effects of GM-foods."[3]

The GM potatoes adversely affected virtually every organ system of young rats—with most changes found after just 10 days. Their brains, livers, and testicles were generally smaller, suggesting disruption of normal growth processes due to either malabsorption of nutrients or unknown toxins. White blood cells responded to a challenge more slowly, indicating immune system damage; and organs related to the immune system, including the thymus and the spleen, also showed changes. The animals had enlarged pancreases and intestines, and partial atrophy of the liver.[4] And in all cases, the GM potato created proliferative cell growth in the stomach and small and large intestines; the lining was significantly thicker than controls (see photo left).[5] Although no tumors were detected, such growth can indicate a precancerous condition.

By contrast, rats fed non-GM potatoes spiked with the lectin were relatively unaffected. Even when rats were fed more than 700 times the amount of the GNA lectin that the GM potato produced (in an earlier study), the impact did not approach that of the GM potatoes.[6] Thus, the damage

to the rats was not caused by the lectin, but apparently by "the genetic modification process itself."[7] This includes disruptions in the potato genome as well as unpredicted effects from additional genetic material inserted with the lectin gene (see section 2). **The study raised serious questions about the safety of *all* GM products on the market**, most of which were created with the same process and the same accompanying genetic material. Under normal circumstances, the disturbing results would be followed up to identify the cause of the problems, evaluate effects on female rats and test GM foods on the market to see if they were creating similar effects. It didn't happen.

Research stopped, scientists gagged

Pusztai was invited to speak on television about GM food. With permission from his director, he was interviewed and spoke generally about his research—without sharing details in advance of publication. For about two days he was a hero at his institute, which was besieged with press. Then, allegedly two phone calls were placed from the UK prime minister's office, forwarded through the receptionist to the director. The next morning, Pusztai was released from his job after 35 years and silenced with threats of a lawsuit, the 20-member research team was disbanded, and the project terminated. A part of the results was eventually published in the *Lancet*. In spite of the preliminary nature of the evidence, it remains the most in-depth GMO feeding study ever published.

Problems may be common in GM crops

It is sobering that these potatoes would have passed the tests used to get other GM crops approved. Stanley Ewen, who identified the proliferative cell growth in the rats, says that if GM foods create such effects in humans, they might increase the incidence of digestive system ailments such as Barrett's esophagus and stomach and colorectal cancer. We don't know if commercialized GM crops have this effect (although a rat study on experimental GM peas did show "significantly enlarged"[8] small and large intestines that might have resulted from excessive cell growth). Consumers in the United States and elsewhere are exposed to GM ingredients everyday, but usually in smaller doses and in more processed formats than was used in this potato study.

1 . 2

Rats fed GM tomatoes got bleeding stomachs, several died

"The data fall short of 'a demonstration of safety' or of a 'demonstration of reasonable certainty of no harm,' which is the standard we typically apply to food additives."[9]

—Robert J. Scheuplein, director, FDA's Office of Special Research Skills

1. Rats were fed the GM FlavrSavr tomato for 28 days.

2. Of the 20 rats, 7 developed stomach lesions (bleeding stomachs); another 7 of 40 died within two weeks and were replaced in the study.

Calgene genetically modified a tomato to look fresh for weeks after being picked. Called the FlavrSavr™, it was the first GM crop approved in the United States. Although the FDA did not require it, Calgene voluntarily conducted three 28-day rat feeding studies and sent the results to the agency in 1993. In one study, 7 of 20 female rats that ate one of the two FlavrSavr tomato lines tested developed stomach lesions—bleeding stomachs; none were found in the male rats or in the controls that ate natural tomatoes. The lab that conducted the study for Calgene wrote in its report, the "transgenic tomato dosed to females did suggest a possible treatment-related mild, focal necrosis of the glandular stomach."[10]

Internal documents show that FDA scientists were concerned. They repeatedly asked Calgene to provide additional data in order to resolve what they regarded as outstanding safety questions. The director of FDA's Office of Special Research Skills wrote that the tomatoes did not demonstrate a "reasonable certainty of no harm,"[11] which is the normal standard of safety. The Additives Evaluation Branch agreed that "unresolved questions still remain,"[12] and the staff pathologist stated, "In the absence of adequate explanations by Calgene, the issues raised by the Pathology Branch … remain and leave doubts as to the validity of any scientific conclusion(s) which may be drawn from the studies' findings."[13]

The full results of the study and the FDA's assessment were made public in 1999, when a lawsuit forced the agency to divulge its internal files. This permitted analysis by independent scientists, who discovered a footnote that had apparently gone unnoticed by the FDA reviewers. It said that 7 of the 40 rats fed the same FlavrSavr line as above died within two weeks and were replaced in the study. One each from the other groups (the other GM variety, a tomato control and a water control) also died and was replaced. The cause of death was summarily dismissed as husbandry error, but no explanation or additional data was provided.

In a follow-up study that Calgene claimed was a "repeat," they used tomatoes from a different batch and changed their preparation. Instead of using frozen concentrate, they freeze-dried the concentrate (which is a form not normally consumed by humans). This time, 1 male rat from the non-GM group of 20 and 2 females from the GM-fed group of 15 showed stomach lesions. Calgene claimed that the necrosis (dead tissue) and erosions (inflammation and bleeding) were "incidental." The FDA staff pathologist, however, responded that "the criteria for qualifying a lesion as incidental were not provided," and the disparity between the studies "has not been adequately addressed or explained."[14]

Furthermore, Calgene failed to look for problems in the intestines, did not increase the number of animals in the experiment, and did not use young (e.g. month-old) or pregnant animals, as is done with pharmaceutical studies. Tomatoes were grown at different locations and harvested at different times, which increases the variability of results. There were also large differences in rat starting weights (130 to 258 g for males and 114 to 175 g for females), which invalidates conclusions of finding no significant differences in weight gain, feed intake, or organ weights between GM and non-GM fed groups. According to a 2002 paper by Arpad Pusztai, the "study was poorly designed and executed and, most importantly, led to flawed conclusions." He said, **the claim that these GM tomatoes were as safe as conventional ones is at best premature and, at worst, faulty.**"[15]

Political appointees at the FDA claimed that the lesions were not related to the GM tomatoes. The bleeding stomachs, they argued, came from mucolytic agents in the tomato (i.e. agents that can degrade the protective layer of the stomach surface), food restriction, and/or stress resulting from animal restraint.[16] Others pointed to stomach lesions in water-fed controls in the follow-up study. But tomatoes are *not* known to contain mucolytic agents, the rats ate as much as they wanted, they were not restrained,[17] and there is no explanation why the GM tomato elicited more effect. Arpad Pusztai said the lesions in the water-fed rats observed in the follow-up study does not adequately account for the high rate of lesions observed in the GM tomato group in the previous study. He also points out, "in humans they could lead to life-endangering hemorrhage, particularly in the elderly who use aspirin to prevent thrombosis."[18]

Calgene chose not to commercialize the tomato line that was associated with the high rate of stomach lesions and deaths. The other FlavrSavr line was commercialized, but has since been taken off the market.

FDA criteria may be illegal

One internal FDA memo implied that the agency may have violated the law in its review. It stated, "It has been made clear to us that this present submission [FlavrSavr] is not a food additive petition and the safety standard is not the food additive safety standard. It is less than that but I am not sure how much less."[19] According to attorney Steven Druker, who is an expert in US food safety law, the FDA's own regulations clearly state that a lower standard cannot be applied in such instances.[20,21] After the FlavrSavr review, no company has presented such detailed GM test data to the FDA (see part 2).

1.3

Rats fed *Bt* corn had multiple health problems

> "I hear the argument of natural variability, but what struck me in this file is the number of anomalies. There are too many elements here where significant variations are observed. I never saw that in another file."[22]
>
> —Gerard Pascal, rapporteur Mon 863, French Commission for Biomolecular Genetics

1. Rats were fed Monsanto's MON 863 *Bt* corn for 90 days.

2. They showed significant changes in their blood cells, livers, and kidneys, which might indicate disease.

3. Although experts demanded follow-up, Monsanto used unscientific, contradictory arguments to dismiss concerns.

Measure	Function	Might indicate	Comments
Increased basophil counts	Creates histamine	Allergic reaction	Other *Bt* corn studies suggest possible allergic reactions.
Increased lymphocytes and white blood cells	Immune reactions to fight infections, etc.	Infections, various toxins, and diseases	Researchers omitted tests to see if the spleen, which creates lymphocytes, was affected.
Decreased reticulocytes	Becomes mature erythrocytes (red blood cells)	Anemia	5% variability is allowable. Astoundingly, Monsanto claimed a 52% decrease was "attributable to normal biological variability."
Decreased kidney weight	To clear waste products	Blood pressure problems	Any inadequacy in kidney function is potentially life threatening.
Increased blood sugar	Energy source	Risk for diabetes	A 10% elevation cannot be written off as insignificant, given the diabetes epidemic.

Mon 863 corn is designed to kill the corn rootworm. It contains a modified gene from a soil bacterium that produces Bt-toxin (Cry3Bb1). During a 90-day rat feeding trial, a group of 20 males and 20 females fed the corn developed multiple reactions. Changes included those typically found in response to allergies, infections, toxins, and diseases including cancer, anemia, and blood pressure problems (see chart at left). Also found were increased blood sugar levels, kidney inflammation, and liver and kidney lesions.[23]

The changes were statistically significant compared to the control group fed non-GM corn from the same "parent line," i.e., the same genetics as Mon 863 before genetic modification. Monsanto defended its corn's safety in ways that disregarded accepted scientific methods and principles:

1. Researchers used six additional control groups, each fed commercial corn varieties with quite different genetics. While such comparisons are suitable for commercial studies, they are entirely inappropriate for safety assessments (see part 3). Nonetheless, Monsanto claimed that since some reactions were no longer significant when compared to these other groups, the changes were unimportant.

2. For some results that remained statistically significant even when compared to these irrelevant controls, Monsanto claimed that the changes fell within a wide range of variability that is normal for rats. Thus, by ignoring the findings of their own study, they declared the reactions irrelevant. They stated, for example, that a 52% decrease in immature red blood cells (reticulocytes) was "attributable to normal biological variability," and a 10% increase in blood sugar levels was biologically insignificant. According to Arpad Pusztai, an allowance of 5% variability is the norm in food experiments and a 10% rise in blood sugar has serious ramifications, given the epidemics of obesity and diabetes. He said, "It is almost impossible to imagine that major lesions in important organs (kidneys, liver, etc.) or changes in blood parameters (lymphocytes, granulocytes, blood glucose, etc.) that occurred in GM corn-fed rats, is incidental and due to simple biological variability."

3. Several changes in the rats were *still* significantly outside the generous range that Monsanto defined as normal and acceptable. For some of these, they claimed that the health effects were not diet-related because the reaction was not consistent between males and females. This flies in the face of scientific understanding. Scientists studying cancer and endocrinology, for example, have established that genders can respond to toxins and disease quite differently.

4. Monsanto dismissed other findings on the grounds that the intensity of reactions was greater in rats fed a diet with 11% of the Mon 863 compared to the group that ate 33%. In endocrinology and immunology research, however, responses are not always consistent with dosage. A small amount of a hormone, for example, can cause a woman to ovulate, while a larger dose can make her infertile.

5. When other excuses failed, Monsanto claimed that with such a large study, one would expect lots of results to fall into the statistically significant category purely by chance. But Monsanto inflated the total number of results by doing a lot of irrelevant statistical tests. According to epidemiologist Judy Carman, this may hide significant results. "Their whole approach to the analysis would fail a basic statistics class." She adds that Monsanto also ignored findings that would make a *clinical* difference to the rats. "These may have reached statistical significance if Monsanto had used more rats," she said.

According to Gilles-Eric Séralini, who reviewed the study as part of the French Commission for Biomolecular Genetics, "Monsanto contradicts itself. The first time around, their studies explain, in a rather amusing manner by the way, that there are 'significant effects without a pathological significance,' and the second time around, their studies say that the effects observed are no longer significant. On top of that, the file was sliced up by examining the problems separately and not in their entirety, which is unacceptable."[24] Seralini says that the response by the rats was similar to reactions caused by pesticides. Although the Bt-toxin is a pesticide, he points out that animal research on pesticide-producing corn is nowhere near as thorough as that required for approval of pesticides.

In addition to criticizing Monsanto for statistical sleight-of-hand, scientists condemned the study as poorly designed and below the standards typically required for publication (see part 3). Follow-up studies on these serious findings were demanded from organizations worldwide. None have been conducted and the corn is approved.

1 . 4

Mice fed GM *Bt* potatoes had intestinal damage

"*Mice fed the delta-endotoxin had hyperplasia and other changes which may signal future cancer.*"

— Judy Carman,
nutrional biochemist and
epidemiologist, director,
Institute of Health and
Environmental Research

1. Mice were fed either GM potatoes engineered to produce the *Bt*-toxin or natural potatoes spiked with *Bt*-toxin.

2. Both diets created abnormal and excessive cell growth in the lower part of their small intestine (ileum).

3. Similar damage to the human small intestine might result in incontinence or flu-like symptoms, and may be precancerous.

4. This study overturns the assumptions that *Bt*-toxin is destroyed during digestion and is not biologically active in mammals.

egulators have allowed *Bt* food crops onto the market based on the assumption that the *Bt*-toxin will not survive digestion in the stomach. They further contend that even if some portion did survive, since "there are no receptors on the surface of mammalian intestinal cells for the [*Bt*] proteins,"[25] the toxin would not react with mammals. The results of this mouse study illustrate that *Bt*-toxin *can* survive digestion and *can* damage mammalian cells. (The ability for *Bt*-toxin to survive and interact with the mouse gut was also demonstrated in subsequent research, in which the toxin (Cry1Ac) bound with surface material in the middle section of the intestine (jejunum).)[26]

Groups of five one-month old male mice were fed for two weeks on either GM *Bt* potatoes, non-GM potatoes mixed with *Bt*-toxin, or non-GM potatoes without *Bt*.[27] Using light and electron microscopes, researchers examined just one portion of the mouse gut, the lower part of their small intestine (ileum). The mice fed GM potatoes or *Bt*-toxin showed significant disruption in the structure and size of their cells. Some cells were damaged, broken off, abnormally shaped, swollen, or had multiple nuclei.

While both of these groups showed statistically significant changes, damage in mice fed potatoes spiked with *Bt* was more pronounced. It is not clear from the study how much toxin was expressed in the GM potatoes and how much was consumed with the *Bt*-toxin diet. The study does, however, indicate that damage to the intestinal cells was due to the *Bt*-toxin.

The extent of the damage after just two weeks was significant enough to suggest that long-term consumption may create serious health problems in the intestines and possibly elsewhere. Some cellular changes, for example, may be precursors to cancer. Since *Bt* crops have been widely grown without long-term safety studies, the results of the mouse research prompted the authors to warn that, "thorough tests of these new types of genetically engineered crops must be made to avoid the risks before marketing."

Changes in the cells (details)

In both the mice fed the GM potatoes and the diet containing *Bt*-toxin, the mitochondria (which are sensitive to toxins) exhibited an abnormal appearance with signs of degeneration. Microscopic projections on the cell surface, called short microvilli, were also disrupted.

Mice fed the *Bt*-toxin diet had an abnormally high number of cells of the intestinal lining (enterocytes per villus were 151.8 in the control group compared to 197 in the *Bt*-toxin fed group). Of the enterocytes, 50% had multiple

nuclei and were larger. In addition, the mean area (105.3 μm^2 in the control group versus 165.4 μm^2 in the *Bt*-toxin group) and perimeter length (23 μm in control group versus 44 μm in *Bt*-toxin fed group) of the enterocytes was highly and significantly increased in the group fed *Bt*-toxin. The enterocytes of this group also had several forms of secondary digestive vacuoles (membrane-covered bubbles with proteins inside). A smaller but still statistically significant increase was also observed with the GM *Bt* potato-fed group in the perimeter length (28 μm). There was also a trend of increasing area and enterocyte number (116.5 μm^2 area and 155.8 respectively). However, these numbers were not statistically significant given the small number of animals used.

There was an injury at several points along the base of digestive cells (basal lamina), and the digestive surface (microvilli) of the gut was also damaged, with fragments broken off. In addition, the secretory (Paneth) cells in the group fed *Bt*-toxin "were highly activated and contained a large number of secretory granules,"[28] suggesting that *Bt*-toxin resulted in the development of proliferative (hyperplastic) cells.

Human health impact could be serious

Similarities between the digestive systems of humans and rodents suggest that *Bt*-toxin should also interact with human gut cells. If humans eating *Bt*-crops have reactions similar to the mice, the damage to their intestines could "cause distress to digestion" and likely be "diagnosed as mild food poisoning or flu,"[29] and possibly fecal incompetence. Furthermore, although cancer of the ileum is rare, it empties into the colon, where cancer is common. If the *Bt* protein made it as far as the ileum, some would likely enter the colon as well. Tests are needed to determine whether ingestions of *Bt* crops has an impact on colon cancer. The risks may be greatest among those populations where a *Bt* crop, such as *Bt* corn in South Africa, is a dominant staple in the daily diet.

1 . 5

Workers exposed to *Bt* cotton developed allergies

> "On the very first day of work at around 4:00–5:00 pm, I had itching all over my body followed by swelling. It was more so in face and hands but not much in covered portions. My eyelids became swollen and felt moderate itching inside my eyes. I continued picking cotton for three days and on the fourth day I could not work further because the symptoms had become very bad. . . . [A doctor advised me to go to] the district Hospital where I remained admitted for nine days and I was given blood, injections, and saline bottles. I had massive swelling, especially of [the] face, and fever."[30]
>
> —35 year-old cotton worker in India

1. Agricultural laborers in six villages who picked or loaded *Bt* cotton reported reactions of the skin, eyes, and upper respiratory tract.

2. Some laborers required hospitalization.

3. Employees at a cotton gin factory take antihistamines everyday.

4. One doctor treated about 250 cotton laborers.

In India, agricultural workers handle cotton during picking, loading, and weighing, and when separating cotton fiber from the seeds (ginning). In 2004 and 2005, several workers complained of allergies associated with *Bt* cotton, but not with other varieties. In a preliminary investigation, 23 laborers from six villages in two districts in western Madhya Pradesh who complained of symptoms were interviewed using a questionnaire. All had handled cotton in the past, but did not show allergic responses for non-*Bt* varieties.

According to investigators, the allergic reaction typically proceeded from "mild to severe itching" with redness and swelling, followed by skin eruptions. "In severe cases the eyes also become red, swollen," with excessive tears, nasal discharge, and sneezing. Specifically, all 23 subjects experienced itching (pruritis), sometimes severe enough to force them to stop working. Twenty had small, solid- or fluid-filled raised lesions (white papulo-vescicular eruptions) mostly on their face and hands. Some also appeared on the feet, back, neck, and abdomen. Nineteen people showed redness of skin (erythema) and 13 experienced facial swelling (oedema). Eleven of 23 had symptoms of the eyes, including itching, swelling, redness, and watering. Nine had nasal discharge and/or excessive sneezing.

Mild reactions were reported by 3 people, 10 were moderate and 10 were considered severe. One woman had to be taken from the cotton field to the hospital, where she stayed for nine days. Another farm worker reported that within one hour of picking *Bt* cotton, "she had itching on the face, followed by burning sensation as if someone had rubbed chilli powder. … The burning was so much that she could not even wash her face. Then for five to six months there was [a] serious discharge from the face. . . The skin became dark, almost black in color."[31]

The reactions among all subjects coincided with the introduction of *Bt* cotton and were not experienced beforehand. Reactions were mostly related to exposure with cotton in the field (78%). The longer the workers stayed in the fields, the worse their symptoms became. Reactions became less severe after they stopped work. Other reactions came from storing *Bt* cotton at home, sleeping on it or even resting on a cotton heap. Some field laborers take antihistamines daily.

After a farmer hired six people to tie cotton into bundles and load a tractor, he reported, "All the workers suffered from itching on hands and feet. The skin became red and there were rashes and there was lot of itching." He said that an antihistamine (Tab Avil) relieved the symptoms.

Reactions are widespread

According to owners of a cotton gin factory, most of the laborers experienced skin-related problems due to *Bt* cotton. Symptoms included "itching, redness of eyes, watering of eyes, and cough." At another factory, itching throughout the body was reported as "very common among laborers who carry *Bt* cotton." Employees take antihistamines daily in order to continue to work there. At a third factory, interviews with six laborers revealed that all had itching problems and two had skin eruptions. They had worked at the factory for two to seven years, but only suffered from the recently introduced *Bt* cotton.

A local doctor reported that he had seen approximately 150 cases of allergies in 2005 from two villages, and about 100 cases in 2004. The symptoms primarily occurred while the villagers picked cotton and for some, while loading it. According to the doctor, the symptoms "begin with itching in all parts of body, followed by red patches, redness of eyes, [and] swelling of [the] face and hands."

All reactions to *Bt* cotton plants were reported to have occurred after the cotton had emerged from the bolls. While *Bt* cotton is supposed to express *Bt* in all cells, including leaves, stems and roots, the lack of allergic responses reported earlier in the growing season may be due to several factors: 1) The exposure of workers to portions of the cotton plant may be substantially increased during picking and processing; 2) Worker's hands may be cut during the picking process, exposing open sores to *Bt*-toxin; 3) The *Bt* expressed by the cotton fiber may be different—in higher concentration or altered—compared to other parts of the plant; 4) According to agricultural scientist, Debashish Banerji, the leaves, stem, and roots have a protective coating that may inhibit exposure of *Bt* to humans. The cotton fiber does not contain such a coating.

No reports of allergic reactions have yet been compiled for the United States, where cotton is harvested mechanically.

Cotton products need testing

Cotton is widely used for clothing. In addition, cotton bandages are exposed to wounds, cotton diapers come in contact with rashes, and cotton feminine protection products used during menstruation contact blood and mucous membranes. It is essential that cotton be tested for the presence of *Bt* and that further tests evaluate its allergenicity, to ensure that large numbers of people are not being harmed.

1 . 6

Sheep died after grazing in *Bt* cotton fields

"The mortality started to occur within a week of continuously grazing on Bt cotton crops-residue." [32]

—Investigative report

1. After the cotton harvest in parts of India, sheep herds grazed continuously on *Bt* cotton plants.

2. Reports from four villages revealed that about 25% of the sheep died within a week.

3. Post mortem studies suggest a toxic reaction.

While visiting the district Animal Health Centre (AHC) in late April 2006, a local president of an Indian shepherd's union looked through the veterinary register and noticed 11 unusual post mortems on sheep. Examinations were conducted during February and March on animals that had grazed continuously in *Bt* cotton fields; they developed unusual symptoms before dying mysteriously. Some notes even gave a tentative diagnosis that *Bt* cotton was the cause. The union organized a fact-finding team, which included veterinary and agricultural scientists from area organizations.

On April 22, 2006, they conducted interviews in four villages located about 20–25 kilometers apart from each other in the Warangal district of Andhra Pradesh.[33] Shepherds and farmers described at least 1,820 deaths among sheep that grazed on *Bt* cotton plants after harvest. In one village, the death rate from 42 herds was 25% (651 out of 2,601). Sheep had grazed on tender leaves and pods of the plants. Within two to three days, they appeared dull or depressed. They developed coughs with nasal discharge, reddish and erosive mouth lesions, bloat, blackish diarrhea and sometimes red-colored urine. Symptoms did not match the usual sheep diseases. Death occurred in five to seven days, primarily among one and a half to two year old adults and three to four month old lambs. One shepherd reported that many of his sheep had died in 2005 after grazing on *Bt* crops. In 2006, he kept them out of *Bt* fields and there was no mortality. In a second village, shepherds "described the identical symptoms." Among 29 herds with 2,168 sheep, 549 animals (25%) died. Visits to two other villages yielded similar reports, with deaths sometimes occurring within four days. Farmers estimated that the total number of sheep deaths in the region was 10,000.

Post mortems and analysis

The AHC conducted post mortems on at least 11 of the sheep and "observed black patches in the small intestines, enlarged bile duct and liver with discoloration, and accumulation of pericardial fluid." Shepherds who did their own post mortems similarly found "black patches in the intestine and enlarged bile duct and black patches on the liver."[34] According to the investigative team, the findings "suggest severe irritation of the intestines and associated organs (bile duct, liver) connected to the absorption and assimilation of food and processing of toxins." Preliminary evidence "strongly suggests that the sheep mortality was due to a toxin. … most probably *Bt*-toxin."

The team said that livestock diets rich in cellulose make the stomach more alkaline, which could prolong the survival of the toxin in its active form. They wrote, "Since the toxin may bind to intestinal proteins,[35] there is a chance that if the sheep were exclusively eating the *Bt* crop matter, they would have in effect concentrated the toxin in their intestines due to the binding properties." They also point to a study in which *Bt*-toxin was shown to create changes in the electrophysiological properties of the mouse intestine, as well as diarrhea and intestinal irritation.[36]

Some Indian officials were quick to deny that GM crops were a factor. They cited a study that found no effect of *Bt* cottonseeds fed to goats and other animals. The quantity of the seed was not disclosed, however, and test conditions did not approximate continuous grazing on *Bt* cotton plants. Officials also referred to an acute toxicity test that showed no reaction, but a single high dose of isolated GM protein given to a rodent also fails to approximate long-term feeding.

The AHC's post mortem notes were also tampered with. In a different pen, comments were later added in an apparent attempt to divert the blame. Phrases indicated, for example, that fields had been sprayed with pesticides or that sheep had also grazed on chili plants. At least three shepherds named on the documents, however, later testified on video that they had never made those statements. The use of pesticides was actually less that year, and no chilis had been grown in the area indicated.[37]

When *Bt* cotton plant samples were tested, they showed only traces of pesticides. Analysis did show higher than normal levels of nitrates. This may have been due to the increased use of chemical fertilizer that farmers in the region say is necessary to get the cotton to perform adequately. The nitrate may be a factor in the sheep ailments.

Additional reports of *Bt*-related sheep deaths have also emerged from the Khammam[38] and Nalgonda districts in Andhra Pradesh and in the Nimad belt of Madhya Pradesh.[39]

Human exposure through oil and meat

The evidence raises questions about the safety of cottonseed oil. Even people who eat meat from animals fed GM cotton may be at risk. In fact, the Indian shepherds said that they discarded meat from the dead sheep, fearing it may cause health problems. One man who ate the meat said he suffered from diarrhea.

1 . 7

Inhaled *Bt* corn pollen may have triggered disease in humans

"*Most of those who planted* Bt *corn did not develop these symptoms after planting the crop. But like me, they felt the symptoms when the* Bt *corn plants were flowering.*"[40]

—Pablo Senon

"*One day the horse ate some of the corn plants and its appetite disappeared. . . . The belly swelled, its mouth started frothing, and it slowly died.*"[41]

—Nestor Catoran

1. In 2003, approximately 100 people living next to a *Bt* cornfield in the Philippines developed skin, respiratory, intestinal reactions, and other symptoms while the corn was shedding pollen.

2. Blood tests of 39 people showed an antibody response to *Bt*-toxin, which supports—but does not prove—a link.

3. The symptoms reappeared in 2004 in at least four other villages that planted the same corn variety.

4. Villagers also attribute several animal deaths to the corn.

Virtually an entire Filipino village of about 100 people living adjacent to a large field of *Bt* corn were stricken by a disease. The symptoms, which appeared at the time the corn was producing airborne pollen, included headaches, dizziness, extreme stomach pain, vomiting, chest pains, fever, and allergies, as well as respiratory, intestinal, and skin reactions.

"There was this really pungent smell that got into our throats," said resident Maryjane Malayon. "It was like we were breathing in pesticides."[42] She and her extended family all became ill, and "within days, people living a little further away ... were experiencing similar symptoms."[43] When her family moved out to stay with relatives, their symptoms abated within a week, but the person who rented their house became ill. At least three other families found that their symptoms disappeared when they moved away and appeared again upon returning. Such a response points to an environmental toxin or allergen, rather than an infectious disease.

Mae-Wan Ho, director of the Institute for Science in Society, interviewed many of the Filipinos in 2006. She reports: "As part of an investigation to determine what made the villagers ill, one of the farmers was 'volunteered' to venture inside the *Bt* maize [corn] field in the presence of more than 10 witnesses, as he explained to me via an interpreter. 'Within five minutes, I could not breathe and felt something extraordinary on my face,' he recalled. The others could see that his face had swollen up and remarked that it was 'very dangerous.' In fact, the farmer is ill to this day. Every now and again, he feels weak in his limbs and numb in his hands and feet. He held up the back of his right hand to show me the index finger. A yellowish-brown discoloration and thickening of the fingernail had developed since he was exposed to the GM pollen. . . .

"Many if not all of the villagers exposed to GM-maize pollen in 2003 have remained ill to this day. Furthermore, there have been five unexplained deaths in the village. In total, 96 people got sick. In addition, nine horses, four water buffalos, and 37 chickens died soon after feeding on GM maize."[44]

Terje Traavik, Director of the Norwegian Institute of Gene Ecology, learned about the incident during the fall of 2003 and arranged for blood samples from 39 individuals to be taken in October. In all cases, IgA, IgG, and IgM antibodies were detected in response to *Bt*-toxin. The IgA and IgM reactions indicate recent exposure to *Bt* within the previous three months and are consistent with an interpretation that the disease might have been created by inhalation of the *Bt*-pollen from the field.

Symptoms reappeared with the same corn

The corn was a hybrid between Mon 810, a *Bt* crop from Monsanto, and the conventional Dekalb 818 variety. It was first introduced to the region in 2003. Although it was not replanted in the stricken village in 2004, other regions on the same island of Mindanao did use the corn variety. Similar reactions were reported in at least four villages, all occurring when the corn was shedding pollen.

In South Sepaka, 31 people said that they fell ill while the corn was pollinating, and in an elementary school in Magallon, approximately 20 children (aged 5–10 years) developed coughs, sneezing, asthma and breathing difficulties.[45] "Thirty-two people in Tuka," according to Ho, "suffered from headache, stomach-ache, dizziness, diarrhea, vomiting, and difficulty in breathing."[46] An advocacy officer for Mindanao, where the villages were located, also reported that people experienced nosebleeds and flu-like symptoms including fever. He said the symptoms "were similar to those experienced" when "the first case of alleged harmful effects of the flowering *Bt* corn was documented."[47] Before they got sick, most residents had not known that the planted corn was *Bt*.

When Traavik's team conducted blood tests in 2003, they also tested how much *Bt*-toxin (Cry1AB) was being produced by the corn. The study, which is not yet published, showed that the levels varied considerably in the kernels, even from the same plant. The levels ranged from 0.014 ug to 0.9 ug, with other kernels expressing levels both above and below the limits of detection for the test. This raises questions about the stability of the transgene or its expression (see section 4.3). It is possible that the particular corn variety had been altered in some way *only in that area*, which may explain why similar results were not reported elsewhere.

The potential dangers of breathing GM pollen had been identified years earlier by the UK Joint Food Safety and Standards Group. In a letter to the US FDA in 1998, they had even warned that genes from inhaled pollen might transfer into the DNA of bacteria that reside in the respiratory system.[48]

When the reports surfaced about the sickness in the Philippines, advocates for GM crops were quick to dismiss them. There has not, however, been a thorough investigation and very little research has been done to follow-up on this significant red flag.

1 . 8

Farmers report pigs and cows became sterile from GM corn

"More than 20 farmers have complained over the last two years about sows that ate the corn developing pseudo pregnancy, exhibiting signs of pregnancy for full term without carrying a fetus."

— Reuters

1. More than 20 farmers in North America report that pigs fed GM corn varieties had low conception rates, false pregnancies, or gave birth to bags of water.

2. Both male and female pigs became sterile.

3. Some farmers also report sterility among cows and bulls.

In the early spring of 2001, the conception rates of sows (female pigs) on Jerry Rosman's Iowa farm dropped from 80% to 20%. Most animals had false pregnancies, some delivered bags of water and some stopped menstruating altogether. Rosman, an animal nutrition consultant, along with veterinarian and a nutritionist, did extensive testing. They ruled out common causes of reproductive problems. Rosman had fed his hogs GM corn since 1997. When he switched to *Bt* Liberty Link varieties from Garst Hybrids in 2000, the problem started. It persisted through most of 2001 with "several brief upswings in pregnancy rates"[49] coinciding with the times when sows were fed the previous year's (1999) corn.

Four nearby farmers told Rosman they too were having hog conception problems and were using Garst corn. Right after the *Farm Bureau Spokesman* ran a story on Rosman in 2002, other farmers called complaining of sterile pigs. As media coverage expanded, so did the calls. USDA microbiologist Mark Rasmussen said, "After Jerry's incident was publicized, about a dozen farmers in the Midwest contacted me to discuss similar problems." Rosman spoke with at least 20. He said many had consulted veterinarians and conducted tests and that sterility affected both males and females. Some noted that the problem went away when they switched corn varieties. Not all were using Garst, but all were GM with similar genetic backgrounds (maturity, height, etc.).

Three farmers reported similar issues with cows. In September 2005, Rosman fed some of the 2000 corn to three cows, just after they gave birth. He said they should have started menstruation after three months and been bred. Eight months later, however, they had not started cycling and were sold. A semen check of the bull fed the same corn showed it was nearly infertile. Rosman also fed 11 heifers the corn after they weaned at eight months. Although they usually start menstruating at nine or ten months, his never started. They were sold at 13 months.

Corn tests show anomalies

Basic toxicity tests on Rosman's corn showed no abnormalities. At one lab, after their standard test for the fusarium mold repeatedly came up negative, they let the test plates incubate for an additional 48 hours. The corn developed huge mold growth colonies of an uncommon strain. Samples from about 15 farms with animal reproductive problems all came up positive for the mold, says Rosman, but the technicians could not identify an associated toxin. Researchers were unsure if the mold was the cause of the problem or a marker for another cause.

Research at Baylor College of Medicine offers another possible explanation. Scientists reported, "Rats in our animal facility neither breed nor exhibit reproductive behavior when housed on corncob bedding."[50] Tests on the material revealed two classes of compounds (tetrahydrofurandiols and leukotoxin diol) which, when isolated, "disrupted endocrine function in male and female rats." They stopped the estrus cycle (similar to menstrual cycle) in females "at concentrations approximately two-hundredfold lower than classical phytoestrogens." One compound also curtailed male sexual behavior and both substances contributed to the growth of breast and prostate cancer cell cultures. The crushed corncob used at Baylor was likely shipped from central Iowa where many of the animal reproductive problems were reported.

Researchers isolated the same compounds from store-bought fresh corn, corn tortillas, and genetically engineered corn. It was not destroyed by pressurized steam (autoclaving) and is believed to be present in corn oil. The amount varied significantly "in different lots or varieties of corncob, and genetically engineered corn." [51] The differences, they say, "may serve to limit or enhance exposure and potential toxicity."[52]

The non-investigation

In the summer of 2001, Garst was given a sample of Rosman's corn for analysis. About six weeks later, Rosman's agronomist was told by Garst that the sample had been regrettably lost. When Rosman offered to furnish more, the company did not return his calls. When the pig sterility story hit the TV news the following year, however, the company announced that they had done an investigation and concluded that their corn was not at fault.

Rosman's corn was collateral for a USDA Farm Service Agency loan. The local office had granted a loan extension, but the local manager told Rosman that the national head of operations ordered that it be confiscated instead. A driver revealed that it was sent to a Cargill plant to be processed for human consumption.

The FSA refused to provide Rosman with the records related to his corn. It took six separate Freedom of Information Act requests, two from Rosman, one from each of three nonprofit organizations and one from a US congressman, for the FDA to turn over part of his file. Several documents omitted important data.

Rosman has declared bankruptcy and no further studies evaluated whether certain GM corn varieties may create reproductive problems in livestock or humans.

1 . 9

Twelve cows in Germany died mysteriously when fed *Bt* corn

> "*After common errors in feeding and infections had by and large been ruled out as the cause of death, the farmer now suspects Syngenta company GM maize … to blame for the sudden death of his cows.*"[53]
>
> — Greenpeace report

1. Twelve dairy cows died on a farm in Hesse Germany, after being fed a diet with significant amounts of a single GM corn variety, *Bt* 176.

2. Other cows in the herd had to be killed due to a mysterious illness.

3. Syngenta, the producers of *Bt* 176, compensated the farmer for part of his losses, but did not admit responsibility for the cow deaths.

4. In spite of demands by the farmer and even public protests, no detailed autopsy reports were made available.

Gottfried Glöckner started growing GM corn variety *Bt* 176 in his fields in Woelfersheim in the state of Hesse, Germany in 1997. He increased the amount over the years and in 2000 and 2001, switched over entirely to the GM variety. "The farmer reports that his cows had become sick more frequently after being fed the maize harvest from the year 2000."[54] Within four months of being fed *Bt* 176 corn and silage (made from corn plants), five cows died in 2001 and another seven in 2002. Milk production also decreased in some cows and others were slaughtered due to an unidentified illness.

The corn plots were part of GM field trials, which were being managed by the Robert Koch Institute on behalf of the corn's producer Syngenta. After reporting the deaths of five cows to the institute, Syngenta gave the farmer 40,000 euros. Although this was to compensate him for the deceased cows, reduced milk, and vet bills, the company did not admit responsibility for the problems. In February 2002, Glöckner stopped feeding his cattle the GM corn, but by October 2002 another seven cows had died. The farmer, "who by this time was over 100,000 euros out of pocket called upon Syngenta and the Robert Koch Institute to conduct a proper investigation."[55]

Unfortunately, the institute did not impound the dead animals or the corn and did not undertake "comprehensive tests on the soil from the farm or any dung samples from the cows in question."[56] Only one dead cow was examined. Although additional tissue samples were sent to the University of Göttingen, "they vanished in unexplained circumstances," according to a Greenpeace report. The report also stated that "common errors in feeding and infections had by and large been ruled out as the cause of death."[57] The institute ended its investigations in December 2002, without identifying the cause of the deaths.

Characteristics of *Bt* 176

According to a press release by the Institute for Science in Society, although *Bt* 176 is engineered to resist the herbicide glufosinate and to produce the *Bt*-toxin Cry1AB, molecular analysis carried out by French and Belgian[58] government scientists suggests that Syngenta may have been wrong about which form of *Bt* their corn produces. The *Bt* gene in *Bt* 176 showed a 94% similarity with a synthetic *cry1Ac* gene, but only 65% with the natural *Bt cry1Ab* gene. The authors also write, "Many *Bt* transgenes are synthetic, including the one in *Bt* 176. They are hybrids of multiple toxins. That means *Bt* transgenes not only risk killing more species of insects than intended, but may also contain previously unknown toxicities for other animals and human beings." They further suggest that the sequence of the multiple transgenes inserted into the *Bt* 176 may be unstable and appear to have rearranged.[59] (See section 4.3)

The *Bt* 176 corn variety has been taken off the market.

1 . 1 0

Mice fed Roundup Ready soy had liver cell problems

> *"Changes in cell nuclear architecture as observed in this study are not random and must reflect some 'insult' on the liver by the GM Soya."*
>
> — Michael Antoniou, molecular geneticist, King's College London

1. The liver cells of mice fed Roundup Ready soybeans showed significant changes.

2. Irregularly shaped nuclei and nucleoli, an increased number of nuclear pores and other changes, all suggest higher metabolism and altered patterns of gene expression.

3. The changes may be in response to a toxin.

4. Most of the effects disappeared when GM soy was removed from the diet.

When a group of 12 female rats were fed Roundup Ready soy, their liver cells underwent substantial changes, indicative of a dramatic increase in the general metabolism of the liver.[60] Changes in the liver are significant for many reasons. The liver "degrades and detoxifies toxic compounds received from the intestines or from the general circulation."[61] The liver also synthesizes material used in the blood and in digestion, and has a significant influence on general metabolism. Increased liver metabolism in GM-fed rats may be a response to elevated levels of toxins, to new toxins, or both. Furthermore, the study points to GM soy as the source of these changes in liver function. This was confirmed after the GM soy was substituted by non-GM soy and most of the changes to the liver cells disappeared.[62]

The GM and non-GM soy diet was first fed to the pregnant mothers of the mice, and then to the mice after weaning. Animals from both groups were sacrificed at one, two, five, or eight months. The size of the nucleus tends to grow with age, but in GM-fed mice, its size was significantly lower than controls at every age studied. At month one, the nuclei of the liver cells from both groups appeared "roundish" with a smooth, regular shape. Beginning at month two, however, "all GM-fed mice showed irregularly shaped nuclei, while control animals generally showed roundish nuclei."[63] According to several studies, "An irregular nuclear shape generally represents an index of high metabolic rate."[64]

In addition, by month one, the GM fed mice had 50% more pores of the cell nuclear membrane, (through which molecules pass in and out of the nucleus) and they remained substantially higher (by 40%–64%) in all subsequent measurements. This suggests increased trafficking of molecules between the nucleus and the rest of the cell in the GM-fed mice and is another indication of increased metabolic activity.

The highly structured nucleus of the cell contains specialized components responsible for DNA expression.[65,66] They are "highly sensitive indicators of cellular activity."[67] Thus, changes in the physical properties of these components reflect alterations in the general metabolic state of the cell.[68,69] One such component is the nucleolus. In the nucleolus, the cell's apparatus to create proteins (ribosomes) is produced. Here again, in mice fed Roundup Ready soy, the shapes of the nucleoli were more irregular. Furthermore, the size and distribution of structures within the nucleoli (the fibrillar centers and dense fibrillar components) had changed significantly. This too suggests an increased metabolic rate.

The GM-fed mice also had more splicing factors in their liver cells. These are the complex molecular machines that process RNA (by removing introns, if present). An increased number of splicing factors suggests increased gene expression, i.e., DNA in the liver is making more RNA copies.

Effects reversed with changed diet

In order to verify that GM soy was the cause of the modifications of liver nuclei, three-month-old (adult) mice that had been fed a diet with GM soy all their lives, switched to non-GM soy for one month. Most nuclear alterations disappeared. Similarly, when adult mice raised on non-GM soy switched to GM soy for the same period, their liver nuclei developed some of the alterations. According to the researchers, "This suggests that the modifications related to GM soybean are potentially reversible, but also that some modifications are inducible in adult organisms in a short time."[70]

Although there were no changes in the levels of major liver proteins found in the mice, biochemical analyses carried out on rabbits fed Roundup Ready soy exhibited altered expression of LDH1 liver isoenzymes. This provides supporting evidence of "a general increase of cell metabolism."[71] (See section 1.13.)

Implications for human health

According to Michael Antoniou, "The long-term health consequences of this type of metabolic and possibly toxic insult on the liver is unknown, but could lead to liver damage and consequently general toxemia."

About 89% of soybeans grown in the United States are Roundup Ready. They are also grown extensively in parts of South America. Most is fed to livestock, but soy and soy derivatives are also used for food. Given our widespread exposure to soy, soy derivatives and animals raised on soy, it is urgent that we track down the reason why the liver reacts as it does.

1 . 11

Mice fed Roundup Ready soy had problems with the pancreas

"*Our data indicate that the reduction in alpha-amylase synthesis and secretion is related to GM food at all ages considered. . . . [A] diet containing significant amount of GM food seems to influence zymogen synthesis and processing.*" [72]

— Manuela Malatesta et al,
Journal of Anatomy

1. Mice fed GM soy showed changes in the synthesis and processing of digestive enzymes.

2. The production of alpha-amylase, a major digestive enzyme, dropped by as much as 77%.

3. This, combined with other pancreatic changes, suggests that GM soy may interfere with digestion and assimilation, as well as alter gene expression.

A structural and chemical analysis of the pancreas demonstrated profound changes in mice fed Roundup Ready soy. Taken together, they indicate changes in gene expression, reduction in enzyme production, and likely hindrance of digestion.

Using the protocol described on the page 41, pregnant mice were fed a diet containing either 14% GM or non-GM soybeans. Their offspring continued the diet beginning at weaning, with 12 female mice per group. These animals were killed and their pancreas was examined at one, two, five or eight months of age.

Starting in month two, the production of alpha-amylase, a major pancreatic enzyme responsible for degrading carbohydrates, dropped in GM-fed mice by an average of 77%. In months five and eight, it remained 75% and 60% lower than controls. The reduced production of the enzyme was confirmed in three places in the cell (the rough endoplasmic reticulum, the Golgi apparatus and within zymogen granules).

Scientists are not clear why or how GM soybeans are responsible for this highly significant drop. "A similar decrease in alpha-amylase ... has been observed under starvation conditions;"[73] however, the mice in this soy experiment had free access to food and water. Reductions in alpha-amylase in the pancreas have also been reported "under diabetic conditions,"[74] but insulin levels and pancreatic function did not indicate the disease. While the mechanism of how GM soy suppressed enzyme production is unclear, such a dramatic drop may certainly create problems with carbohydrate digestion.

One-month-old GM-fed mice also produced less zymogens, but the differences became negligible in subsequent ages. Zymogens are digestive enzymes in a pre-active state, which become active when released into the intestine by the pancreas. Until that time, they are held in the pancreas in zymogen granules. The size of these granules was consistently smaller in GM-fed mice, with the highest difference of 39% in month five.

Researchers also noted differences in the nuclei of the pancreatic cells. (The nuclei from GM-fed mice had a more roundish shape, decreased pore density and reduced amount of splicing factors.) The changes suggest that consumption of GM soy reduced the processing of RNA and/or reduced the number of molecules that passed from inside the nucleus into the rest of the cell.[75]

The reason for all these changes is unclear, but their size, consistency, and highly significant correlations demonstrate that consumption of GM soy is the cause. Further analysis demonstrated that, as with the liver, pancreatic modifications disappear after removing the GM soy from the diet.[76]

Reduced enzymes might impair digestion and cause problems

Enzymes secreted by the pancreas are responsible for the breakdown of food within the small intestine. Any restriction of these enzymes might result in impaired digestion and a shortfall of nutrient assimilation. If carbohydrates are not properly degraded in the small intestine, (as may occur with reduced alpha-amylase), they may be broken down by bacteria in the large intestine, which can produce gas. If protein digestion is inhibited, (which may occur with reduced zymogens), it may increase the chance of allergic reactions to protein fragments. The pancreas may also be forced to produce and excrete more protein digesting enzymes, which might put undue pressure on the organ.

1.12

Mice fed Roundup Ready soy had unexplained changes in testicular cells

---

> "In the testes of young and adult mice fed on GM soybeans, both spermatocytes (precursors of sperm cells) and Sertoli cells (their nurse cells) show reduced nuclear activity, especially RNA production. Structures involved in lipid metabolism and detoxification are also enlarged in Sertoli cells. We are investigating to see if these affect sperm formation and fertility."
>
> — Manuela Malatesta, biologist, University of Verona

1. The structure and gene expression pattern of testicle cells of mice fed Roundup Ready soybeans changed significantly.

---

2. The cause for the changes is unknown, but the testicles are sensitive indicators of toxins.

---

3. Some of the changes might possibly influence adult fertility as well as the health of the offspring.

---

4. Mouse embryos from GM-fed mothers did show a temporary decrease in gene expression.

Using the same protocol as the previous two studies (using 12 *males*), researchers examined components within testicle cells of mice fed Roundup Ready soybeans (14% of diet). Observations were made after one, two, five, and eight months (using immuno-electron microscopy.)

Changes were found in both spermatocytes and Sertoli cells. Spermatocytes develop into sperm cells. Their health and proper functioning can impact fertility, as well as the health and viability of offspring. Sertoli cells nurture the developing sperm cell and are critical in their proper development and maintenance. Components in both had altered structures. In particular, apparatus involved with gene expression and RNA processing were significantly affected.

Testicular cells are sensitive indicators of toxins. They have been used, for example, to monitor heavy metal pollution.[77] Changes resulting from GM soy may be an impairment of gene expression due to toxins in the soy or it may be the cells' attempt to protect itself in response to toxins. In any case, findings are preliminary and require follow-up studies to determine what component of the GM soy (or herbicide residue) is the cause and if the changes impair fertility or offspring health.

Changes in Sertoli cells

Sertoli cells are known as the "nurse" cell of the testicles. "Sertoli cells from GM-fed mice of all ages showed enlarged vesicles of the smooth endoplasmic reticulum (SER)."[78] The SER is involved in metabolizing lipids and detoxification. Its increased size suggests an increase in one or both of these functions. It is not clear if this interferes with the Sertoli cells' support of sperm development.

In two- and five-month-old GM-fed mice, "The nucleoli appeared larger and more reticulated"[79] (network-like). Nucleoli contain genes that produce the RNA used in ribosomes. Ribosomes are the protein-synthesizing machines of the cell. The changes suggest that the cell is producing larger quantities of ribosomes and is operating at a much higher metabolic state, perhaps in response to stress.

Changes in Sertoli cells and spermatocytes

"At all the ages considered, a statistically significant increase in perichromatin granules (PGs) was observed not only in Sertoli cells but also in spermatocytes of GM-fed mice."[80] PGs are small particles that contain (pre)messenger RNAs.[81] Accumulation of PGs in the nucleus may have several causes. It may be due to higher levels of gene expression—genes that are normally active in the cell might have increased production, or the GM soy caused silent genes to become active. Or it may be that (pre)messenger RNAs are no longer being adequately processed or their normal export from the nucleus into the cytoplasm is being inhibited. Such interference with normal gene expression may result in unhealthy Sertoli cells or spermatocytes, either of which might interfere with sperm health or quantity.

As in the case of pancreatic cells in the previous study, "A decrease in the number of nuclear pores (NP) was also detected in GM soy fed mice."[82] Pores are the gateway through which RNA and proteins move in and out of the cell nucleus. Their reduced number in Sertoli cells and spermatocytes suggests lower molecular trafficking. This supports the notion above that RNA accumulates within the PG because its transport out of the nucleus is inhibited.

Finally, components involved in either gene expression (RNA Polymerase II) or RNA processing (Sm antigen, hnRNPs, and SC35) were "decreased in two- and five-month-old GM-fed mice, and … restored to normal at eight months."[83] This implies that components in the GM soy diet resulted in lower metabolic activity in Sertoli cells and spermatocytes during the early stages of adulthood of the mice.

Although there is no clear explanation for these changes, the authors speculate that there is a reduction of transcription (from DNA to RNA) that "takes place in parallel with a decrease in NP density." This results in "accumulation of RNAs in the form of PG" within the nucleus. This explanation is similar to a feedback mechanism that was observed in another study, in which the accumulation of PG in the nucleus was observed in response to stress factors and to drugs that inhibit translation of RNA into proteins.[84] If such a mechanism is operating here, it points to an imbalanced pattern of gene expression, an imbalanced pattern of proteins and an unhealthy cell.

Although the far-reaching implications of this study imply that GM soy might impact male fertility and the health of human offspring, such speculation is premature without substantial follow-up research. The researchers did, however, conduct a study in which they found an overall reduction in the level of gene expression inside early stage (four to eight cells) mouse embryos from parents fed GM soy. They identified "a temporary decrease in the transcription and maturation of [messenger] RNA."[85] More work will be needed to see if this carries any health risks.

1.13

Roundup Ready soy changed cell metabolism in rabbit organs

> "*An increased activity of LDH1 occurred in three organs from GM-fed rabbits.*"[86]
>
> — R. Tudisco, et al., *Animal Science*

> "*Any significant change in organ-specific enzyme activity during a feeding trial is cause for concern.*"
>
> — David Schubert, molecular biologist and protein chemist, Salk Institute for Biological Studies

1. Rabbits fed GM soy for about 40 days showed significant differences in the amounts of certain enzymes in their kidneys, hearts, and livers.

2. A rise in LDH1 levels in all three organs suggests an increase in cellular metabolism.

3. Changes in other enzymes point to other alterations in the organs.

Roundup Ready soybean meal was added to the diet of 10 30-day-old rabbits. After about 40 days, measurements of enzyme activity in organs showed significant differences in the kidney, heart, and liver, compared with organs of control rabbits fed non-GM soy meal.[87]

Enzymes in the kidney showed the greatest difference, with the levels of three enzymes significantly higher (alanine aminotransferase, lactic dehydrogenase, and gamma glutamyltransferase). According to the researchers, "Such a result seems to indicate that some alteration occurred in [the] kidney." One of the three enzymes, lactic dehydrogenase (LDH), also increased significantly in the heart. The authors noted that this shows "that the local production of LDH altered in two of the most important organs of the body."

Subtle changes in LDH

LDH is divided into five different protein fractions, called isoenzymes. They are labeled LDH-1 through LDH-5 and their concentration tends to vary per organ type. Tests that measure changes in the relative levels of these isoenzymes are used to evaluate the presence of certain diseases or injuries. In the GM-fed rabbits, LDH-1 levels in the kidneys were 20% higher. In the heart, LDH-1 levels were 25% higher and LDH-2 levels were 69% higher.

In the liver, although the overall LDH levels were not significantly different, LDH-1 was significantly higher (by 16%) and LDH-4 was significantly lower (by 46%). This "shift supports the hypothesis that some metabolic changes occurred in the liver." According to the authors, the increased levels of LDH-1 found in all three organs "should indicate a general increase of cell metabolism." According to molecular geneticist Michael Antoniou, it also indicates changes in the underlying pattern of expression of the LDH genes.

The rabbits showed no signs of any particular disease as a result of this short 40-day diet. There were indications, however, that the diet caused changes in the cell metabolism in key organs. While the particular patterns are not known to be a precursor of illness, the effects indicate that the rabbit physiology reacts differently to GM soy; long-term impacts may result. The indication of increased metabolic activity, according to the authors, is consistent with the apparent increase in liver metabolism in mice fed GM soy, noted in section 1.10. Further study is needed to evaluate whether such changes are indicative of a toxic reaction or some other health problem.

1 . 1 4

Most offspring of rats fed Roundup Ready soy died within three weeks

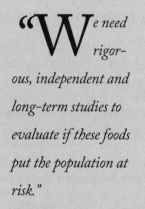

"*We need rigorous, independent and long-term studies to evaluate if these foods put the population at risk.*"

—Jim Willoughby, past president of the American Academy of Environmental Medicine, which passed a resolution asking the US National Institutes of Health to sponsor a follow-up of this rat study

1. Female rats were fed Roundup Ready soy starting before conception and continuing through pregnancy and weaning.

2. Of the offspring, 55.6% died within three weeks compared to 9% from non-GM soy controls.

3. Some pups from GM-fed mothers were significantly smaller and both mothers and pups were more aggressive.

5. In a separate study, after a lab began feeding rats a commercial diet containing GM soy, offspring mortality reached 55.3%.

6. When offspring from GM-fed rats were mated together, they were unable to conceive.

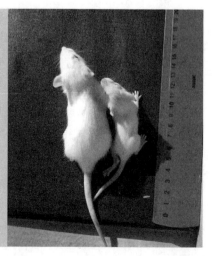

The smaller rat is 20 days old, while the larger is 19 days old. The mother of the smaller rat was fed GM soy.

A leading scientist at the Institute of Higher Nervous Activity and Neurophysiology of the Russian Academy of Sciences (RAS) conducted research in 2005, which if confirmed, suggests that GM soy fed to mothers may significantly harm the health and viability of offspring.

Flour from Roundup Ready GM soy was added to the diet of female rats. Other females were fed non-GM soy or no soy at all. The diet began two weeks before the rats conceived and continued through pregnancy and nursing. After weaning (at 13–14 days), the rat pup's diet was also supplemented with soy flour.

High mortality and illness

Within three weeks of birth, 25 of the 45 (55.6%) rats from the GM soy group died, compared to only 3 of 33 (9%) from the non-GM soy group and 3 of 44 (6.8%) from the non-soy controls. The timing of the deaths for the GM soy group was also more spread out: 14 occurred in week one, 6 in week two, and 5 in week three. Among the non-soy controls, all three deaths occurred during week one, and in the non-GM soy group, two deaths were in week one, and one was in week two.

Pups from the non-GM soy group weighed, on average, 13% more than those whose mothers consumed GM soy. Many from the GM group were quite small. At two weeks, 36% weighed less than 20 grams, compared to about 6% from the other two groups (see photo at left). The stunted growth was not likely due to a limitation in the quantity of mothers' milk. Because of the high death rate in the GM-soy litters, the mothers presumably had *more* milk available per pup, not less (assuming the GM soy diet did not reduce milk production).

The livers, lungs, hearts, kidneys, spleens, and testicles from the GM-group were tiny compared to the other groups. The brain was not substantially smaller, suggesting that its size is primarily dictated by age. Researchers also noted "a high level of anxiety and aggression" in both the "females and young pups from GM groups. … They attacked and bit each other and the worker." In another unpublished study on male rats, aggressive behavior was also noted in the GM-fed group.[88]

When the offspring of GM-fed rats in Ermakova's study were mated, they did not produce offspring. This apparent sterility persisted whether or not they continued to feed on GM soy. When the female offspring were mated with male controls, they did conceive. The size of the litters, however, was about 25% less than controls.

The study's author, Irina Ermakova, notes that, "The morphology and biochemical structures of rats are very similar to those of humans, and this makes the results we obtained very disturbing."[89]

Repetitions yield similar results

The data presented above, which was published in the Russian peer-reviewed journal *Ecosinform*,[90] was actually derived from two successive experiments conducted in June–July and August–September, 2005. Ermakova, who is now the vice president of the Russian National Genetic Safety Association, also repeated it a third time in September–October. The combined results for all 221 rat pups used in the three experiments yielded an offspring mortality rate of 51.6% for the GM soy group, 10% for non-GM soy, 15.1% for GM soy protein isolate and 8.1% for non-soy controls. "High pup mortality was characteristic of every litter from mothers fed the GM soy flour."[91]

As there was no detailed analysis of the feed, it is possible that substances such as mycotoxins had contaminated the GM soy flour and were responsible for the damage to the offspring. More recent events from the same laboratory, however, suggest that whatever caused the high mortality is not unique to the one batch of GM flour used in the experiments.

In November 2005, the supplier of rat food used at the RAS laboratory began using GM soy in the formulation. The presence of GM soy in the diet of all rats housed there disallowed further repetitions of the mortality study. After two months, however, Ermakova inquired of other scientists about the mortality rate of rat offspring used for other experiments. It turned out that 99 of 179 (55.3%) rat pups whose parents were fed GM soy-based rat chow had died within the first 20 days.[92]

Follow-up is urgently needed

This is the only published research in which female rats were fed GM feed prior to conception. Other studies introduced GM feed during pregnancy, which may miss toxic effects to reproductive organs, eggs, and sperm.

The study is preliminary, the number of rats was small, the feed was not evaluated, and the organs were not analyzed. But given the enormous implications, immediate replication, and expansion of the study is the only responsible option. According to Ermakova, however, she and her colleagues were forced to stop all GMO studies by the institute's administration, who were put under pressure by the Presidium of the Russian Academy of Sciences.

1 . 15

Soy allergies skyrocketed in the UK, soon after GM soy was introduced

> *"Their findings provide real evidence that GM food could have a tangible, harmful impact on the human body."*[93]
>
> — Daily Express

1. In a single year, 1999, soy allergies in the United Kingdom jumped from 10% to 15% of the sampled population.

2. GM soy was imported into the country shortly before 1999.

3. Antibody tests verify that some individuals react differently to GM and non-GM soy varieties.

4. GM soy also has an increased concentration of a known allergen.

In March 1999, researchers at the United Kingdom's York Laboratory tested 4,500 people for allergic reactions and sensitivities to a wide range of foods. In previous years, soy had affected 10% of consumers. In 1999, that figure jumped to 15%. Soy entered the "Top Ten" list of allergens for the first time in the 17 years of testing. The United Kingdom's *Daily Express* wrote, soy "moved up four places to ninth and now sits alongside foodstuffs with a long history of causing allergies, such as yeast, sunflower seeds, and nuts."[94]

Reactions included irritable bowel syndrome, digestion problems, skin complaints including acne and eczema, chronic fatigue, headaches, and lethargy. Blood tests confirmed an antibody reaction to soy.

Roundup Ready soy had recently entered the United Kingdom from US imports. The soy used in the study was also largely GM. John Graham, spokesman for the York laboratory, said, "We believe this raises serious new questions about the safety of GM foods."[95]

GM soy has unique allergic response

Remarkably, no follow-up tests to the UK allergy study were conducted at the time to see if individuals reacted differently to GM and non-GM soybeans. A study published six years later, however, verified that the immune system of some individuals does react differently to the two soy types. Using a skin prick test of 49 subjects, 13 exhibited positive reactions to non-GM soybeans while 8 reacted to GMO soybeans. "One patient had a positive skin test result to GMO soybeans only."[96] Geneticist Joe Cummins says, "The GM-soy-only individual stands out and should have triggered a review"[97] by regulators.

Tests verified that GM soy contained proteins that the natural soy did not have, and vice versa. Furthermore, an antibody related to allergies (IgE) had strong binding with one protein in the GM soy (at 25 kDa), while the non-GM variety had a "moderately strong" reaction to proteins of a different weight (30-36 kDa). Although further tests are needed to verify if this protein is unique to GM soy and not an artifact of a particular growing condition, this demonstration "of an extra IgE/binding protein allergen in Roundup Ready soybean," says biologist Arpad Pusztai, "is highly significant per se. And again it shows the superficiality of the risk assessment studies done by the Monsanto scientists."[98]

GM process can boost allergencity

There are many other possible reasons why GM soy may provoke increase allergic responses. The transgenic protein, which has amino acid sequences identical to known allergens (see section 3.2), might cause a reaction. The damaged sections of its DNA may participate in creating allergens (see section 2.9). And altered levels of gene expression due to the process of genetic transformation might introduce a new allergen or increase levels of a known allergen. Indeed, according to a study by Monsanto, Roundup Ready soybeans contain 27% more trypsin inhibitor, a known allergen, compared to matched non-GM soy. Once heated, however, that difference jumped to threefold and sevenfold in the two Roundup Ready soy lines tested. This suggests that the allergen in GM soybeans does not break down as readily by heating (see section 2.11). (Monsanto had left out this comparison from its published report, but it was later recovered in the journal archives by an investigator.)

There is also cross-reactivity between proteins in natural soybeans and in peanuts.[99] Unpredicted changes in GM soybeans might increase the amount or power of this potentially dangerous allergen as well. If so, it might have contributed to the doubling of peanut allergies among children in the United States from 1997–2002. GM soy was introduced into the US food supply in late 1996.

It is not confirmed that the GM soy caused the rise in UK soy allergies. The suspicious timing of the increase, combined with the multiple ways that GM soy might increase allergen production, however, demands further study. In the meantime, many people are not waiting to take steps to protect themselves.

Physician John Boyles, an allergy specialist from Ohio, says, "I used to test for soy allergies all the time, but now that soy is genetically engineered, it is so dangerous that I tell people never to eat it—unless it says organic."[100]

1.16

Rats fed Roundup Ready canola had heavier livers

"We are concerned that ANZFA may be comfortable with the possibility of a significant number of people suffering a hepatitis-like illness as a result of a food that ANZFA has assessed to be safe."[101]

— Public Health Association of Australia

1. The livers of rats fed GM canola were 12%–16% heavier than those fed non-GM varieties.

2. The liver is a chemical factory and primary detoxifier for the body.

3. Heavier livers may indicate liver disease or inflammation.

4. If this were caused by oil-soluble toxins, they may be present in canola oil.

In Monsanto's application for their Roundup Ready (GT73) canola, rats were fed ground canola and processed canola meal (toasted and defatted) for four weeks. Oddly, researchers used a mixture of the variety being studied, GT73, with another GM variety, GT200. The male rats gained significantly less weight than those fed the non-GM canola and meal. Differences in the amount of food consumed, however, did not account for this result.

In a second test, rats were fed only processed canola meal. In the group that was fed the pure GM variety (GT73), both sexes had livers that were 12%–16% heavier compared to controls. "This time, non-significant differences were observed in body weights and body weight gain."[102]

The researchers attributed the heavier livers to a higher level of glucosinolates in the GM canola, which they said would not appear in the oil portion consumed by humans. They did not, however, actually investigate to see if rats fed similar levels of glucosinolates had comparable abnormalities; thus, their conclusion remains an unsupported assertion.

Even the UK Government scientific advisors, known for their staunchly pro-GM stance, wrote, "ACRE and ACAF are not satisfied that the notifiers have supported the hypothesis that increased liver weight in rats fed GT73 compared with controls is attributed to higher glucosinolate content levels in the test material. A satisfactory explanation for this potentially adverse response observed in the rat feeding study is required."[103]

The level of glucosinolates in the GM canola meal was only about one-third the limit determined as safe for animal feed according to CODEX, a global United Nations agency for setting food standards. If such a low level was the actual cause for the heavier livers, then this study provides evidence that the CODEX limit is too high and should be lowered to a level *below* that found in the GM canola. Since canola meal is routinely fed to animals, admittance that the GM meal contains levels of glucosinolates sufficient to increase liver size by such a margin is paramount to declaring the GM brand unsafe.

In reality, the glucosinolate limit set by CODEX is probably not so dramatically flawed. Rather, the liver changes likely resulted from something else present in the GM canola.

The size of the liver is normally very stable. Such an increase in weight is unusual and implies a disturbance in its function. It may be due to increased cell numbers or inflammation. The condition known as Fatty Liver (Steatosis), usually due to alcohol consumption, can increase liver weight, as can hepatitis. Unfortunately, since no detailed analysis of the liver and no follow-up studies were conducted, the cause of the weight gain remains speculative.

That researchers did not undertake additional studies to verify the cause of the rats' heavier livers is a dangerous omission. If the condition had been created by a fat-soluble compound that is present in canola oil, it might adversely affect liver function in humans.

1.17

Twice the number of chickens died when fed Liberty Link corn

> "*Mortality was twice as high amongst those fed the GM maize as amongst those fed non-GM maize.*"[104]
>
> — Eva Novotny, astrophysicist, report for the UK Chardon LL hearing

1. The death rate for chickens fed Chardon LL GM corn for 42 days was 7%, compared to 3.5% among controls.

---

2. GM-fed chickens also had more erratic body weight and food intake, and less weight gain overall.

---

3. The study was designed so that only huge differences would be statistically significant.

---

4. The results were therefore dismissed without follow-up.

Chardon Liberty Link corn, engineered to withstand the herbicide glufosinate ammonium, was tested on chickens for 42 days.[105] One hundred and forty chickens were divided into four pens of 35 chickens each and fed as much of the GM corn as they wanted. Chickens in four other pens were fed a commercial corn diet. Ten chickens (7.14%) from the GM group died, while only 5 died (3.57%) from the non-GM group. The UK industry average was 4%. The GM-fed group also gained less weight and had far greater body weight variability. Their feed intake was also more erratic.

The Public Health Association of Australia (PHAA) pointed out that "Although birds who died underwent post mortems, no data on what was done, what was found, or any statistical differences were given."[106]

Veterinary scientists Steve Kestin and Toby Knowles testified in a hearing in the UK[107] that the study had major flaws. Most especially, the number of chicken pens was so small that the differences in death rates and weight gain were not statistically significant. The study could only demonstrate a "trend." Kestin and Knowles calculated that with such a poor research design, statistical significance would only be identified for very large differences, such as a "huge" weight difference. Using such insufficient numbers of pens (replicates), they said, is "one of the best methods" to "show no effect," if that is the aim.

They testified that the study was "inadequate in terms of providing any evidence or conclusions" and "not of a standard that would be acceptable for publication in a scientific journal." It had inadequate controls and insufficient reporting. "If anything," they concluded, "the results as reported arouse suspicions of real differences between the treatments. This should act as a spur to further investigation."

Although the study was not followed up, a related study also showed lower weight gain and erratic feeding. Rats were not fed Liberty Link corn; they were fed either high or low doses of the transgenic protein (PAT protein) that the GM corn was designed to create. According to a detailed analysis, "The slow rates of gain in weight of several of the animals eating PAT-protein indicate that they are not thriving as well as the rats in the control groups. Unusual patterns in the average food intake of animals consuming PAT-protein also suggest that the diet does not suit them." Here, like in the chicken study, the "data are not conclusive because too few animals (five per gender per group) were studied over too short a time." (13 days).[108]

It is interesting to note that the corn's producer claimed that the increased death rates were not significant because the research institute where the study took place typically has death rates of 5%–8%. Not only was this contention unsupported with data, it is largely irrelevant. Comparison with data collected from other studies is not a valid means for determining biological significance. Appropriate comparisons in animal feeding studies are between experimental and control groups using identical conditions (see part 3). In fact, this study should not have fed controls a commercial diet, but rather used Liberty Link's parental line, i.e., identical genetics (isogenic) prior to the insertion.

Liberty Link corn is currently marketed by Bayer CropScience. Without adequate tests, we do not know if the weight differences or higher death rate is significant and might impact human health. The lack of follow-up, however, shows a profound lack of rigor in the safety assessments and requirements for approval.

1.18

GM peas generated an allergic-type inflammatory response in mice

"*This is probably the single most important study published to date showing the potential dangers of GE crops because allergens can be dangerous at incredibly low levels and most if not all GE proteins have antigenic properties that are different from their normal counterpart.*"

— David Schubert, molecular biologist and protein chemist, Salk Institute for Biological Studies

1. In advanced tests not normally part of GM crop evaluations, protein produced by GM peas generated a dangerous immune response in mice.

2. That "same" protein, when produced naturally in beans, had no effect.

3. The GM peas produced a subtle, hard-to-detect difference in the way sugar molecules attached to the protein, which likely caused the problem.

4. The response in mice suggested that the GM peas could provoke inflammatory or allergic reactions in humans; commercialization of the peas was therefore cancelled.

5. This type of subtle but dangerous change in the GM protein would rarely, if ever, be detected in the safety assessments typically used to approve GM crops.

In the mid-1990s, Australian scientists at the Commonwealth Scientific and Industrial Research Organization (CSIRO) began research into manufacturing a GM pea that would be resistant to a pest known as the pea weevil. They inserted a gene from the kidney bean, which produces an antinutrient (alpha-amylase inhibitor) that interferes with the weevils' digestion—starving them to death. The natural protein in beans, when fully cooked, is safe for humans.

As part of the pea's safety assessment,[109] groups of mice were fed a commercial diet and also given GM peas, non-GM peas or kidney beans, twice a week for four weeks. The mice were then put through a battery of immune response tests that are considered predictive of human allergenicity. Only mice that were fed GM peas developed a reaction. Specifically, injections of the GM protein into the footpad resulted in significant swelling. When introduced into the trachea, it caused mild lung damage and tissue inflammation (similar to asthma in humans). Lymph nodes also responded to the GM protein.

In addition, mice fed GM peas became more sensitive to other substances. They reacted to egg albumin, for example, while those fed non-GM peas did not. Even GM peas that had been boiled for 20 minutes and were no longer effective at protecting against weevils still caused an immune response in mice. The findings suggested that both raw and cooked GM peas might cause allergic or inflammatory reactions in humans, as well as promote reactions to a wide range of other foods.

Subtle protein changes may be dangerous

The alpha-amylase inhibitor protein produced in GM peas had the same amino acid sequence as the protein produced in kidney beans. But only the GM protein created an immune response. Using an advanced test (MALDI-TOF), researchers identified subtle differences in the sugar chains (glycosylation patterns) that were attached to the protein. Since glycosylation is known to impact allergenicity, they concluded it was the likely cause.

The study reveals that when genes are passed between even closely related species, subtle and unpredictable changes in the protein can make it dangerous – even deadly. This information contradicts industry's assumptions that differences in glycosylation patterns are irrelevant and can be ignored. Their safety assessments don't adequately test for these types of changes in the protein. In fact, if those GM peas had been evaluated by tests *normally* used to assess the allergenicity of GM proteins (e.g. comparing amino acid sequences to known allergens and testing sta-

bility of the protein in a simulated digestive solution), they would have passed.

The mouse test that alerted researchers about the dangers of their peas is typically used to test medicines. It had never before been used on an approved GM crop. Furthermore, the MALDI-TOF test that precisely identified the glycosylation patterns is almost never used on GM crops. Instead, the test normally relied on to examine protein structure, the SDS gel test, is not as sensitive; it does not give any molecular detail of the glycosylation patterns. According to former EPA scientist Doug Gurian-Sherman, those subtle differences in glycosylation patterns found in the pea study "would not be detected by the tests that are currently required by US regulatory agencies." In fact, in the 1990s, when the GM peas were tested with an inferior "gel test" method that is sometimes used in GM food assessments, researchers didn't see any difference between the GM and non-GM proteins. The peas had passed this test. Thus, normal testing protocols are not adequate to identify potential allergenic crops (see part 3).

Cooked GM food may cause allergies

One argument used to defend the safety of GM crops is that cooking will change the shape (denature) the protein so that it will not be allergenic. Advocates assert, for example, that when *Bt* crops are cooked, the *Bt*-toxin is denatured and will no longer act as a pesticide. They claim, without evidence, that it would also lose any potentially allergenic properties. The pea study refuted this assumption. The cooked GM pea was denatured and no longer effective as a pesticide, but it was still able to create an immune response in the mice.

Approved crops may have similar problems

If the GM peas had been commercialized in Australia, they would have been widely consumed in India where they may have caused dangerous allergic reactions. The GM crops on the market, however, contain novel proteins derived from bacteria or viruses. When expressed in a plant, they also may undergo unintended modifications with unknown consequences. These transgenic proteins have never been tested with the same rigor as the peas and may be harmful.

1.19

Eyewitness reports: Animals avoid GMOs

"If a field contained GM and non-GM corn, cattle would always eat the non-GM first."[110]

— Gale Lush, Nebraska

"A neighbor had been growing Pioneer Bt corn. When the cattle were turned out onto the stalks they just wouldn't eat them."[111]

— Gary Smith, Montana

"While my cows show a preference for open-pollinated corn over the hybrid varieties, they both beat Bt corn hands down."[112]

— Tim Eisenbeis, South Dakota

1. When given a choice, several animals avoid eating GM food.

2. In farmer-run tests, cows and pigs repeatedly passed up GM corn.

3. Animals that avoided GM food include cows, pigs, geese, squirrels, elk, deer, raccoons, mice, and rats.

Avoiding GM soybeans

A flock of geese visit an Illinois pond each year and feed on soybeans from a nearby 50-acre field. The year the farmer planted GM soybeans on half the field, he was shocked to discover that the geese ate only from non-GM side. There was a line right down the middle of his field with the natural beans on one side and the genetically engineered beans, untouched by the geese, on the other. Agricultural writer C.F. Marley reported, "I've never seen anything like it. What's amazing is that the field with Roundup Ready beans had been planted with conventional beans the previous year, and the geese ate them. This year, they won't go near that field."[113]

A herd of about 40 deer ate organic soybeans from one field, but avoided the Roundup Ready variety across the road.[114]

Avoiding GM corn

In 1998, Iowa farmer Howard Vlieger filled one side of his sixteen-foot trough with the *Bt* corn and dumped non-GM corn on the other. When he let his cows into the pen, they all congregated on the side with the natural corn. When it was gone, they nibbled a bit on the *Bt*, but quickly changed their minds and walked away.[115]

Inspired by this story, several farmers in Northwest Iowa conducted their own tests. They let two or three cows into the feeding area at a time. The cows came to the first trough containing *Bt* corn, sniffed it and withdrew. They then walked over to the next trough and finished off the non-GM corn. Some would then go back for a sniff or taste of the *Bt* variety, but then walk away. This same scenario was repeated by both cows and pigs over and over again on six or seven farms in 1998, and again in 1999.[116]

After a 2000 campaign speech to farmers by Al Gore, Vlieger told the presidential candidate about his cow's preference for non-GM corn. Gore asked if other farmers noticed that their animals responded differently to GM food. About 12 to 15 hands went up.[117]

Cattle even broke through a fence and walked through a field of Roundup Ready corn in order to consume the non-GM variety on the other side.[118]

A retired Iowa farmer fed squirrels through the winter months by placing corncobs on feeders. One year, he put non-GM corn in one feeder and *Bt* in another about 20 feet away. The squirrels ate all the corn off the natural cobs but didn't touch the *Bt*. Each time the farmer refilled the feeder with natural corn, it was soon gone. The *Bt* remained untouched. Out of curiosity, he didn't refill the natural corn. During the coldest days of winter, the *Bt* cob remained in-

tact. After about 10 days, the squirrels ate about an inch off the tip of an ear, but that's all. The farmer felt sorry for the squirrels and put natural corn back into the feeders, which the squirrels once again consumed.[119]

Raccoons devoured organic corn, but didn't touch the *Bt* variety growing down the road.[120] Mice consumed a pile of non-GM corn in a barn in Holland, but left the GM pile nearby untouched.[121] A couple in Minnesota reported, "A captive elk escaped and took up residence in our crops of organic corn and soy. It had total access to the neighboring fields of GM crops, but never went into them."[122]

A Dutch undergraduate student offered mice a choice between GM and non-GM mixture of corn and soy. Over a nine-week period, the mice consumed 61% non-GM and 39% GM food. (When he forced half the mice to eat only GM and the other half to eat non-GM, the GM group ate more food, gained less weight, and "seemed less active while in their cages." When picked up to be weighed at the end of the experiment, he said the GM-fed mice were "more distressed. … Many were running round and round the basket, scrabbling desperately in the sawdust, and even frantically jumping up the sides, something I'd never seen before.")[123]

Avoiding GM tomatoes

The Washington Post reported that rodents, usually happy to munch on tomatoes, turned their noses up at the genetically modified FlavrSavr tomato that scientists were so anxious to test on them. Calgene CEO Roger Salquist said of his tomato, "I gotta tell you, you can be Chef Boyardee and . . . [they] are still not going to like them."[124] These were the rats described in section 1.2. They were force-fed the tomato through gastric tubes. Several developed stomach lesions; 7 of 40 died within two weeks.

1.20

A GM food supplement killed about 100 people and caused 5,000–10,000 to fall sick

"*Impurities in Showa Denko's genetically "engineered" tryptophan happened to cause an illness—EMS— which was novel. The surge of numbers therefore stood out and got noticed. If [Showa Denko's] poison had caused the same numbers of a common illness instead, say asthma, we would still not know about it. Or if it had caused delayed harm, such as cancer 20–30 years later, or senile dementia in some whose mothers had taken it early in pregnancy, there would have been no way to attribute the harm to the cause.*"[125]

*— L. R. B.` Mann, et al.,
"The Thalidomide of
Genetic Engineering"*

1. One brand of the supplement L-tryptophan created a deadly US epidemic in the 1980s.

2. The company genetically engineered bacteria to produce the supplement more economically.

3. Their product contained many contaminants, five or six of which were suspected as the cause of the disease.

4. Discovering the epidemic required multiple coincidences, suggesting that adverse reactions to GM foods may be hard to identify.

In the 1980s, thousands of individuals in the United States contracted a disease that physicians could not at first identify. The symptoms varied by patient and included swelling, coughs, rashes, physical weakness, pneumonia, breathing difficulties, hardening of the skin, mouth ulcers, nausea, shortness of breath, muscle spasms, visual problems, hair loss, difficulty with concentration or memory, and paralysis. The one symptom shared by all was intense debilitating muscle pain (myalgia). The patients' levels of white blood cells, called eosinophils, also skyrocketed, suggesting a severely disrupted immune system.

After several years, a series of coincidences allowed doctors to identify that an epidemic of a new disease was taking place and that all victims had consumed the food supplement L-Tryptophan (LT). LT is an essential amino acid found in turkey, milk, and other foods. It is a precursor to the neurotransmitter serotonin and had been taken as a supplement for stress, insomnia, and depression.

The disease was named eosinophilia myalgia syndrome (EMS). Trace-back studies revealed that only one of the six LT brands imported into the United States caused EMS. The brand contained five or six unique contaminants, one or more of which was likely to be the cause. The Japanese manufacturer, Showa Denko, had taken precautions against contaminants entering the production process. They were, however, the only company that had genetically engineered their bacteria to produce LT. And starting in 1984, as they progressively added more genes to their bacteria, there was a corresponding increase in contamination levels. The final strain, which caused the most illness, contained five separate transgenes.[126]

There are several ways in which genetic engineering could have produced the contaminants. Unintended changes in the DNA might create unintended proteins or shift proportions of naturally occurring ones. Showa Denko's bacteria produced enzymes in higher than normal concentrations, which might interact in unpredictable ways to produce contaminants.

In addition, if LT molecules were changed in structure or concentration, they might produce additional problems. For example, LT is toxic to the bacteria that create it. Thus, the bacteria might have modified the more concentrated LT, or itself, or the environment, as a means of self-preservation. Also, LT is one of the inputs used by organisms to produce niacin. During this process, a number of intermediate substances are created, which help regulate immune system responses. An altered LT could theoretically produce a change in these immune regulators, causing significant disruption of the immune system.

Alternative causes unsupported

Several alternative explanations attempt to shift blame away from genetic engineering. Some are based on the misconception that the first GM strain of bacteria was introduced in December 1988. Proponents argued that since some EMS cases had been contracted from LT manufactured prior to that point, "there would have to be a cause other than just the mere engineering of the strains."[127] Since four earlier GM strains had been used during the four years prior to December 1988, this theory is baseless.

Similarly, some had blamed the epidemic on a change in the filter used at the factory to purify the LT. But the filter change occurred in January 1989, years after EMS had been first contracted. (It is interesting to note that after being filtered, the LT was still more than 99.6% pure—passing US pharmaceutical standards. The suspected toxins were present at less than 0.1% of the final product.)

Some, including the FDA, argued that LT itself was dangerous and responsible for EMS. According to epidemiologist Edwin Kilbourne who investigated EMS while at the Centers for Disease Control (CDC), if this were true, then "all tryptophan products of equal dose produced from different companies should have had the same [effect]."[128] Kilbourne insists that no evidence supports this. In fact, EMS investigator William Crist revealed that in every case where the origins of EMS-associated LT were identified, Showa Denko was the source. EMS expert Gerald Gleich says, "Tryptophan itself clearly is not the cause of EMS in that individuals who consumed products from companies other than Showa Denko did not develop EMS. The evidence points to Showa Denko product as the culprit and to the contaminants as the cause."[129]

Sobering lessons

According to CDC officials, the GM supplement killed about 100 people and caused 5,000–10,000 others to fall sick or become disabled. There are still no special safeguards for GM-produced supplements. If that same LT were first introduced today, it could get on the market.

The epidemic took years to identify. It was discovered only because the disease was rare, acute, came on quickly, and had a unique source. If one of these four attributes were not present, the epidemic might have remained undiscovered. Similarly, if common GM food ingredients are creating adverse reactions, the problems and their source may go undetected.

"*The products of genetic engineering today are still at the level of a dinosaur technology. We use genes, which are foreign to a species, not knowing where they are inserted or what else will change in the whole chain from gene to protein.*"[1]

—Cesare Gessler, The ETH Swiss Federal Institute of Technology

"*The default prediction for the impacts of expression of a new gene (and its products) within a transgenic organism would . . . be that this expression will be accompanied by a range of collateral changes in expression of other genes, changes in the pattern of proteins produced and/or changes in metabolic activities.*"[2]

—The Royal Society of Canada

SECTION 2:

Gene insertion disrupts the DNA

The process of genetic engineering results in widespread mutations—within the transgene, in DNA flanking the transgene and in hundreds or thousands of locations throughout the genome. These disruptions, which are usually overlooked by scientists and regulators,[3] are "far greater than previously thought," says molecular geneticist Michael Antoniou, who warns that they can lead "to the generation of novel toxic effects, allergies, and altered nutritional value."

Research on these mutations overturns the central arguments by biotech advocates—that the technology is precise, predictable, and safe, and that current studies are adequate.

2.1

Foreign genes disrupt the DNA at the insertion site

> "Widespread use of transgenic crops carrying insertion-site mutations of this magnitude will, in our opinion, lead sooner or later to harmful consequences. Nevertheless, detailed inspection has shown that mutations such as these would almost certainly pass unnoticed through both the molecular and phenotypic characterization stages of the regulatory systems of both the European Union and the United States."[4]
>
> —Allison Wilson, et al,
> *Nature Biotechnology*

1. When genes are inserted at random in the DNA, their location can influence their function, as well as the function of natural genes.

2. "Insertion mutations" can scramble, delete or relocate the genetic code near the insertion site.

3. Evaluation of insertion sites have shown relocations of up to 40,000 DNA base pairs, mixing together of foreign and host DNA, large scale deletions of more than a dozen genes and multiple random insertions of foreign DNA fragments.

Inserting transgenes usually disrupts sections of plant DNA near the insertion site. Called insertional mutagenesis or insertion mutation, this effect has been known for years, but it wasn't until 2003 that a large systematic analysis was done. Scientists looked at 112 plants (*Arabidopsis thaliana*) engineered with the *Agrobacterium* method.[5] Only plants with single copies of the transgene were used. (Most commercialized GM crops have single copies.) Of 112, 80 (71%) had small mutations near the insertion site, including deletions of 1-100 base pairs and/or insertions of 1-100 extraneous base pairs. The extra base pairs came from the transgene, other parts of the plant's DNA or the circular (plasmid) DNA used in the *Agrobacterium* insertion process. The remaining 32 plants (29%) appeared to have large-scale insertions, rearrangements, duplications, and/or deletions. In two, parts of whole chromosomes broke off and translocated next to the inserted gene.

In a study of the same plant species, a section of at least 40,000 base pairs long had translocated from one chromosome to another. In fact, it had been duplicated, since it was also found intact in its original position.[6] A third study identified a deletion of 75,800 base pairs—approximately 15 genes.[7]

These three studies used *Agrobacterium* insertions. The very few that analyze insertion mutations from the gene gun method consistently demonstrate large-scale DNA disruptions. According to a comprehensive review, "The majority of transgene insertion events created by particle bombardment are complex, having multiple copies of the transgenic DNA integrated at a single [insertion-site]."[8] They contain large amounts of extraneous DNA, including multiple fragments of the transgene and/or small or large fragments of plant DNA interspersed with inserted genes. One study found 155 separate breaks, indicating recombinations of the inserted genetic material.[9] In rare cases where only a single copy of the foreign gene is inserted, they "turn out to contain fragments of superfluous DNA and/or they appear to be associated with large deletions and/or rearrangements of the target plant DNA."[10]

In a study of an oat plant, for example, the host DNA contained the full sequence of the foreign gene (plasmid), *plus* a small stretch in which oat DNA was mixed with foreign plasmid DNA, *plus* a partial copy of the plasmid, *plus* another section with oat and plasmid sequences scrambled together.[11] DNA on either side of the insertion appeared to contain rearrangements or deletions. Two additional insertions were also identified elsewhere in the DNA. One had a rearranged section of the plasmid (296 base pairs), scrambled plant DNA on both sides, and a deletion of 845 base pairs. The study employed DNA sequence analysis, the most thorough method for evaluating insertion mutations. Genetic engineers, however, usually rely on the less precise Southern blot test, which picks up only major changes. When this test was applied to the oat DNA above, it indicated the presence of only a single intact inserted gene. It missed all of the mutations and fragments as well as the two additional insertions. **This means that on the whole, biologists who create GM plants and the regulators that approve them have no idea of the extent of DNA damage or the associated unintended effects.**

Transgene location can cause problems

Scientists cannot "aim" the transgene into the DNA and they rarely conduct tests to find out where it ends up. But its placement has a "position effect," which can determine the level and reliability of transgene expression as well as the severity of unpredicted side effects.

Even though only about 1–10% of plant DNA constitutes actual genes, *Agrobacterium* insertions in the most commonly studied GM plants disrupt known gene sequences between 27%–63% of the time.[12] (The percentage using gene guns is unknown, but probably similar.) One reason is that in order for transgenes to function, they need to be located within "active" regions of the host DNA, which are more densely populated with functioning genes. If inserted into inactive sections, transgenes and marker genes would not function. (When antibiotic was applied, the cell would die because the antibiotic resistant marker would be inactive. Those cells would not be grown into GM plants.)

Transgenes can alter host gene expression when they land inside of or next to genes, or when they disrupt related genes (most genes operate in coordinated clusters). Protein production can be increased, decreased, or shut off. According to the FDA, transgene location might cause "the food derived from the plant to have higher levels of toxins than normal, or lower levels of a significant nutrient."[13] New or increased levels of allergens and antinutrients are also possible. According to a 2005 study sponsored by the UK's Food Standards Agency, "Information on the genomic location of transgenes would seem to be essential to any safety assessment."[14]

2 . 2

Growing GM crops using tissue culture can create hundreds or thousands of DNA mutations

"Insertional mutation damages the target genome in unpredictable ways, rendering literally unforeseeable the many properties of any surviving GM-cells. The unforeseeability is compounded by somaclonal variation in the GM-progeny: plants grown from single cells."[15]

—Robert Mann, biochemist, University of Auckland

1. The process of growing plant cells into GM plants may create hundreds or thousands of mutations throughout the genome.

2. While a change in a single base pair may have serious consequences, widespread changes in the genome can have multiple, interacting effects.

3. Most scientists working in the field are unaware of the extent of these mutations, and no studies have examined genome-wide changes in commercialized GM plants.

In order to create a GM plant, scientists first isolate and grow plant cells in the laboratory using a process known as tissue culture. After transgenes are inserted and the transformed genes are selected (e.g. using antibiotics) they use tissue culture, again, but change the nutrient medium in which the cells grow. The new conditions facilitate differentiation, allowing cells to develop roots and shoots. When ready, they are placed into soil and grown into plants. Tissue culture may be used a third time, to multiply a single GM plant into many others with identical DNA. Thus, GM plants are clones from a single GM transformed cell.

Unfortunately, the tissue culture method of plant propagation results in widespread mutations throughout the genome, called somaclonal variation. In fact, *tissue culture is sometimes used specifically to create mutations* in plant DNA, although the mechanics of how this occurs is not yet clear. Changes range from small deletions or base changes, to entire translocation of chromosomes from one region of the DNA to another. These mutations can influence the crops' height, resistance to disease, oil content, number of seeds, and many other traits.[16]

In some cases, cells that undergo tissue culture *and* genetic modification will have significantly more genome-wide mutations than cells just grown by tissue culture. It is unclear why gene insertion has this effect, but scientists speculate that it may, in part, come from unsuccessful insertions or insertions of small fragments of GM plasmid DNA that are sometimes scattered throughout the genome. Some mutations may also be due to the added stress from infection by agrobacteria, bombardment of particles or exposure to antibiotics.[17]

Taken together, the process of gene insertion combined with tissue culture typically results in hundreds or even thousands of mutations, including small deletions, substitutions, insertions, or large chromosomal rearrangements in the genetic code. The changes are vast. Two studies suggested that 2%-4% of the random stretches of DNA sampled from tissue culture samples were different than non-GM controls.[18,19] Furthermore, estimates are based on detection methods that may miss many mutations, such as short deletions and insertions, and most base pair substitutions. Thus, the actual degree of gene disruption is probably greater. These genome-wide mutations are found in every GM plant analyzed and are greater in number than mutations produced by transgene insertion. Studies in 2005 confirmed that the production of RNA, proteins and metabolites are significantly influenced by tissue-culture-induced changes,[20] and one concluded that "somaclonal variation may be an underestimated source of compositional variation."[21] These types of mutations, however, are not evaluated in commercially released GM food crops.

If the original GM plant is crossed (mated) through many generations with the parent or other lines, many (but not all) of these small, genome-wide mutations may get corrected. It is unknown, however, how many crossings have been conducted on food crops and how many mutations persist. Furthermore, certain plant species are propagated vegetatively—they don't cross with other plants. These plants would retain the vast number of mutations created during the GM transformation process. The GM potato that was on the market years ago and the papaya currently on the market are examples of GM crops that are propagated vegetatively and therefore pose greater risks as a result.

Mutations carry serious consequences

Mutations and extraneous insertions might permanently turn genes on or off, alter their function, and/or change the structure or function of the proteins they create. Even a single base pair change may result in serious consequences. Because of our limited understanding of the DNA, even if we knew which parts were disrupted, we would not necessarily know the impact.

In reality, many biotech scientists are unaware of the massive quantity of mutations that are generated by the GM transformation process (gene insertion and tissue culture). In fact, the regulatory agencies that approve GM foods operate as if the insertion process has no impact on safety.[22,23] They do not require extensive evaluation of the mutations and therefore the extent of these in approved GM food crops has not been identified. The few studies that have been conducted revealed many significant problems. GM varieties contain truncated or multiple fragments of the inserted gene and extraneous or scrambled DNA. One GM corn variety (*Bt* 11) contained a fragment from a gene that was supposed to be inserted into a different GM variety (E 176).

Advocates of biotechnology often defend the safety of their products by claming that modern methods of plant development *other* than genetic engineering, such as exposure to radiation, are used on a wide scale, have a history of safe use and create comparable mutations. This is pure speculation. There is *no* evidence that these modern methods are used widely, are consistently safe or create mutations of the same kind or frequency as genetic engineering.[24]

2 . 3

Gene insertion creates genome-wide changes in gene expression

---

1. One study using a micro-array gene chip found that 5% of the host's genes changed their levels of expression after a single gene was inserted.

---

2. The changes, which are in addition to the deletions and mutations already discussed, are not predictable and have not been fully investigated in the GM crops on the market.

---

3. These massive changes may have multiple health-related effects.

Gene chips allows scientists to monitor the expression levels of nearly all the genes in an organism's DNA simultaneously. They identify changes in messenger RNA levels, from which we can infer changes in their corresponding proteins, affording a more holistic evaluation of the gene function. This is a fairly new technology and has not been widely used in plant biotechnology. In fact, there are no records of these gene chips ever being used by a biotech company with the GM crops currently on the market.

Scientists studying cystic fibrosis (CF) inserted a gene that regulates the passage of chloride into human cells.[26] After the insertion took place, the gene chip revealed that up to 5% of the levels of messenger RNA that were monitored either increased or decreased. Extrapolated to the number of active genes in plants, a single insertion might change the expression of hundreds, possibly thousands of genes. The authors wrote, "This is a remarkable and somewhat unexpected finding in view of the implicit assumption that gene transfer . . . ought only to have the consequence of increasing the level of functional . . . protein in the target cell. Instead, we find here that many changes occur."[27]

According to the Royal Society of Canada, "Thousands of genes are being expressed in a plant in an orchestrated manner at any given time. The rate and timing of transcript expression from any given gene in any particular cell represents an integrated response to many factors, internal and external, that impinge on that cell. The pattern of expression of all transcripts is thus an exquisitely sensitive monitor of cell and tissue status. . . . Carefully controlled DNA microarray analysis has the potential to reveal significant shifts in the overall pattern of gene expression associated with transgene insertion."[28]

Thus, the impact of gene transfer, whether in human gene therapy or transgenic plants, is holistic; gene regulation is an integrated affair. The huge number of changes will alter the types and levels of proteins in significant, but entirely unpredictable, ways. In the cystic fibrosis study, the scientists were at a loss to determine the impact. "In the absence of more biological information," they wrote, "we cannot discern which directions are better or worse, since any of these may have positive or negative effects on the physiology of the CF cell."[29]

It is expected that the genes in a corn or soybean plant may react on a similar scale to the insertion of a transgene. The changes may result in the "synthesis of toxic, carcinogenic, teratogenic [causing changes in the fetus], or allergenic compounds," or inhibit "the synthesis of a beneficial plant molecule." [30] Even if we monitored all the changes in protein levels in GM plants (which we don't), it would be impossible to predict the impact of a single protein on the cell since they act differently depending on the cell type, organism and circumstance. For example, the "the over-expression of a gene involved in pectin synthesis had no effect in tobacco, but caused major structural changes and premature leaf shedding in apple trees."[31] Newly introduced enzymes could create unexpected, even totally new products, by interacting with other enzymatic pathways.

While evaluating the impact of a few new proteins or enzymes is difficult or impossible, consider the complex interaction of hundreds of thousands of changed protein levels that may result from gene insertion. According to Schubert, "While these types of unpredicted changes in gene expression are very real, they have not received much attention outside the community of the DNA chip users. Furthermore, they are not unexpected." [32]

2 . 4

The promoter may accidentally switch on harmful genes

"The activity of the CaMV promoter is itself unregulated, acting something like an out-of-control flywheel that drives whatever gene(s) it lands closest to, without consideration of the balance, integration, and co-ordination that regulate gene function in a normal plant."[33]

— E. Ann Clark, crop physiologist, University of Guelph

1. Promoters are switches that turn on genes.

2. The promoter used in nearly all GM crops is designed to permanently turn on the foreign gene at high output.

3. Although scientists had claimed that the promoter would only turn on the foreign gene, it can accidentally turn on other natural plant genes—permanently.

4. These genes may overproduce an allergen, toxin, carcinogen or antinutrient, or regulators that block other genes.

Although the plant genome contains tens of thousands of genes, they are not all active at the same time; sets of genes are switched on at different times and locations. The amount of RNA and proteins that each gene produces, if any, is normally determined by the needs of the cells or tissues. This is ultimately accomplished through the action of promoters, genetic sequences located immediately next to the gene, which dictate its level of expression. (The DNA sequence of the promoter is able to bind with certain proteins, which in turn attract another protein complex called RNA polymerase. The more RNA polymerase that is recruited to a promoter, the more RNA is transcribed from the DNA.) The effectiveness of the promoter can be greatly magnified by other genetic sequences called enhancers. The enhancers can be located much further away from a gene, and can multiply the gene expression tens, hundreds, or even thousands of times.

Genetic engineering places new genes into the DNA of the host, which have not evolved as a part of the organism and are not turned on based on the needs of the cell. In most cases, therefore, scientists attach to the transgenes a powerful promoter (usually with associated enhancer sequences) designed to permanently switch genes on. Thus, transgenes operate independently of the cells' self-regulatory mechanisms. They are artificially stimulated to continuously produce large quantities of proteins.

A significant risk of inserting a transgene into a genome is that the new promoter (or its enhancers) might unintentionally either switch on inactive genes or increase the expression of already active genes present in the host DNA. If this happens, then the natural genes are no longer under the cells' control, but are forced to overproduce proteins without a break.

A tragic example of this mechanism occurred in the treatment of boys with Severe Combined Immune Deficiency type X, known as X-SCID. Scientists inserted the gene that was missing in the boys' DNA. It cured their condition but three of the boys developed leukemia. It is believed that the enhancer, that was part of the inserted therapy gene unit, stimulated a nearby promoter, which switched on a gene permanently. The gene made a growth regulator (LMO2). Expression levels went up one-thousandfold. T-cells grew out of control and caused cancer.[34]

The promoter can switch on host genes

The powerful promoter used in nearly all GM crops is called the cauliflower mosaic virus (CaMV) 35S promoter. It originates from the cauliflower mosaic virus, but is altered in several significant ways.

Advocates of the promoter insisted that it would only turn on the transgene to which it was attached. Studies show, however, that the CaMV 35S promoter can and does switch on other natural genes. Ann Clark notes, "The 35S viral promoter can force hyperexpression of wholly unrelated genes, not just the original transgene."[35]

Another popular defense of the CaMV 35S promoter is that since it is found naturally in a plant virus, infected plants like cauliflowers are regularly exposed to the virus in nature; its promoter must not be harmful. But in its natural state, writes geneticist Joseph Cummins and others, the promoter "is a stable, integral part of the virus, and cannot be compared to the 35S promoter in artificial transgenic constructs."[36] The virus normally replicates in the cytoplasm of the cell—not in the nucleus. Thus, the natural virus promoter would not even be in the vicinity of the host plant's genes. With genetic engineering, however, the promoter is integrated into the genome, next to genes. According to Pusztai and Bardocz, it is "unacceptable to expect that the behavior and the potential hazard of the CaMV 35S promoter incorporated into the chromosome of transgenic plants is the same as the replication and behavior of the virus whose DNA possibly never integrates into the chromosomes of the infected plant cell."[37]

Switching on genes at random may produce toxins, carcinogens, allergens, antinutrients, enzymes that stimulate or inhibit hormone production, RNA that silences genes, or changes that will affect fetal development. In many experimental GM crops, the insertion sites have been mapped and scientists can speculate whether the foreign promoter may be impacting a dangerous gene in the host DNA. But with commercialized GM crops, no studies have actually looked at this potentially lethal problem.

2 . 5

The promoter might switch on a dormant virus in plants

"A possible scenario, in the case of the CaMV promoter, is for a sleeping pararetrovirus that has lost its promoter, to recombine with the CaMV promoter to give an infectious recombinant virus."[38]

—Mae-Wan Ho, et al, *Microbial Ecology in Health and Disease*

1. When certain viruses infect an organism, they splice themselves into the host's DNA.

2. These embedded viral sequences can be passed on to future generations and even inherited by future species.

3. Most ancient embedded viral sequences become mutated over time, but some may be intact, just not switched on.

4. If the GM promoter is inserted in the vicinity of a dormant virus, it might switch it on, resulting in virus production and a potential catastrophe.

Certain viruses splice themselves into the DNA of organisms they infect. Once integrated into the DNA, these viral sequences, called proviruses, can synthesize genetic material to produce new viruses. Since proviruses are embedded in the DNA, they can be inherited by offspring and are even passed on to future species. Thus, the DNA of many organisms, including plants, animals and humans, contain ancient viral sequences.

Most of these proviruses have become non-functional due to eons of mutation. In some cases, however, the virus-producing sequence may be intact, but the accompanying promoter or enhancer is no longer functioning. In theory, a GM promoter or enhancer might be inserted near such a provirus, causing it to produce potentially dangerous viruses.

Reactivation of dormant (endogenous) retroviruses has been observed in many different kinds of cells. To guard against this, all GM crops should have the insertion site mapped and sequenced to make sure that the transgene has not been inserted near known proviral genetic material. Such mapping is simple and takes only a few days, but is not generally done.

It is true that the chance of waking a dormant virus is quite small. There are presumably very few intact proviruses and billions of possible locations where a transgene might end up. But the potential severity of activating an ancient virus if it *were* to occur, demands investigation. Even a miniscule but finite possibility, given enough time, becomes a certainty.

2 . 6

The promoter might create genetic instability and mutations

"The CaMV 35S promoter sequence contains a "recombination hot-spot," meaning it is especially prone to breaking and rejoining with other DNA. Herein lies the potential for unintended side effects."[39]

—E. Ann Clark,
crop physiologist,
University of Guelph

1. Evidence suggests that the CaMV promoter, used in most GM foods, contains a recombination hotspot.

2. If confirmed, this might result in breakup and recombination of the gene sequence.

3. This instability of the inserted gene material might create unpredicted effects.

Recombination hotspots are genetic sequences that attract enzymes, which then cut the nearby DNA and reconnect it in different combinations. This recombination is often done for repair purposes but is sometimes destructive. Researchers identified such a hotspot in a 19 base pair sequence within the CaMV 35S promoter, which is used in most GM foods.[40] In their study, they identified seven places in the promoter where the DNA had recombined; six out of the seven were found near the hotspot. Another study also found that fragmentation and recombination of genetic sequences occurred frequently within the promoter.[41]

Instability of the CaMV 35S promoter may help explain a study that was reported in 2003. Scientists analyzed the transgene sequence of five GM crop varieties. In each case, the sequence identified was not the same as had been registered with the European Union by the biotech company.[42] This suggests instability and spontaneous rearrangements. According to Mae-Wan Ho, director of the Institute of Science in Society, "Many of the breakpoints for rearrangement involve the CaMV 35S promoter, as can be predicted from its known recombination hotspot."[43]

The scale of genetic instability caused by CaMV is unknown, but there is certainly a limit. If it recombined too extensively, it would quickly self-destruct and no longer switch on the transgene. GM crop developers verify that their introduced traits are stable over several generations prior to commercialization. But small scale, localized recombinations that do not switch off gene expression may be a greater concern, because the mutated transgene may continue to create unintended RNA and proteins.

There is also evidence that other genetic elements inserted into plants "may act as 'hotspots' and elicit recombination at high frequencies (the Ti plasmid of *Agrobacterium tumefasciens* and the NOS terminator)."[44]

2 . 7

Genetic engineering activates mobile DNA, called transposons, which generate mutations

"*After common errors in feeding and infections had by and large been ruled out as the cause of death, the farmer now suspects Syngenta company GM maize as to blame for the sudden death of his cows.*"[53]

— Greenpeace report

1. In plant DNA, mobile elements called transposons move from place to place and can lead to mutations.

2. The tissue culture process used in genetic engineering activates transposons, and is a major factor for the resulting genome-wide mutations.

3. Transgenes in commercial GM crops tend to be inserted near transposons.

4. This insertion might alter the transgene expression.

Throughout the genome of plants are virus-like DNA sequences called transposons. Under conditions of stress, transposons are activated and make RNA. Their RNA, however, produces DNA, which then reinserts itself back into the genome in a new location. This reinsertion causes a mutation at the insertion site and may disrupt gene expression in some way.

Under normal conditions, transposons are rarely activated. During tissue culture, however, they are widely activated, which helps explain the extensive DNA mutations associated with this method. According to biologist David Schubert, "This is the biggest single source for mutations in genetic engineering."[45]

Based on analysis of six transgene insertion sites, four (corn varieties T25, Mon 810, GA21, and *Bt* 11 corn) appeared to be in or near transposons.[46] "This poses additional risks."[47] The promoter (and enhancers) that accompany the transgene may cause the transposons to become more active and mobile. In addition, the strong promoters that are often associated with transposons may increase the expression levels of the transgenes. According to Traavik and Heinemann, "All these events may have unpredictable effects on the long-term genetic stability of [GMOs], as well as on their nutritional value, allergenicity, and toxicant contents."[48]

Biophysicist and geneticist Mae-Wan Ho points out another risk of transgene insertion near transposons. She says that the transgene may become mobile with the transposon and deposit additional copies of itself in other locations in the DNA, also resulting in further genome scrambling.

[Some advocates of GM crops argue that transgene insertions act just like transposons in the DNA, and therefore GM technology is nothing new or special. According to Freese and Schubert, "This natural process, however, is very distinct from GE gene insertion." Transposons do not have a "viral promoter to drive continuous expression" and "while the transposon event in wild-type plants is rare and subject to natural selection," the GM insertion is artificially selected by the scientist. In addition, the "sites of transposon insertion are not completely random throughout the chromosome, and may be quite distinct from the insertion sites of engineered genes."[49]]

2 . 8

Novel RNA may be harmful to humans and their offspring

"The creation of novel RNA molecules by insertion of DNA into the maize genome could create species of RNA that are harmful to humans, possibly through food. . . . There is also evidence in animal studies that some small RNA molecules can be transmitted through food, causing lasting, sometimes heritable, effects on consumers and their children."[50]

—New Zealand Institute of Gene Ecology

1. Small RNA sequences can regulate gene expression, most commonly by silencing genes.

2. RNA is stable, survives digestion and, can impact gene expression in mammals that ingest it.

3. The impact can be passed on to future generations.

4. Genetic modification introduces new DNA combinations and mutations, which increase the likelihood that harmful regulatory RNA will be accidentally produced.

RNA has a far more important role in controlling gene expression and cellular processes than previously thought. Consider that 63% of the mouse genome is transcribed into RNA, while only about 1%–2% of the genome actually codes for proteins.[51] "The newly revealed ferment of RNA transcription," according to *Nature*, combined with the finding that 'microRNAs' and other RNA molecules are "now known to be vital in controlling many cellular processes in plants and animals . . . contributes to the view that RNA actively processes and carries out the instructions in the genome."[52] In fact, "well over one-third of human genes appear to be" regulated by double stranded RNA (dsRNA).[53]

One of the best known functions of regulatory RNA is to silence genes. This is typically accomplished by very small RNA molecules, e.g. less than 30 nucleotides,[54] usually in the form of double-stranded RNA. "Silencing instigated by dsRNA occurs in organisms of all biological kingdoms."[55]

According to the Centre for Integrated Research on Biosafety (INBI), "Once introduced into a model plant or animal, the effect of dsRNA is systemically spread throughout the organism and persists through the entire developmental period. Uniquely in humans, so far as is known from tissue culture experiments, [dsRNA species longer than 50 nucleotides cause a complete cessation of all gene expression[56] (and thus effectively kill human cells)."[57]

RNA effects can transmit through food and then be inherited by the next generation in many different organisms (although this has not been demonstrated in humans).[58] When worms were fed bacteria engineered to produce dsRNA, for example, the dsRNA survived digestion and penetrated into the worms' gut cells and deeper tissues. It silenced the corresponding gene in the worm *and in the offspring for at least two generations.*[59] In other studies, inherited RNA apparently silenced a gene in mice[60] and repaired an abnormal DNA sequence in a plant.[61]

GM crops raise RNA risks

Changes produced by GM transformation might create harmful RNA in many ways. A segment of the transgene may be nearly identical to a sequence of the plant genome. This increases the likelihood that they will together form dsRNA. Shorter regulatory RNA may also be produced when transcription stops before the full gene is read (called an aborted transcript), and RNA sequences can be further rearranged by the cell after transcription. The probability of randomly producing dangerous RNA is increased because regulatory sequences can be very short.

Activation or interference with a pseudogene can also impact RNA regulation. "A pseudogene is a gene copy that does not produce a functional, full-length protein. The human genome is estimated to contain up to 20,000 pseudogenes. . . . Their biological roles remain largely unknown."[62] A study in *Nature* confirmed that a gene insert into mouse DNA altered the expression of a nearby pseudogene, which in turn altered the activity of regulatory RNA.

According to INBI, "The same dsRNA can have physiologically different effects[63] at different concentrations."[64] It is not always clear in advance which gene the dsRNA will affect. "The potential to inadvertently create novel RNA regulatory molecules, usually in the form of dsRNA, is too high by chance to ignore."[65] They say it is "imperative" to find out if and how much regulatory RNA is produced by GM crops and how this might influence the plant, wildlife exposed to the plant (by "grafting or pollination"), and humans who consume it.[66]

Regulators rely on obsolete assumptions

Regulators dismiss concerns about RNA based on obsolete assumptions. FSANZ, for example, said "RNA is rapidly degraded even in intact cells. Following harvest, processing, cooking, and digestion, it is unlikely that intact RNA would remain. Even if it did, it is very unlikely that it would enter human cells and be able to exert effects on endogenous genes." INBI points out that dsRNA is, in fact "stable enough in mammalian cells to be routinely used as gene regulators. . . . It is transmitted through food in other animals, where it survives degradation in bacteria producing the molecule and digestion in the animal gut. The medical literature is already exploring the use of exogenously developed dsRNA as therapeutics.[67] Delivery mechanism in mammals include through food[68] and injection.[69] Injection of dsRNA into the tail of a mouse affects gene expression in broadly distributed organs,[70] thus demonstrating its stability and transmissibility inside mammals."[71]

INBI further cites a study in which "Mice were fed *E. coli* expressing dsRNA. . . . The bacteria were nonpathogenic but engineered to invade human cells.[72] What the study demonstrates is that dsRNA is stable in *E. coli*, stable in the human stomach under some conditions, survives the intestine, and is biologically active in intestinal cells. *The dsRNA was transmitted to the animal through oral ingestion, as if it were food.*"[73]

2 . 9

Roundup Ready soybeans produce unintentional RNA variations

"The NOS terminator signal of transcription introduced into the genome in [Roundup Ready soy] is (at least in part) ignored, resulting in the production of an over-length transcript. Furthermore, this transcript was found to be processed . . . resulting in the production of different RNA variants. . . . Since the nos terminator was introduced as regulatory region in several other GMOs, read-through products and RNA variants might be transcribed in these transgenic crops as well." [74]

—Andreas Rang, et al, *European Food Research and Technology*

1. A "stop signal" is placed after the transgene, telling the cell, "STOP TRANSCRIBING AT THIS POINT."

2. The stop is ignored in GM soy, resulting in longer than intended RNA.

3. It is transcribed from a combination of the transgene, an adjacent transgene fragment, and a mutated sequence of DNA.

4. The RNA is further rearranged into four variations, any of which may be harmful.

5. The faulty "stop" signal may have triggered the rearrangements.

6. The same "stop" signal is used in other crops, and might lead to similar "read-throughs" and RNA processing.

nserted promoters instruct the cell, "START READ-ING THE TRANSGENE FROM HERE." Another genetic sequence, called the stop signal or stop sequence, is located on the opposite side of the transgene. It tells the transcription mechanism, "STOP READING AT THIS POINT." The promoter and stop signal, therefore, set the length of the RNA that is transcribed from the DNA. The terminator used most often in GM crops is called the NOS terminator.

In 2000, years after GM soybeans were introduced, scientists discovered two extra Roundup Ready transgene fragments in the soy DNA. One of these fragments (254 base pairs) was located immediately after the NOS terminator.[75]

A 2005 study further determined that the NOS terminator was not functioning as expected. The stop signal was ignored and the cell continued to read the DNA "resulting in the production of an over-length transcript." The resulting RNA combined sequences from both the transgene and the adjacent transgene fragment. But it didn't stop there. It also contained sequences from plant DNA located downstream from the fragment.[76] That plant DNA was actually part of a section (534 base pairs) that had been significantly mutated[77] (probably due to insertion mutation) and was unlike any known natural soy sequence.

To complicate things further, for some unknown reason this longer-than-intended RNA strand was processed by the cell into four different variations. Four sections of the code, ranging from 368 to 413 bases, were deleted and the remaining RNA was reattached into four strands of varying lengths.

The splicing and rearranging of RNA is a common feature in gene expression. It allows a gene to produce more than one protein. Indeed, the authors state, "As deduced from our data, the RNA variants described in this study may code for as yet unknown … fusion proteins." In this case, the fusion protein includes amino acids translated from three sources: the transgene, transgene fragment and mutated plant DNA. It is unknown if the proteins would be harmful.

The four RNA variants present another risk. Sections may turn out to be regulatory RNA, which might silence a gene in the plant or even in humans who consume the soy. The Centre for Integrated Research on Biosafety (INBI) says that the "post-transcriptional processing" of RNA into the four variants "could signal entry into pathways that produce regulatory RNAs."[78] No one has yet studied this possibility.

Problems may be common to GM crops

The authors speculate that sequences within the NOS terminator may "be responsible for processing the RNA" into four variants. Furthermore, "Since the NOS terminator was and still is commonly used" in GM crops, "read-through products and RNA variants could also be expressed in these plants."[79] In other words, because of an unreliable NOS terminator, GM crops might regularly create over-length RNAs, which are then spliced into various sizes. These, in turn, might create dangerous regulatory RNA or fusion proteins.

Monsanto offers baseless denials

In response to the 2001 study that identified the location of the gene fragment and scrambled plant DNA in GM soybeans, Monsanto boldly assured everyone that "no new mRNA transcripts or proteins are produced from the newly described DNA."[80] Monsanto's assurances notwithstanding, the mutations and extra transgene sequences do produce new transcripts and may in fact lead to unknown proteins.

Monsanto also claimed in 2002 that RNA "is generally recognized as safe (GRAS)," and thus "the presence of . . . secondary RNA transcripts themselves raises no safety concern."[81] As for being safe, INBI says that "such claims are incongruous with the literature on small RNA molecules and gene silencing effects."[82]

2.10

Changes in proteins can alter thousands of natural chemicals in plants, increasing toxins or reducing phytonutrients

"Of particular concern in plants is the potential for induced alterations in their secondary metabolite patterns."[83]

—Royal Society of Canada

"It is the alterations in the synthesis of low molecular weight toxins, mutagens and carcinogens caused by GE that has the potential to be the single greatest long-term health risk entailed by this technology."

— David Schubert, molecular biologist and protein chemist, Salk Institute for Biological Studies

1. Plants produce thousands of chemicals which, if ingested, may fight disease, influence behavior or be toxic.

2. The genome changes described in this section can alter the composition and concentration of these chemicals.

3. GM soybeans, for example, produce less cancer-fighting isoflavones.

4. Most GM-induced changes in these natural products go undetected.

Most plants "make a unique mixture of chemicals" [84] called natural products (also known as secondary metabolites). About 100,000 natural products have been identified and researchers say there may be more than half a million.[85] A single plant can produce more than 5,000.[86] Proteins provide inputs for biochemical pathways that create natural products. "When you insert a foreign gene, you are changing the whole metabolic process," says horticulture professor Sharad Phatak. "You just don't change one thing. Each change is going to have an effect on other pathways."[87] According to a UK government funded study, changes "to a specific biochemical pathway can result in unintended effects to related and unrelated pathways."[88] This can be triggered by the GM protein and by unintended changes in gene expression due to genetic engineering.

Toxins may increase

"Most of mankind's staple food plants were once low yield and very pest resistant," says microbiologist Mark Rasmussen. "Pest resistance was due to the presence of a wide array of defensive chemical compounds within the plant."[89] According to the Royal Society of Canada, "These 'secondary' metabolites represent an extraordinarily rich chemical arsenal that enables plants to survive as immobile organisms in a challenging environment."[90]

Many plant compounds are toxic or carcinogenic. Some, called excitotoxins, can cause neurological damage.[91] Through selective breeding over centuries, harmful compounds in food have been suppressed. These include crops that have been genetically engineered, e.g. corn, soybean, canola, tomato, alfalfa, and potato.[92] "However, secondary metabolism is highly plastic," warns the Royal Society, and "changes in enzyme levels" and/or other input levels "can have a marked effect[93] on the final metabolite profile." It is "important to establish that transgene insertion has not significantly altered the secondary metabolite profile."[94]

In fact, "in most advisory reports it is stated that the possibility of altered levels of natural toxins and important nutrients should be investigated."[95] Unfortunately, adequately safeguarding against toxic natural products may be impossible at this point. "Every plant and microbial species will possess a unique spectrum of chemicals," says natural products specialist Richard Firn. "Natural product metabolism is predictably unpredictable." He says that a gene that codes for an enzyme used to create a natural product "might be producing several unknown new structures. Looking for unknowns is a challenge and determining the structures of these new chemicals is an even greater challenge." Extracting or synthesizing sufficient quantities of the chemicals for toxicological studies may be impossible and there is no reference data to determine if slight changes in the chemicals produced in GM plants would be harmful. Furthermore, the production of natural products varies with temperature, water, insects, infection, and many other factors. "Consequently, any analysis that is undertaken of the natural product composition of a plant really only applies to the conditions used," Firn says. "Studies of the composition of plants grown under a range of conditions, with and without infestations and infections, would be required to provide meaningful conclusions."[96]

Rasmussen, who was formerly with the USDA, says that long-term, "full life cycle" feeding studies, which include reproduction analysis are "the best, if not the only means by which to identify those plant modifications with unexpected or novel toxins."[97] But David Schubert points out, "Even extensive animal testing might not detect the consequences of deficiencies in beneficial plant products."[98] In any case, extensive animal testing is not done for GM crops.

Beneficial compounds may change

A new science has emerged to study useful phytonutrients. A USDA Website reported, "On the cusp of the millennium, researchers are busily uncovering a host of beneficial compounds in plant foods. …They apparently reduce risks of diseases of aging. For example, the isoflavones in soy products may reduce the risk of heart disease, osteoporosis, and several types of cancer."[99] Antioxidants found in grape skins may also fight cancer and reduce heart disease and the pigment in blueberries may revive the brain's neural communication system. "Plants make a very large variety of nutrients and antioxidants whose loss or reduction could have serious adverse consequences for human health."[100] But unpredicted changes due to genetic modification might eliminate important ones before they are identified. Researchers have already shown that some Roundup Ready soy varieties contain 12%–14% less of the cancer-fighting isoflavones touted by the USDA. The levels in GM soy were also more variable.[101]

A study in *Science* in December 2002 described that "food molecules act like hormones, regulating body functioning and triggering cell division. The molecules can cause mental imbalances ranging from attention-deficit and hyperactivity disorder to serious mental illness."[102] Preliminary evidence of changed behavior in GM-fed animals was presented in section 1.14 and 1.19.

2.11

GM crops have altered levels of nutrients and toxins

> "No one can scientifically claim to be able to predict all consequences of the presence and functioning of a new gene (and even less for several) in a genome which has never been exposed [to] or contained this gene. The potential hazard here is not a consequence of the action of modification [of] the plant genome, but of the fact that it generates high levels of unpredictability."[103]
>
> — European Commission

1. Numerous studies on GMOs reveal unintended changes in nutrients, toxins, allergens, and small molecule products of metabolism.

2. These demonstrate the risks associated with unintended changes that occur due to genetic engineering.

3. Safety assessments are not adequate to guard against potential health risks associated with these changes.

Previous pages in this section describe how the GM transformation process may alter the composition of GM crops. Unfortunately, biotech companies avoid using modern techniques to identify and quantify many known nutrients, antioxidants, mutagens, carcinogens and toxins in plants. Instead, they typically measure only a few items at a gross compositional level (e.g. total protein, total carbohydrates) rather than specific components (e.g. what proteins, what carbohydrates). Furthermore, studies are designed to make it difficult to identify significant differences (see part 3).

Reviews of safety assessments for GM crop approvals in the United States[104] and Europe[105] show that compositional analyses are highly inconsistent between submissions. In several, "no declarations even on essential inherent plant toxins and antinutrients could be found."[106] Reviewers call for "consistent guidelines" that specify harmful compounds to be evaluated for each species[107] and the US National Academy of Sciences recommends "the establishment of a database for natural plant compounds of potential dietary or other toxicological concern."[108] Even without consistent and meaningful measurements, there is plenty of evidence of unexpected compositional changes in experimental and commercialized GMOs.

Changed metabolites

Metabolites are small molecules that are the intermediate and end products of metabolism. They can be beneficial or harmful (e.g. nutrients or toxins). In four lines of potatoes engineered to alter sugar metabolism, scientists measured the presence of 88 metabolites. Most levels had been changed and 9 of the 88 were only present in the GM potatoes—not controls.[109] David Schubert writes, "Given the enormous pool of plant metabolites, the observation that 10% of those assayed are new in one set of transfections [GM transformation events] strongly suggests that undesirable or harmful metabolites may be produced and accumulate."[110]

In most cases, changed metabolites in GM crops are not measured. By knowing which major compound has been altered, sometimes one can infer changes in intermediate products. For example, the stems of Bt-corn varieties MON 810 and Bt-11,[111] as well as Roundup Ready soybeans, have markedly increased levels of lignin (by 20%)—a woody, non-digestible compound.[112] Lignin is produced through a complex series of steps, which also create other important plant constituents. Since lignin has increased, the amount of the other related compounds may have changed. According to David Schubert, "Components of

this same biochemical pathway also produce both flavonoids and isoflavonoids that have a high nutritional value, and rotenone, a plant-produced insecticide that may cause Parkinson's disease."[113,114] No tests have been done to evaluate changes in these other components. In fact, even the increased lignin content in corn was not discovered until the varieties had been on the market for five years. The higher lignin in soybeans was only identified after the stems of plants inexplicably split in the heat at the height of the growing season.

It is odd that lignin increased in three separate GM products. Schubert and Freese write, "Normally, one would expect that each non-repeatable, unique transformation event [gene insertion] would yield unique unintended effects." They suggest that an increase in lignin, and possibly other undetected effects, may be an unintentional response to the insertion of a unique gene, as opposed to the usually random mutations caused by the genetic engineering process.

Examples of unpredicted changes

Tobacco: When genes were inserted into tobacco to produce a particular acid, the plant also created a toxic compound not normally found in tobacco.[115]

Yeast: Yeast DNA was inserted with multiple copies of its own genes in order to increase alcohol production. This unexpectedly raised levels of a naturally occurring toxin and potential carcinogen by 40 to 200 times. The authors said that their results "may raise some questions regarding the safety and acceptability of genetically engineered food, and give some credence to the many consumers who are not yet prepared to accept food produced using gene engineering techniques."[116]

Potatoes: When Oxford University scientists attempted to suppress a potato enzyme, the starch content increased substantially. Plant scientist Chris Leaver said, "We were as surprised as anyone. . . . Nothing in our current understanding of the metabolic pathways of plants would have suggested that our enzyme would have such a profound influence on starch production."[117] In other potatoes inserted with a soybean gene (glycinin), some vitamins were reduced and dangerous toxins (solanine and chaconine) increased. And although the insertion was designed to increase protein content, the transgenic version has *less* protein than the controls.[118]

Potatoes engineered to produce an insecticide (GNA lectin), contained 22% less protein than their own parent line. And the nutritional content of two different GM potatoes from the same parent line grown in identical conditions was significantly different. Other GM potato varieties had problems with tissues[119] and carbohydrate processing.[120]

Wheat: One GM wheat variety showed lesions,[121] another variety had higher levels of toxicity.[122]

Rice: One GM rice unexpectedly produced 50% more vitamin B6.[123] Another designed to produce vitamin A altered other compounds (carotenoid derivatives).[124]

Peas: GM pea varieties showed a fourfold increase in lectins and a doubling of trypsin inhibitor.[125]

Squash: A USDA-approved GM squash contains 67 times less beta-carotene and 4 times more sodium than non-GM squash.[126]

Soy: Monsanto's own study on Roundup Ready soy showed significant differences in the ash, fat, and carbohydrate content as well as a 27% increase in trypsin inhibitor,[127] a known allergen. Additional differences (which Monsanto had omitted from their paper but were later recovered in journal archives) showed that GM soy had significantly lower levels of protein, a fatty acid, and phenylalanine (an essential amino acid). The toasted GM soy meal contained nearly twice the amount of a lectin, which may interfere with assimilation of nutrients.[128]

There was also a disturbing finding related to trypsin inhibitor. Cooking normally breaks down (denatures) this potential allergen, making it safer to consume, but "heat treatment appeared to have a far lesser denaturing effect on the trypsin inhibitor content of the GM lines."[129] The cooked soy had nearly as much trypsin inhibitor as the uncooked variety—as much as seven times more than non-GM soy.

In the same study, both rats and catfish fed various lines of Roundup Ready soybeans exhibited different growth rates, suggesting that the nutrition content of the soybeans varied significantly. Also, cows fed GM soy produced milk with a higher fat content than those fed non-GM soy.[130]

In a 2004 study, cooked soybean meal from Argentina had about 18.5% less protein than meal from China and India. US soybean meal had about 8.5% less. These differences might be attributable to the genetic modification. At the time of the study, soy from Argentina was almost all GM, while soy from the United States was mixed. Soy from China and India, which had the higher protein content, was non-GM.[131]

Corn: In *Bt*-corn MON 810, 8 out of the 18 amino acids measured (44%) were significantly different than the controls. The Public Health Association of Australia (PHAA) points out that the expected new protein created from the transgene "constitutes less than 0.001% of the total protein ... the change in amino acid profile cannot be at-

tributed to the presence of this new, expected protein in the plant. It indicates that other proteins may have been produced, which may be potentially toxic."[132] The calcium and beta tocopherols levels were also significantly different.[133]

Roundup Ready corn varied significantly in five amino acids. As amino acids may form potentially harmful proteins, the PHAA, said it was "of concern that these results have not been followed-up with experiments of the whole food to determine if any new, unexpected substances are present which may cause disease."[134]

In Liberty Link corn, two of six fatty acids, 7 of 18 amino acids, and calcium, phosphorus, protein, and carbohydrate levels were statistically different. (Calcium was down 64%.)[135]

A high-lysine corn under review for commercialization "had higher levels in all of the 18 measured amino acids among the four commercial varieties used as references."[136] (115.17 mg/g compared to an average of 77.8 mg/g.)

Canola: Although the vitamin A (carotene) content of canola seeds was successfully increased (50-fold) with the addition of a bacterial gene, there was an unexpected and significant decrease in vitamin E (tocopherol). The fatty acid composition was significantly altered and chlorophyll levels were also reduced.[137]

Monsanto's Roundup Ready Canola line Gt173 has significantly higher levels of amino acids compared to its parent line. The increase is greater that the additional protein produced from the inserted genes and, according to the PHAA, should have been further evaluated for possible toxicity.[138] The canola also had a significantly altered fat content.[139]

Unexpected agricultural performance

In addition to lab tests, we can infer other compositional differences based on varied agronomic performance of GM crops and the reactions of plants to various conditions of disease and stress. The levels of certain toxins in potatoes (sesquiterpenes and the glycoalkaloids—PGAs), for example, differed between GM potatoes and non-GM potatoes, after they were exposed to a variety of stresses in the field and at the store.[140]

GM cotton has greater susceptibility to nematodes[141] and other pests, and in various conditions, dropped their cotton bolls, died on contact with the herbicide they were engineered to tolerate, succumbed to disease or drought, failed to germinate, or had smaller cotton bolls and poorer cotton quality. Monsanto paid millions in settlements with farmers.[142]

Yields of GM Roundup Ready soy have been on average 7%–10% less than equivalent conventional varieties.[143]

Furthermore, a study consisting of side-by-side field trials over a two-year period at four different locations of GM and equivalent non-GM varieties of glyphosate-resistant (GR) soybean cultivars concluded that, "Yields were suppressed with GR soybean cultivars. ... The work reported here demonstrates that a **5% yield suppression was related to the gene or its insertion process** and another 5% suppression was due to cultivar genetic differential."[144] Given that yield is dependent on the overall physiological condition of the plants and not just on the function of a single gene, the results from these controlled studies demonstrate the general disruptive effect that the GM transformation process has on the genome and consequent biochemical functioning as a whole.

In spite of the overwhelming evidence of substantial compositional changes in GM crops, advocates continue to deny the presence of these unpredictable, potentially harmful changes. In a 2002 article, for example, the authors claimed that "transgenic varieties expressing a single agronomic trait (are) not expected to (have an) altered nutrient composition."[145] According to Pusztai and Bardocz, "It would be helpful in the interests of science to generally recognize and accept that views such as that . . . fly in the face of the facts and published data."[146]

New studies reveal more unknowns

Modern techniques can provide data on a full range of RNA transcripts, proteins, and metabolites (transcriptome, proteome, and metabolome) that are produced by an organism. Scientists have been calling for GM foods to be submitted to these analyses for some time. A 2005 UK government-funded study concluded that "a combination of proteomic, metabolomic, and genomic approaches would seem to be necessary for any safety assessment to be as comprehensive as possible."[147]

Recent studies using these techniques demonstrated that the impacts of the GM transformation process vary considerably from one "event" to another, producing both intended and unintended effects. In one study, the expression of "up to 58 genes" was increased or decreased "more than fivefold."[148] Another study concluded that "the unintended effects" of GM transformation were greater than the natural biological variation of the plant, when comparing plants grown under a specific experimental condition.[149]

Using these techniques to quantify how many proteins change and by how much, is limited by our lack of understanding of biochemical pathways. In a study of GM potatoes for example, researchers found that only 9 of the 730 proteins they analyzed showed significant differences. But

they were at a loss to explain how such small differences could result in some potato lines being extremely stunted with low tuber yield.[150]

Scientists have been cataloging various enzymes and their effects in their native organism for years. But according to Richard Firn, this "is only partly useful because it is the properties of the enzyme in its new biochemical environment that will determine which chemicals it transforms and at what rate."[151] Similarly, the European Commission says that "Even if a given protein per se does not represent an allergen, its expression in another host organism may indirectly upregulate the expression of potential allergens."[152]

Our lack of understanding of the effects of transporting material between species is compounded by our inability to grasp the holistic complexity at work inside plants and animals. "If a biologist is shown a map of all known biochemical pathways," says Firn, "they are unlikely to see any patterns—to most biologists it is just a collection of names and arrows. There is much knowledge, and some understanding, of many individual enzymes and most biochemical pathways, but how and why has evolution shaped biochemistry as an entity? If we cannot answer that question how can we confidently predict the outcomes of attempts to change an organism's biochemical repertoire by genetic manipulation?"[153]

The quest to understand these mechanics at work in plants is made more complicated by the finding that patterns of gene expression vary considerably due to changing environmental conditions. Variations in response to the environment, according to recent studies, were "generally greater than the effect of the genetic transformation."[154] This doesn't minimize the potential harm that can arise from the GM transformation process. Quite the contrary; changes due to genetic engineering would be added onto—and possibly interfere with—changes caused by the environment. For example, suppose that a gene or gene cluster designed to protect the plant from a specific infestation is disabled. If an infestation occurs, the plant may compensate by producing compounds that are toxic to humans. Safety assessments of GM crops grown only under a narrow range of conditions would overlook this risk and might not even identify that the genes were impaired.

"We have such a miserably poor understanding of how the organism develops from its DNA that I would be surprised if we don't get one rude shock after another."[1]

—Professor Richard Lewontin, professor of genetics, Harvard University

The protein produced by the inserted gene may create problems

Many safety assessments focus solely on the health implications of the GM protein created by the transgene and ignore the potential for widespread damage in the DNA, presented in the previous section. Even if we limit our focus to the narrow evaluation of these single proteins, however, there are significant health risks.

3 . 1

A gene from a Brazil nut carried allergies into soybeans

"In trying to build a better soybean the company had made a potentially deadly one."[2]

—*Washington Post*

1. A gene from a Brazil nut was inserted into soybeans.

2. When tests verified that people allergic to Brazil nuts would react to the GM soy, the project was canceled.

3. This research verified that genetic engineering can transfer allergenic proteins into crops.

Pioneer Hi-Bred wanted to create a soybean that had a more complete balance of protein. They inserted a gene from a Brazil nut into soy DNA to increase production of an amino acid (methionine). Although the soy was planned for use in animal feed, some would certainly end up in the human food chain. Since some people are allergic to Brazil nuts, the company had the soybean tested for allergenicity.

"I didn't think we'd find anything interesting,"[3] said scientist Steve Taylor, who figured that Brazil nuts produce thousands of proteins. The chances were quite small that the one created by the inserted gene was allergenic. Nonetheless, three separate tests (radioallergosorbent testing, immunoblotting, and skin-prick testing) all demonstrated that the soy did in fact cause reactions in people allergic to Brazil nuts.[4] The study, which was published in 1996 in the *New England Journal of Medicine*, confirmed that genes inserted into crops can carry allergenic properties.

New proteins are hard to test for allergies

Allergic reactions develop over time with repeated exposure. The above study had the advantage of using test subjects who had been exposed to Brazil nuts in the past and had developed confirmed allergic reactions. If they had tested the GM soy on people who had never before been exposed to the Brazil nut protein, their blood and skin would not have reacted.

This illustrates the problem with allergenicity testing in the current GM crops. Their DNA is inserted with genes from bacteria, viruses, and other organisms. The proteins they create have never before been part of the human food supply. People will not react to the protein in the first exposure and no one knows how many will develop allergies over time.

The FDA acknowledged this difficulty. Agency toxicologist Louis Pribyl wrote, "there are very few allergens that have been identified at the protein or gene level."[5] The FDA's 1992 policy states, "At this time, FDA is unaware of any practical method to predict or assess the potential for new proteins in food to induce allergenicity and requests comments on this issue."[6] Part 3 of this book reveals that the methods used still offer no guarantees and expose the population to significant allergy risks.

Avoiding GM allergens is difficult

People with food allergies often read labels carefully and interview restaurant wait staff to avoid allergens. Imagine what might have happened if Pioneer Hi-Bred's Brazil nut soybean were produced in the United States, where GM foods are not labeled. Those with Brazil nut allergies might have reacted to a wide range of foods containing soy derivatives without any understanding of the cause. A similar situation may already be occurring with GM foods on the market. A percentage of the population may have allergic reactions without a clue as to the origin of their condition.

Even if a country had strictly enforced mandatory labeling, there is always a threshold level below which GM content does not have to be labeled. Since some allergens can elicit responses at very low levels, reactions to small amounts of GM content are possible. Furthermore, GM content can vary with each shipment. Thus, people's reaction to a food may vary from day to day or brand to brand, making it difficult to identify the allergen.

3 . 2

GM proteins in soy, corn, and papaya may be allergens

> "While the EPA ostensibly 'requires' data on these three parameters for all Bt crop proteins 'to provide a reasonable certainty that no harm will result from the aggregate exposure'[7] to them, in practice it has simply not collected pertinent studies, accepted substandard ones, or ignored relevant evidence."[8]
>
> —William Freese and David Schubert, *Nature Biotechnology*

1. Tests cannot guarantee that a GM protein will not cause allergies.

2. The WHO and FAO offer criteria that help minimize the likelihood that allergenic GM crops are approved.

3. GM soybeans, corn, and papaya fail those criteria.

4. The GM proteins from these foods are too similar to known allergens.

5. This evidence was ignored by regulators, who approved the crops.

Although tests cannot verify that a novel GM protein won't cause allergies, the World Health Organization (WHO) and UN Food and Agriculture Organization (FAO) offer criteria to reduce the likelihood that allergenic GM crops are approved.[9] This includes examining GM protein for 1) similarity of amino acid sequences to known allergens, 2) digestive stability, and 3) heat stability. These three aren't *predictive* of allergenicity, but according to experts, their presence should be sufficient to reject the crop or at least require more testing. GM soy, corn, and papaya fail the WHO/FAO criteria, but all have been approved without follow-up testing.

GM proteins fail allergy tests

Crop developers search databases to see if the overall amino acid sequence of their GM protein is similar to known allergens. WHO/FAO also recommends comparing each segment of six amino acids with sections (epitopes) from known allergens where IgE antibodies (Immunoglobulin E) are known to attach.[10] IgE binding is required for a common type of allergic reaction to take place.

This method offers no guarantees. 1) Not all allergenic sequences have been identified. 2) Once the protein is folded, the exposed amino acid sequences are reconfigured anyway. 3) This method ignores allergies and food sensitivities that are unrelated to IgE. For these and other reasons, allergenic proteins can pass undetected using this method (see part 3).

Ironically, proteins that *have* been identified as having similarities to known allergies have been approved without regulators even officially acknowledging this red flag. In 1998, for example, an FDA researcher discovered that the Cry1Ab protein created in *Bt* corn shared a sequence of 9–12 amino acids with vitellogenin, an egg yolk allergen. The study concluded that "the similarity . . . might be sufficient to warrant additional evaluation."[11] No evaluation took place, however, and in 2001, the EPA re-registered the corn variety for an additional seven years.[12]

The two herbicide-resistance proteins produced by Roundup Ready crops were found to have sequences identical to those found in a shrimp allergen and a house dust mite allergen. This was discovered years after Roundup Ready soybeans were on the market. The protein in GM papaya also possesses allergen look-alike sequences.[13]

Since many food allergens are stable during digestion (giving people more time to get a reaction) a second test evaluates GM protein stability. Rather than using animal or human subjects to see if their proteins survive digestion,

safety assessments rely on an inferior, but less expensive method. They put GM protein into test tubes with digestive enzymes (pepsin) and, acid and measure how quickly the protein is broken down.

Test tube studies, however, do not accurately predict what happens inside the human gut. Several animal studies demonstrate that GM proteins, which break down quickly in test tubes, survive much longer in the actual digestive system.[14] Research also showed that these test tube studies cannot accurately distinguish between known allergens and non-allergens.[15,16]

In addition, companies manipulate results by using a stronger pH and more enzymes to breakdown their protein more quickly. Monsanto, for example, "used 2000 times the amount of pepsin by weight recommended in the WHO/FAO protocol,"[17] and a pH of 1.2, rather than the recommended 2.0. The EPA's Scientific Advisory Panel also concurred that "The normal population has a relative higher gastric value than the pH 1.2 or 1.5," and that using lower values does "not mimic the physiological state."[18]

The *Bt* protein Cry1Ab,[19] found in Monsanto's Yield Guard and Syngenta's *Bt*-11 corn varieties, fails the WHO/FAO criteria. It is particularly resistant to digestion—nearly as stable as the *Bt* found in the unapproved corn variety StarLink. One test tube study reported that 10% of Cry1Ab survived for one to two hours.[20] At two hours, there were still protein fragments of substantial size—within the range considered typical of food allergens (15 kilodaltons). If the conditions used were those specified by the WHO/FAO, the protein would have lasted even longer. (By contrast, Monsanto used so much pepsin and acid that they reported over 90% degradation in just two minutes.) Animal studies demonstrated that "Cry1Ab protein is 92% indigestible in pigs."[21] Similarly, after calves were fed *Bt*-11, undigested Cry1Ab was found in the stomach, intestine and feces.

A third test for allergenicity measures how well the protein survives heat treatment. This not only indicates general stability, it also suggests how well the protein might survive food processing. In one study, Cry1Ab was described as having "relatively significant thermostability . . . comparable to that of . . . Cry9C protein" found in StarLink corn. Although the study did not provide any additional measurements for Cry1AB, it did report that Cry9C protein was stable for 120 minutes at 90°C.[22] Here again, the EPA failed to collect the required heat stability data on Cry1Ab from Monsanto on its MON 810 corn variety.[23]

3 . 3

Bt crops may create allergies and illness

> *"The findings on Bt-toxins have been completely ignored in a regulatory process that can only be described as a sham."[24]*
>
> —Mae-Wan Ho and Joseph Cummins, Briefing to Parliament

1. Soil bacteria (*Bt*) create a natural pesticide that has been used in spray form for years.

2. Genes from the bacteria are inserted into crop DNA, so the plant produces *Bt*-toxin.

3. Approvals of *Bt* crops are based on the claim that the spray is harmless and *Bt*-toxin does not react with mammals.

4. In reality, *Bt* spray is linked to allergies and illness in humans and mammals.

5. *Bt*-toxins also elicit immune responses in mice.

Bt (*Bacillus thuringiensis*) is a soil bacterium that produces a pesticide. Solutions containing the bacteria (including spores and protein crystals) are sprayed on plants as a method of insect control, used by organic farmers. Scientists altered the sequence of the gene that produces *Bt*-toxin and inserted it into plant DNA. Very few studies have assessed the health effects of *Bt* crops. Instead, justification for their approval is largely based on the argument that *Bt* sprays have a history of safe use and that the *Bt*-toxin does not react with mammals. Research contradicts both arguments.

Bt spray is dangerous to humans

When *Bt* was sprayed over areas around Vancouver to fight gypsy moth infestations, nearly 250 people reported reactions—mostly allergy or flu-like symptoms. Spraying over Washington resulted in more than 250 health complaints; six people had to go to the emergency room for allergies or asthma.[25,26] Workers who apply *Bt* sprays reported eye, nose, throat, and respiratory irritation. The frequency of symptoms correlated with the degree of exposure.[27] The allergic symptoms associated with *Bt* spray exposure (allergic rhinitis (sneezing, running nose, watery eyes), dermatitis (skin inflammation), pruritis (itching), swelling, erythema (redness) with conjunctival infection (red eye), exacerbations of asthma, angioedema (facial swelling), and rash)[28] are nearly identical to those of *Bt* cotton workers in section 1.5.

One farmer who splashed a liquid *Bt* formulation in his eye developed an infection and an ulcer on his cornea.[29] Another splashed a *Bt* solution on his face and eyes and developed skin irritation, burning, swelling, and redness.[30] A woman exposed to *Bt* from spray drift went to the hospital due to burning, itching, and swelling of her face and upper chest. She later had a fever, altered consciousness, and seizures.[31] In one study, two farm workers exposed to *Bt*-toxins by inhalation, skin contact, and possibly ingestion had "indicators" of allergenicity. (Protein extracts of *Bt* pesticides containing Cry1Ab and Cry1Ac elicited positive skin tests and IgE antibody responses.) Although the workers did not have allergic reactions, they were tested after only one to four months. "Clinical symptoms would not be anticipated unless there was repeated long-term exposure."[32] In addition, the "healthy worker effect" might have biased the results, i.e., workers who were allergic to *Bt* may have already quit.

"People with compromised immune systems or preexisting allergies may be particularly susceptible to the effects of *Bt*."[33] Before a *Bt* spray program, the Oregon Health Division advises that "individuals with . . . physician-diagnosed causes of severe immune disorders may consider leaving the area during the actual spraying."[34] A spray manufacturer warns, "Repeated exposure via inhalation can result in sensitization and allergic response in hypersensitive individuals."[35] And injections of natural *Bt* were considerably more lethal to mice with reduced immune function compared to healthy mice.[36,37]

Bt-toxin is dangerous to mammals

Although inert chemicals added to *Bt* sprays may contribute to adverse reactions, isolated *Bt*-toxin clearly has an impact. In a series of mouse studies, for example, researchers demonstrated that *Bt*-toxin elicited an immune response throughout the system ("an intense systemic antibody response") as well as in localized areas ("the secretion of specific mucosal antibodies").[38] The immune response to *Bt*-toxin was "as potent as cholera toxin." In addition, the *Bt*-toxin caused the immune system to become overly sensitive to other compounds (eliciting systemic and mucosal adjuvant responses).[39] This suggests, for example, that *Bt*-toxin might make a person more susceptible to allergic reactions from a wide range of substances. These studies administered the *Bt*-toxin (Cry1Ac protoxin and toxin) by injection (intraperitoneally) and ingestion (intragastrically). In another study, *Bt* exposure via the nose and rectum induced antibody responses ("IgM, IgG, and IgA in all the mucosal surfaces analyzed").[40]

Expert advisors to the EPA said that the mouse and farm worker studies above "suggest that *Bt* proteins could act as antigenic and allergenic sources. ... Only surveillance and clinical assessment of exposed individuals will confirm the allergenicity of *Bt* products."[41]

GMO proponents claimed that since mammals (including humans) don't have receptors in their gut for *Bt*-toxin, it will not create a reaction. A 2000 study, however, confirmed that a *Bt* protein binds to surface proteins in the mouse's small intestine, with corresponding "changes in the electrophysiological properties" of the organ.[42] The form of the *Bt* protein used (Cry1Ac) is quite similar in structure to the *Bt* protein used in most *Bt* corn varieties (Cry1Ab). Binding tests on Cry1Ab have yielded ambiguous results. Cry1Ab created from GM *E. coli* did not show binding in rats, while test tube studies using tissue from the cecum and colon of rhesus monkeys did show some binding.[43] In addition, research presented in section 1.4 verified that *Bt*-toxin not only interacted with the small intestine (ileum), it caused abnormal and excessive cell growth.

3.4

The *Bt* in crops is more toxic than the *Bt* spray

"*It is very important to be aware of the fact that the Bt-toxins expressed in [genetically engineered plants] have never been carefully analyzed, and accordingly, their characteristics and properties are not known. What is clear from the starting point, however, is that they are vastly different from the bacterial Bacillus thuringiensis protoxins, used in organic and traditional farming and forestry for decennia.*"[44]

—Terje Traavik and Jack Heinemann

1. *Bt*-toxin in GM crops is more harmful than *Bt* spray due to differences in the concentration and form of the protein.

2. *Bt* sprays are used intermittently and degrade in the environment.

3. The *Bt*-toxin in crops is thousands of times more concentrated and is continuously produced in every plant cell.

4. The form of the *Bt*-toxin protein in GM crops is also more toxic.

Not only is *Bt* spray associated with allergies and immune responses, the *Bt* in GM crops is far more dangerous, based on the total exposure and the form of the protein.

Bt-toxin is more concentrated in crops

Bt spray is applied in organic agriculture only during high insect infestation emergencies. It is applied on the plant's surface and the concentration of the toxin quickly dissipates. "There is a rapid decline in the ability of the bacteria to infect insects within 12 to 48 hours after it is applied."[45] Furthermore, it is broken down within a few days to two weeks upon exposure to UV light from the sun.[46] "It is also degraded rapidly by high temperatures and substances on plants' leaves. It is also washed from leaves into the soil by rainfall"[47] or can be washed off by consumers.

A *Bt* crop, however, makes the toxin in every cell on a continuous basis. The concentration does not dissipate by the weather and it cannot be washed off.

It is estimated that the plants produce 3,000–5,000 times the amount of toxin as the sprays, but it varies with plants. Mon 810, for example, had 1,500–3,000 times the level found in sprayed plants. Since the *Bt*-toxin is exempted from the requirement of a tolerance, there are no legal limits as to how much can be expressed in food.

The higher concentration of *Bt*-toxin is by design. It is believed that by making the dose acutely toxic to pests, it will slow development of pest resistance to *Bt* crops.[48] As newer *Bt* crop varieties enter the market, the trend is to increase the amount of *Bt* protein even further. For instance, Mycogen/Pioneer's Herculex Cry1F corn, registered in 2001, expresses at least 10 times more Cry protein in kernels than MON 810.[49]

The *Bt* levels are therefore much higher for consumers. Farm workers exposed to corn dust and workers in mills and other processing plants would conceivably have an even greater risk.

The *Bt* protein in crops is more toxic

Bt sprays contain bacterial spores and the *Bt*-toxin protein—primarily in an inactive crystalline form (protoxin). The shape of the inactive protoxin does not necessarily alert the immune system that a toxin is present. Once inside the alkaline gut of an insect, the crystalline form becomes soluble and enzymes cut off a portion of the protein. When the extra amino acids are removed, the *Bt* becomes active.[50] It changes into a new shape that sounds the immune system's alarm.

When scientists engineer *Bt* crops, however, they usually remove the part of the gene that codes for the extra amino acids that make the toxin inactive. Thus, *Bt* crops such as *Bt*-11 corn, produce *Bt*-toxin which is immediately active without the need for an alkaline gut or further processing. Evidence suggests that these *Bt*-toxins will elicit a greater immune response in mammals than the natural inactive protoxin state.

Studies also demonstrate that that the toxin produced in *Bt* plants can be more deadly to insects than the natural bacterial variety. For example, when green lacewings consume lepidopterans that had previously consumed *Bt*-toxin, the chances of the green lacewing dying or suffering delayed development is greater if the lepidopterans had consumed *Bt* corn (containing Cry1AB) than if it had consumed much higher levels of natural *Bt*.[51]

When people eat *Bt* corn, they consume *Bt*-toxin in every bite. **It is remarkable that regulators have allowed this into our food based on obsolete assumptions that *Bt* sprays are harmless and that the form and exposure level of GM *Bt* is equivalent to sprayed *Bt*.** It is particularly alarming in light of consistent reports of immune system responses in lab animals and humans exposed to *Bt*, in animals fed *Bt* crops and in humans handling *Bt* cotton or breathing *Bt* corn pollen (see section 1).

3 . 5

StarLink corn's built-in pesticide has a "medium likelihood" of being an allergen

"Based on reasonable scientific certainty, there is no identifiable maximum level of Cry9C protein that can be suggested that would not provoke an allergic response and thus would not be harmful to the public."[52]

— EPA's Scientific Advisory Panel

1. StarLink corn, considered potentially allergenic by the US EPA, was approved as animal feed but not for human consumption.

2. The tiny amount planted in the United States nonetheless contaminated the food supply, prompting massive food recalls.

3. Thousands reported health effects, including life-threatening episodes they thought may be related to StarLink.

4. The FDA was unable to create a test to rule out allergenicity and experts say it has a "medium likelihood" of being an allergen.

5. A small amount remains in the food supply.

The *Bt* protein in StarLink corn (Cry9C) was designed to be more stable to enhance its ability to kill pests. As a result, it took longer to break down by heat and simulated gastric juices than other *Bt* proteins. Concerned that it may cause allergies, the EPA did not approve the corn for human consumption. They did approve StarLink as animal feed.

The agency told the seed's producer that farmers must sign statements that any StarLink they grew, plus any corn grown within 660 feet of it, was to be used for animal feed or industrial (fuel) purposes—not for human food. In spite of the rules, many farmers and grain elevators were never informed. Some StarLink seed tags even *stated* that the corn was suitable for "food, feed, or grain processing."[53]

In 1999, StarLink was planted on well under 1% of US corn acreage (247,694 acres). At least 60% was likely used for animal feed or ethanol.[54] But by the time a coalition of environmental groups discovered StarLink in store-bought taco shells in September 2000, StarLink was throughout the food chain. It was identified in 22% of the corn samples tested by the USDA. US shipments of corn were halted, the price of US corn dropped and over 10 million individual food items were subject to recall.[55] The debacle cost about $1 billion and exposed tens of millions of people to the potential allergen.[56]

Thousands complain of reactions

When the StarLink contamination was reported in the US media, thousands of people complained to food companies of reactions. It is not clear how many, if any, were StarLink-related, as neither the companies nor the FDA followed up. Hundreds contacted the FDA directly, but only 51 individuals bothered to fill out the paperwork necessary to officially register their reaction with the agency. Symptoms "varied from just abdominal pain and diarrhea [and] skin rashes to . . . a very small group having very severe life-threatening reactions."[57]

Prior to its discovery, people may have been having allergic reactions to StarLink for months without knowing the cause. In April 2000, for example, five months before the StarLink recall, one person "experienced immediate respiratory failure after ingesting two taco products."[58] He had a heart attack and died soon after. No one at the time knew to question whether the corn was the culprit.

It took the FDA nine months to develop and execute a test to see if StarLink's *Bt* protein was a human allergen. Even then, officials claimed that it wasn't definitive. A scientist working for StarLink's producer, Aventis, acknowledged that there is no way to ensure that a novel protein is not an allergen, other than "giving it to a lot of people and seeing what happens."[59]

The FDA's test found no positive reactions to StarLink's protein, but allergy experts on the EPA's Scientific Advisory Panel (SAP) said the test was so poorly designed (see part 3), its conclusions should not be accepted. They wrote, "The test, as conducted, does not eliminate StarLink Cry9C as a potential cause of allergic symptoms."[60] The SAP's final determination was that StarLink had a "medium likelihood" of being an allergen.

The panel also rejected a request by Aventis to allow a 20 parts per billion tolerance for Cry9C. The SAP stated that "smaller doses are more likely to sensitize the immune system than to induce tolerance." (Billionths of a gram of peanut allergen can provoke an allergic response.)

Although EPA's Stephen Johnson said it "would require many months or years of continued scientific evaluation to answer the question of allergenicity,"[61] the agency is not pursuing further study. The SAP recommended that allergy testing be expanded to include all GM foods, but this too is not being done. StarLink was officially withdrawn from commercial production, but continues to show up in corn around the world.

The StarLink affair brought to light several issues: 1) There is no secure way to segregate varieties of GM crops that look the same; 2) Even a small amount of dangerous GM foods could create a massive health and economic catastrophe; 3) Health effects from dangerous GM crops can go unidentified (if it hadn't been for a privately funded effort by Friends of the Earth and others, StarLink might still be on the market); 4) Testing procedures have not yet been designed to adequately verify that GM crops are free from allergens.

The criteria used by the EPA to ban StarLink from human food also raise questions about the allergenicity of other *Bt* proteins. StarLink's Cr9C protein was not approved for human consumption primarily because it broke down slowly in simulated gastric fluid. But according to industry research, the Cry1Ab protein that is still on the market "was digested at a similar, if slightly faster, rate than the *E. coli*-derived Cry9C protein in simulated gastric fluid."[62]

Allergies have skyrocketed since GM crops have been on the market. Without post-market surveillance or better allergy screening methods, GM crops must be considered a suspect for contributing to this situation.

3 . 6

Pollen-sterilizing barnase in GM crops may cause kidney damage

"In its consultation with Aventis on the company's GE male-sterile corn, the FDA apparently raised no concerns about Aventis' failure to test for possible expression of the pollen-sterilizing GE toxin . . . in kernels, leaves, or other non-pollen corn tissues, . . . despite evidence that bacterial barnase causes kidney damage in rats."[63]

—William Freese and David Schubert, *Nature Biotechnology*

1. Corn and canola are engineered to produce a pollen-sterilizing toxin called barnase.

2. Barnase is toxic to human cells and causes kidney damage in rats.

3. Although the GM plants were designed to produce the toxin in a non-food portion of the plant, some of the toxin is likely produced in all parts of the plant.

As part of the process of breeding hybrid corn, Aventis (now Bayer CropScience) developed male-sterile corn (MS6) that is incapable of producing viable pollen—it will not out-cross or self-pollinate.* This was accomplished by inserting a gene from a bacterium that creates the enzyme barnase.

Barnase is a known toxin. It degrades single-stranded RNA, is toxic to a variety of human cell lines,[64] and can destroy plant cells in which it is expressed.[65] When injected into rats, it causes kidney damage.[66]

Although the barnase gene is present in all cells of the corn plant, the company hoped that the toxic enzyme was produced only in the anther—the pollen-bearing part of the stamen. They therefore used a promoter to switch on the barnase gene which is "tissue-specific," normally activated in the anther.

According to Freese and Schubert, "It is well-known that so-called tissue-specific promoters drive production of low levels of transgenic protein in non-target tissues."[67] Thus, it is likely that low levels of barnase are created in the edible portions of the corn plant as well.

In 2002, three years after the USDA approved its male-sterile corn, Aventis was granted a patent on a new method for creating male sterile plants, one that used both the barnase gene and a "barstar" gene. In its patent application, the company admitted that the barnase gene can be expressed at low levels "in tissues other than the stamen cells," including "somatic cells of the plants or seeds." They therefore added barstar, a barnase inhibitor, "to counteract the undesired effects of possible low level expression of the male-sterility gene (e.g. comprising the barnase DNA)."[68]

Aventis did not elaborate on the nature of the "undesired effects" of barnase in its 2002 patent, yet the very existence of the patent suggests that the effects were serious enough to take measures to counteract them. But what about the MS6 (barnase only) line approved three years earlier? According to their application, *Aventis did not even test for the presence of barnase in the MS6 corn kernels.* Instead, they made the claim—without research to back it up—that any level of barnase in the corn plant would create "abnormal plant growth." Since they didn't *see* any growth problems, they argued that there was no toxic barnase produced in the corn plant other than in the anther. Three years later, however, they acknowledged that barnase could be produced in the kernels.

The MS6 corn line also had a PAT gene inserted to confer tolerance to the herbicide glufosinate. It is interesting to note that Aventis did test their corn for the presence of the PAT enzyme but not for barnase. Why did they omit such an obvious test? According to William Freese, "One possible explanation is that the company realized that barnase would be found in corn kernels, and that this would raise food safety concerns that it preferred not to deal with."[69] Regardless of Aventis' motivation, it is remarkable that the US regulatory agencies accepted the company's unsupported claim that the corn was safe.

GM canola also produces toxic barnase

The same company inserted a barnase gene in canola. When the Australia New Zealand Food Authority accepted company claims that the canola was safe, the Public Health Association of Australia wrote, "This GE plant has this gene in every cell of the plant and in the seeds produced by the plant. As it is such a comprehensive cell poison, it is of concern that it is being placed in plants that enter the human and animal food supply. … There is no guarantee that it will remain unexpressed in these plants or during digestion by animals or humans."[70]

Barnase may damage human health

Because barnase is known to cause kidney damage in rats, degrade RNA, and be toxic to human cells, its presence in food may lead to a wide range of potential problems. "During seed production," says Joe Cummins, "barnase may be present in dust and debris from the crop and surface along with groundwater may be contaminated with the toxin. Humans or animals breathing the plant material may experience severe toxicity."[71] The toxin might also theoretically have effects on offspring (by transmission through the placenta and via damage to the parents' sex cells), as well as effects via milk or meat from animals exposed to barnase, and honey from bees in contact with the pollen may also be toxic. Cummins adds, "There is strong evidence that barstar induces a strong immune response."[72]

---

* This is not a "terminator" crop with sterile seeds, though the same genes have been used in terminator crops.

3 . 7

High lysine corn contains increased toxins and may retard growth

> *"A change in the lysine concentration may generate new classes of toxins, or new concentrations of toxins that are presently extremely rare in our diets."[73]*
>
> — Centre for Integrated Research on Biosafety

1. Monsanto produced corn with higher levels of lysine.

2. If consumed in high quantities, the elevated lysine may adversely affect human health in unpredictable ways.

3. The corn also contains increased amounts of known toxins and other potentially harmful substances.

4. The growth rate of chickens fed high-lysine corn was less than those fed corn plus lysine.

Monsanto is seeking approval to market high lysine corn (LY038), the first GM crop designed to deliver "enhanced" nutrition. The corn is designed to be used as animal feed, where it may reduce the cost for lysine supplementation (which accelerates growth rate). But as StarLink contamination made clear (see section 3.5), any GM corn intended for animal feed will certainly be consumed by humans as well. Not wanting to make a similar mistake, Monsanto applied for approval of the high lysine corn as a human food, so that its inevitable contamination into the food supply will not be grounds for recalls or trade disruptions.

Increasing the amount of a single amino acid may alter growth and metabolism in unpredicted ways. In a chicken feeding study, the addition of lysine resulted "in a growth rate defect and a reduction in breast muscle creatine."[74,75] High amounts of lysine in the diet of rabbits increased serum cholesterol and phospholipids in the liver.[76] Elevated levels of lysine may be a health consideration, particularly in cultures where corn is a staple.

Lysine normally increases the weight of chickens. During tests of high-lysine corn, however, their increased growth rate during the first 21 days was significantly less than that obtained from regular corn with lysine supplements. According to the Centre for Integrated Research in Biosafety (INBI), "This result suggests that there may be an unexpected and unexplained negative factor acting on broilers fed GM lysine-producing corn that prevented them from reaching the same growth rates as broilers fed conventional corn."[77] Unfortunately, the researchers did not provide blood or organ weight data which might have isolated the mechanism for this difference.

Huge exposure to an unusual protein

The gene that is inserted into the corn creates an enzyme (DHDPS) that is necessary for the synthesis of lysine. Under natural conditions in plants, when the desirable level of lysine is reached, DHDPS production is inhibited. The gene inserted into the corn, however, is taken from soil bacteria. The bacterial version of this enzyme ignores the feedback and continues to produce lysine.

Food Standards Australia New Zealand (FSANZ), which is reviewing Monsanto's application, maintains that the enzyme has a history of safe use and therefore does not require any special evaluations. INBI points out, however, that the structure and quantity of the enzyme is unprecedented in human food.

DHDPS is highly unusual in that the bacterial form is substantially different than the plant variety normally found in corn. When the bacterial enzymes join together, their combined three-dimensional structure (quaternary structure) is entirely different than the plant form. Since different structures can turn a benign protein into an allergen, it makes sense to carefully evaluate the impact of the bacterial enzyme. This is particularly important because of the quantities involved. People normally consume only minute amounts of bacterial DHDPS when they ingest soil residues on food. INBI compared the estimated intake via soil with the amount of the enzyme that an average US citizen would eat if all of their corn were the high-lysine variety. The exposure to the bacterial enzyme increases 30 billion to 4 trillion times.

Toxic components increased

When lysine is produced in corn, other by-products of lysine metabolism are also formed. In high lysine corn, the amount of these by-products increases substantially, including those with known toxic effects. Alpha-aminoadipic acid, which is at least ten times higher in LY038 corn, has a neurotoxic activity.[78] Pipecolic acid, which is at least double in quantity, is "considered to be a neurotransmitter or neuromodulator"[79] and may promote brain and nervous system damage that result from liver disorders (chronic hepatic encephalopathy). And cadaverine can promote allergic reactions by inhibiting the breakdown of histamine. Symptoms are "expressed as mild skin discomfort to nausea, vomiting, and diarrhea"[80] There are also "indicators that elevated levels of cadaverine in corn could have physiological consequences altering other nutrient levels or in the creation of potential food hazards."[81] Cadaverine levels have not been reported for Monsanto's corn, but are expected to be higher.

FSANZ argues that people are already exposed to these byproducts of lysine in commonly available foods. According to the INBI, however, "these other foods do not have the same concentration of other metabolites as corn, are not eaten or prepared in precisely the same ways as corn, or eaten in the same quantities." For example, high lysine corn contains at least 50 times the amount of a lysine byproduct called saccharopine, compared to normal corn. Based on the average corn consumption in the United States, high lysine corn could boost the average exposure to saccharopine fifteenfold. Each of these components must be evaluated, not only in raw corn, but as the next section makes clear, health effects should be tested after cooking the corn as well.

3 . 8

Cooking high lysine corn may create disease-promoting toxins

"There is overwhelming reason to suspect that LY038 will produce an entirely unique spectrum of food hazards when cooked or processed. These hazards will be completely beyond what can be predicted from raw LY038 corn or raw or cooked conventional corn."

— Centre for Integrated Research on Biosafety

1. A GM corn variety is engineered to produce high levels of lysine.

2. When cooked and processed, it may produce toxic compounds associated with symptoms of Alzheimer's, diabetes, allergies, kidney disease, cancer, and aging.

When certain foods are roasted or baked, they turn brown or golden and their taste and aroma are enhanced. This is from the Maillard reaction, which occurs when amino acids are cooked in the presence of carbohydrates (particularly reducing sugars such as glucose). This reaction can produce compounds called advanced glycoxidation endproducts (AGEs), which are of significant concern.

AGEs are linked to cancer and "enhanced cancer progression,"[82] diabetes, kidney disease, aging,[83] and neurodegenerative diseases such as Alzheimer's.[84] AGEs are also implicated in slower healing of wounds in diabetics[85] as well as diabetes-related autoimmunity.[86] AGEs may reduce nutritive value,[87] as well as increase protein stability, and therefore allergenicity. Higher levels of AGEs are also detected in patients with Creuzfeldt-Jacob Disease (CJD), but it is not clear if they contribute to the disease.[88]

Corn contains protein, carbohydrates, and amino acids—components of the Maillard reaction that can create AGEs. The most significant amino acid is lysine. It is particularly reactive, capable of producing many toxic products,[89] and is often a major component of the first stage of the reaction.[90] In one study, for example, up to half of the corn's lysine was incorporated in a Maillard reaction that can occur spontaneously with stored corn.[91] In this process, known as stackburn, the corn turns brown due to the build up of heat and can become significantly less nutritious. Stackburn takes place with non-GM corn "at temperatures much milder than those that may be used during processing and cooking for human foods."[92]

Monsanto's high lysine corn, however, presents greater risks. Not only does it contain substantial amounts of carbohydrates with reducing sugars, it contains much higher concentrations of total lysine and free lysine (not part of a protein), as well as other related compounds that may produce AGEs (e.g. saccharopine, α-aminoadipic acid, cadaverine, and pipecolic acid).[93] According to the Centre for Integrated Research in Biosafety (INBI), "There is overwhelming scientific reason . . . to believe that LY038 composition is likely to yield Maillard reaction products, including anti-nutrients and AGEs, and that it will produce these compounds in higher quantities than conventional corn and many other foods with comparable total lysine."[94]

Assessments ignore cooking hazards

In Monsanto's submission for approval of their high-lysine corn to Food Standards Australia New Zealand (FSANZ), the company not only failed to address the Maillard reaction, they did not offer a single test result based on cooked corn. The Codex Alimentarius Commission acknowledges that heating or processing a GM food might create toxins and asks regulatory agencies to consider related information.[95] Nonetheless, FSANZ "made no attempt to assess food hazards resulting from cooking or processing"[96] and has deemed Monsanto's submission as adequate and worthy of approval.

FSANZ says that there are other food products in the diet, such as meat and eggs, which have higher levels of total lysine than the GM corn. INBI points out, however, that "conventional foods with high lysine levels are extremely low in carbohydrates" and "are usually extremely low in free lysine"[97]—both part of the Maillard reaction. High lysine corn accumulated more than 50 times more free lysine than control corn.[98] The ratio of free lysine to total lysine is also a significant factor determining the reaction rate and byproducts.[99] That ratio in LY038 is between 19 and 70 times that of other foods whose ratios have been published.[100] Thus, Monsanto's high lysine corn may be uniquely suited to add significant levels of toxic and disease-related products into our diet from the Maillard reaction.

Children's risk is higher

Infant formula (e.g. Enfamil) contains corn and corn-derived products and is one-hundredfold higher in AGE content compared to human or bovine milk.[101] INBI writes, "The use of infant formula has been associated with a rise in childhood autoimmune diseases. . . . There can be no justification for increasing higher concentrations of glycation reactants [AGEs] in infant formula." [102]

Children also eat plenty of corn products. According to an article in the *Journal of the American Dietetic Association*, "Processing of some ready-to-eat cereals, which includes heating at temperatures over 230°C, may explain the high AGE content of these products. Also, many cereals and snack-type foods undergo an extrusion process under high pressure to produce pellets of various shapes and densities. This treatment causes major chemical changes . . . all of which can promote glycoxidation [AGEs]."[103]

Those with wheat allergies (e.g. Celiac disease) use corn as an important substitute. Since AGEs may cause allergic reactions, those with the disease may become "sensitized to AGEs in high lysine corn that [make] them allergic to all corn, effectively removing this important food source from their already limited diets."[104] Those who inhale corn flour are also at risk of an allergic response.

3 . 9

Disease-resistant crops may promote human viruses and other diseases

"The public has always been assured that only well-understood proteins would ever be inserted into transgenic plants, yet new functions are continuously being discovered for plant viral proteins—including some that appear to have implications for human health."

—Jonathan Latham, molecular biologist and plant virologist, Bioscience Resource Project

1. Viral genes inserted into disease-resistant crops produce "viral" proteins.

2. Consuming these may suppress the body's defense against viral infections, particularly in the gut.

3. The proteins may also be toxic and lead to disease.

4. Viral transgenes produce RNA that might influence gene expression in humans in unpredicted ways.

Virus-resistant crops comprise less than 1% of GM acreage worldwide. Three varieties are on the market: zucchini, crookneck, squash and Hawaiian-grown papaya. Virus-resistant potatoes were withdrawn in 2001. To understand the unique risks that these crops pose, it is important to review some basics of plant viral defense.

Although some viruses are DNA-based, most plant viruses are RNA strands. When an RNA virus attacks a cell, it typically produces an enormous number of copies of itself. These copies produce viral proteins, which can help disable the cell's defenses to viruses.

Plants have evolved a gene silencing mechanism to fight back. The mechanism recognizes an RNA virus, cuts its double-stranded RNA (dsRNA) into short pieces and strips it into a single strand. That strand is then used as a reference to "find" other RNA with identical or similar sequences, which are then destroyed or degraded.

The gene inserted into crops produces a piece of viral RNA as reference material. Thus, it arms the gene silencing mechanism to be on the lookout for a specific target virus. This transgenic RNA may also produce viral proteins in every cell.

Viral proteins may increase viral infections

Viruses create proteins that not only attack the cell's defense against that specific virus, but more than 100 studies have shown that viral proteins can promote infections by related and unrelated viruses.[105] (Nearly every type of virus protein has this ability: viral coat proteins,[106] viral movement proteins, [107] viral replicase proteins,[108] viral proteins involved in overcoming host defenses,[109] and miscellaneous viral proteins.[110]") Since important viral defense mechanisms in plants (such as gene silencing) are very similar in humans, proteins that work in plants may also disable human defenses. GM crops that produce viral proteins in every cell expose us to unprecedented levels. This could weaken our resistance to viral infections, particularly in the gut, where viral proteins circulate after a meal. (The gut is an important entry point for infections by viruses.) The mouth is also at risk, and the nose and lungs may be impacted if protein is expressed in GM pollen.

We do not understand all the ways in which plant viruses overcome host defenses and we do not know which viral proteins are involved. Thus, we cannot identify in advance which viral transgenes are hazardous.

Viral proteins may be toxic

In addition to disturbing viral defenses, viral proteins are often toxic to their hosts. They attack fundamental processes, such as the cycle by which a cell divides and the mechanism for creating proteins from RNA.[111] If these were damaged in human beings, it could have serious consequences and may cause disease. (Disrupting the cell cycle, for example, can lead to cancer.)

Since these metabolic activities are similar in plants and humans, a toxic viral protein that disables them in crops might attack that same process in people. Viral proteins from one kingdom have in fact been shown to be toxic to organisms from other kingdoms. Plant viral proteins can affect yeast and some human viral proteins can disrupt plants. According to molecular biologist and plant virologist Jonathan Latham of the Bioscience Resource Project, "There is no good reason why it should not happen the other way round." According to Latham, the proteins produced in GM crops have never been properly evaluated for human toxicity.

If GM viral proteins disrupt plant metabolism, the impact might be obvious and the variety would not be used. But this might not always be the case. Humans may be more sensitive than plants to the effects of the protein. Also, the quantity of viral protein produced in a GM plant can significantly increase in certain circumstances (e.g. when the plant is infected with a non-target virus).

Government agencies claim that people have eaten virus-infected food for a long time, so these viral proteins must be safe for humans. Latham points out that this reasoning "is a half-argument. The other half requires reliable evidence that people who ate the virus-infected crops were absolutely fine in every way." He says that "an experiment is only as good as its controls, but in this 'experiment' there were none, because no one was found who hadn't eaten viruses."[112]

Similarly, in response to a virus-resistant plum developed by the USDA, geneticist Joe Cummins says, "The fact that people may have eaten virus-infected plums does not really indicate that the transgenic plum that resists virus infection in a novel way is safe for people."

Virus-resistant GM crops are engineered to create large quantities of small regulatory dsRNA. As described in section 2.8, regulatory RNA can influence gene expression, even in future generations. Cummins says, "It is not unreasonable to suggest that a unique interfering plum RNA may be active in humans and animals." Although this proposition is speculative, Cummins says that "common sense requires adequate safety experiments," and calls for "fuller testing of the small silencing RNA" used in transgenic crops.[113]

"By transferring genes across species barriers, which have existed for aeons between species like humans and sheep, we risk breaching natural thresholds against unexpected biological processes. For example, an incorrectly folded form of an ordinary cellular protein can under certain circumstances be replicative and give rise to infectious neurological disease."[1]

—Dr. Peter Wills,
theoretical biologist,
Auckland University

SECTION 4:

The foreign protein may be different than what is intended

There are four fundamental ways in which the structure of a protein can influence its function and impact health:

1. The amino acid sequence of the protein;
2. How the protein is folded;
3. How proteins interact and create aggregate shapes; and
4. The content, shape, and location of other molecules, such as sugars, phosphates, or lipids, that become attached to the proteins.

This section shows how each of these structural aspects of proteins may be altered in GM crops in unpredictable ways.

4.1

GM proteins may be misfolded or have added molecules

"*Slight structural changes may occur depending on the producing organism. These can affect the primary sequence of the protein due to point mutations . . . or can be due to post-translational modifications, i.e., variations in the glycosylation or phosphorylation levels. Such modifications may have an incidence on the immunoreactivity of the protein.*"[2]

—J. M. Wal, food scientist, French National Institute of Agricultural Research

1. Proteins expressed in a GM plant may be processed differently than in the donor organism.

2. Those changes, which could include misfolding or molecular attachments, can be harmful in unpredicted ways.

3. Current studies do not adequately test for these changes.

Proteins are not wholly characterized just by amino acids. The sequences do not necessarily reveal their structure, function, biological activity, stability, and uniqueness. **Characteristics of proteins can vary between species and even between different cells in the same species. The bacterial and viral genes put into GM foods, however, cross entire kingdoms.** It is unclear how plants might alter the bacterial or viral proteins. According to David Schubert, "A toxin that is harmless to humans when made in bacteria could be modified by plant cells in many ways, some of which might be harmful."[3]

GM proteins can become harmful

Depending on where a protein is produced, molecular chains, such as sugars, phosphate, sulfate, or lipids, can become attached to the protein and alter its function. Doug Gurian-Sherman, a plant pathologist who formerly evaluated GM crops at the EPA, says "Such alterations may change the structure, allergenicity, and other properties of a protein."[4] Schubert adds, "With our current state of knowledge . . . there is no way of predicting either the modifications or their biological effects."[5]

Several studies confirm that when sugar chains become attached to proteins, this process, known as glycosylation, can turn a harmless protein into a dangerous allergen.[6] Although bacteria do not add sugar molecules to proteins, plants do. It is possible that a bacterial protein expressed in a GM plant can be glycosylated.

Peas were inserted with genes from kidney beans. The glycosylation pattern in the kidney bean protein, which was apparently harmless, underwent subtle, unpredicted changes when expressed in the pea plant. Researchers believe this surprising difference found between closely related species, was responsible for the pea becoming a potential allergen. (See section 1.18.)

A protein's shape also determines its effect. According to cellular biologist Barry Commoner, "The newly made protein, a strung-out ribbon of a molecule, must be folded up into a precisely organized . . . structure." He points out that according to the old theory of genetics, the protein "always folded itself up in the right way once its amino acid sequence had been determined. In the 1980s, however, it was discovered that some . . . proteins are, on their own, likely to become misfolded—and therefore remain biochemically inactive—unless they come in contact with a special type of 'chaperone' protein that properly folds them."[7]

For millions of years the chaperone folders have evolved along with the proteins they fold. When a foreign bacterial protein comes in contact with a plant's chaperone folders, it is not clear what the results will be. If the protein becomes folded differently, it might create problems. According to the Centre for Integrated Research on Biosafety (INBI), "proteins derived from natural sources generally regarded as safe can be [toxic to cells] if allowed to re-fold under different conditions."[8]

Sometimes, refolding can result in groups of proteins aggregating into shapes with harmful consequences. INBI points out that certain aggregations of "proteins that have sustained mutations or have been misfolded" (amyloid fibrils) are involved in a variety of medical conditions such as Alzheimer's and Parkinson's diseases."[9] "Studies indicate that any protein can adopt" the amyloid configuration[10] upon exposure to appropriate environmental conditions."[11] Consumption of GM crops with misfolded proteins could theoretically trigger diseases, since "hazardous aggregates of proteins survive digestion and are distributed throughout the human body." A difficulty in safety assessment of GM crops is that "exposure to some aggregated proteins in the amyloid form can take decades to produce an effect."[12]

One of the most well-known examples of dangerous misfolded aggregated proteins are prions (proteinaceous infectious particles), responsible for mad cow disease (bovine spongiform encephalopathy) and the deadly Creutzfeld-Jacob disease in humans. Prions cause other healthy proteins to also become misfolded. Over time, they cause holes in the brain, severe dysfunction, and death. Prions survive cooking and are believed to be transmittable to humans who eat meat from infected "mad" cows. The disease may incubate undetected for about two to eight years in cows and up to 30 years in humans.

Although we do not fully understand prions, it is not expected that protein from bacteria, viruses or plants can infect humans or animals. Therefore, it is unlikely that misfolded proteins in current GM food crops would pose such a threat. When human or animal genes are inserted into plants, however, the possibility that the proteins may become prions is more of a concern. This type of human/plant combination has been used with some experimental crops, including those designed to produce drugs.

4 . 2

Transgenes may be altered during insertion

"*Rearrangement of the nucleotide sequence of a gene often occurs during the insertion of that gene into the genome of the recipient plant, . . . Even single nucleotide changes can alter a protein's amino acid sequence and affect the protein's properties. . . . FDA provides little guidance for assuring that potentially deleterious changes have not occurred in the transgene, and consequently to the GE protein, due to transformation of the plant.*"[13]

— Doug Gurian-Sherman, former EPA scientist

1. During insertion, the transgene may become truncated, rearranged, or interspersed with extraneous pieces of DNA.

2. The transgene in MON 810 corn was truncated; the protein it produces is derived from a combination of the transgene sequence and the corn's own DNA.

3. Proteins produced from altered transgenes may have unpredictable harmful effects.

The transgene sequence determines the amino acids of the protein it produces. This sequence, however, can get mixed up when the gene is inserted into DNA.[14] Genes spliced into soybeans and corn, for example, were mutated, fragmented, or truncated. The amino acids that they produce, therefore, may be quite different from those that were intended.

Fusion proteins

Scientists put stop signal sequences at the end of their transgenes, so that transcription ends at that point. If this signal is lost during insertion, transcription may continue, resulting in a "fusion protein" made from both the transgene and plant DNA. This happened in an herbicide (glyphosate) tolerant sugar beet developed by Monsanto and Novartis. Only 69% of the transgene made it into the DNA."[15] The protein it produces combines amino acids made from the inserted gene with "43 amino acids from sugarbeet DNA."[16]

In Monsanto's MON 810 corn,[17] the genetic construct also broke apart during insertion. Only about 70% of the intended gene, (which codes for Cry1AB) was incorporated into the corn DNA. The NOS terminator stop signal was lost. As a result, when the plant creates a GM protein, two additional amino acids are created from the host corn, not the transgene.

Extraneous DNA fragments

Transgenes are multiplied prior to insertion, often as part of a circular piece of bacterial DNA called a plasmid. These days, extraneous bacterial DNA from the plasmid is usually removed prior to insertion. But most GM crops on the market were inserted with plasmid DNA. Fragments of this plasmid can get mixed up into host DNA and into the transgene sequence.[18] This could alter the amino acids of the GM protein. In addition, multiple or partial copies of the transgene can get inserted, as happened with Roundup Ready soybeans. Two transgene fragments were discovered after the crop was commercialized. Syngenta's *Bt*-176 "contains five to six entire pieces of the transgenic DNA."[19]

Mutations

When a transgene is inserted, a significant number of mutations and rearrangements can occur.[20] Transgenes can become reversed, broken up, or mixed up. In one analysis, researchers identified a huge amount of scrambling of transgene and plant genomic sequences with 155 "break points."

Commercialized GM crops also contain significant mutations. In MON 810 corn, for example, the promoter sequence (that turns on the foreign gene) was only partially incorporated into host DNA. The transgene in MON 863 corn underwent some degree of mutation as well,[21] and Syngenta's *Bt*-176 corn was supposed to create the Cry-1Ab form of *Bt*, but according to a report by Mae-Wan Ho, analysis "carried out both by French and Belgian government scientists" showed that the transgene had only a 65% similarity to the intended protein. She believes that the company may have "misreported or misidentified the transgene" since it actually "showed 94% similarity with a synthetic construct of *crylAc* gene"—a different form of the toxin.[22]

Sometimes the insertion process results in a change of a single base in the transgene (point mutation), which in turn can alter a single amino acid in the protein. Studies show that these point mutations can change the protein's immunogenicity and allergenicity.[23]

Assessments miss these problems

Regulatory agencies do not require companies to check the gene and amino acid sequences to see if unpredicted changes have occurred. The US National Academy of Sciences advised the FDA to "require reporting of full DNA sequences of transgenes as they are integrated into the plant genome unless the applicant can provide scientific justification not to do so."[24] But an analysis of 14 submissions to the FDA revealed that none included sequences.[25] Similarly, sequencing amino acids has been recommended by several bodies,[26] but companies typically provide just 5 to 25 amino acids even if the protein has more than 600 in total. The EPA's review of Cry1F corn, for example, states: "sequencing of five [amino acids] determined that the microbial and plant expressed protein maintained this sequence intact."[27] In fact, it is common for scientists seeking permission to study a GM crop to have to pledge that they will not sequence the protein.[28]

A rearranged protein could be quite dangerous. In lieu of sequences, evaluators sometimes look at the molecular weight of the protein to see if the size matches expectations. For certain *Bt* proteins, the weight varies significantly from what was expected.[29]

4.3

Transgenes may be unstable and rearrange over time

"*French government scientists examined five GM varieties already commercialized, and found all the GM inserts had rearranged themselves. Belgian government scientists confirmed those results, and found some of the [changes in the] GM varieties were also non-uniform.*"[30]

—Mae-Wan Ho, biophysicist and geneticist, director, Institute of Science in Society

1. At least two studies showed that the sequence of inserted genes was different than what was described by the company.

2. This suggests that transgenes are unstable and spontaneously rearrange.

3. The GM protein may therefore change, with unpredictable consequences for health.

4. If so, safety assessments conducted on the original protein do not apply to to the new version.

In 2003, two French laboratories analyzed the inserted genes in five GM varieties.[31] In each case, the genetic sequence was different than that described by biotech companies years earlier. In Liberty Link corn by Bayer, a "sequence [was] missing,"[32] a second truncated and rearranged promoter (CaMV 35S) was added to one side of the gene cassette, and additional sequences were added to the other. In Mon 810 (YieldGard) by Monsanto, the NOS terminator and other portions were not present in the gene cassette, but the terminator was "detected elsewhere in the genome, indicating that it has moved from its original position."[33] In Monsanto's Roundup Ready soybeans, a 254 base pair fragment of the herbicide-tolerant gene, plus a 534 base pair section of unknown DNA was added to one end. In Bt-176 corn by Syngenta, "the differences are even more drastic as three rearranged fragments were detected."[34] Each contained a promoter (CaMV), as well as other sequences from either the gene cassette or unknown material. A second inserted gene sequence, which confers an additional trait, was not analyzed, but "at least three integration sites were detected."[35] Roundup Ready corn contained three complete cassettes, along with partial ones. Analysis verified deleted sequences, including missing stop signals in two cassettes.

It is not clear from these results alone whether the transgene rearrangements were made during the insertion process or afterwards, due to genetic instability. But results obtained in Belgium by the Scientific Institute of Public Health (IPH) and presented at a meeting of the Belgian Biosafety Advisory Council, provide evidence of transgene instability. Their study, which compiled data from various institutes, papers, and applications, reviewed sequences from six GM lines, four that the French labs had examined and two they had not. (In the latter group, Syngenta's Bt-11 corn not only showed rearrangements, but appeared to be contaminated with sequences from Bt-176.) Among the four lines in common, the Belgian "reports found evidence of genetic instability similar to those described in the French study. However, there are small and large discrepancies when the two sets of data are compared."[36] Differences ranged from variations in small sequences to differences in the number of transgenes present in the genome. These differences among the same GM crop varieties not only suggest that transgenes are unstable after insertion, but that their changes are non-uniform, i.e., they can mutate in different ways. It also means that GM crops may create new proteins that were never intended or tested.

Traavik and Heinemann summarize the rearrangements in the five most thoroughly studied GM crop varieties. "Deletions (Mon 810, GA21, Bt 176), recombination (T25, GTS 40-3-2, Bt 176), tandem or inverted repeats (T25, GA21, Bt 176) as well as rearranged transgenic fragments scattered through the genome (Mon 810) have been reported."[37,38] They say that "transgenic modification techniques are prone to introduce such rearrangements because exogenous [foreign] DNA transfer in plants elicits a 'wound' response, which activates nucleases and DNA repair enzymes. This may result in either degradation of the incoming DNA, or insertion of rearranged copies into the plant DNA."[39,40]

Stability is necessary for safety and approvals

According to Ho and Cummins, "Transgenic instability is a key safety issue. A GM variety that has changed its identity since characterized by the company invalidates any safety tests or assessments that may have been done."[41] If the transgene or its protein changed enough, than it would not be possible to identify a GM variety after it is released. Identification is essential for implementing remedial action in case of harm, or for assigning liability."

According to a 2001 European Directive (2001/18/EC), it is a requirement that GM crops are stable. So far, regulatory agencies have largely ignored the evidence above. If they officially acknowledged that GM crops were unstable, it would likely force their withdrawal.

Instability may account for hazards

Section 1 reported various problems linked to GM crops, including sterile pigs, dead cows and sheep, a mysterious disease in the Philippines, high offspring mortality among rats, and allergic reactions among Bt cotton workers. In general, follow-up studies are not carried out. If they were, then the element of instability adds a serious complicating factor. Are the adverse findings generic to the GM variety or have they resulted from GM crops that had "gone bad" due to genetic rearrangements? In the case of the latter, follow-up research might not be able to replicate the problems unless the exact same GM plants are used.

4.4

Transgenes may create more than one protein

"The fact that one gene can give rise to multiple proteins . . . destroys the theoretical foundation of a multibillion-dollar industry, the genetic engineering of food crops."⁴²

—Barry Commoner, biologist, Center for the Biology of Natural Systems at Queens College

"Genes can be 'ambiguous' in the sense that each of them can use differently its information to give more than one protein. This can be done through differential 'reading' the genetic message starting and ending at different points of the sequence, or through alternative splicing, i.e. shuffling of RNA exons giving rise to different mature RNAs from the same initial gene transcript."⁴³

—Marcello Buiatti, geneticist, University of Florence

1. Genetic engineering technology was created based on the outmoded notion that a single gene will create only a single protein.

---

2. Due to a process called alternative splicing, a single gene can produce many different proteins.

---

3. Although the bacterial genes used in GM crops will not, in their natural state, be alternatively spliced, scientists modify the sequence in a way that may facilitate this.

The old theory of genetics asserted that each gene is coded to produce one single unique protein. On this basis, biologists predicted that there would be about 100,000 genes in human DNA to account for the various proteins. When the number of human genes was reported on June 26, 2000 as approximately 30,000, it exploded the myth of one-gene, one-protein. In reality, the vast majority of genes can encode for more than one protein; some can produce several.

Splicing RNA produces new proteins

In organisms that have cells with a nucleus (eukaryotes), most genes include two types of sequences. Sections that code for proteins are called exons. Sections located between exons but do not create proteins are called introns. After the gene creates a replica of itself in RNA, molecules called spliceosomes can cut out the introns and leave just the exons intact to create their protein. But spliceosomes can also cut out one or more sections of exons, resulting in altered RNA sequences. These in turn create proteins with different amino acid sequences. This process is known as alternative splicing and can rearrange a single RNA code in numerous ways, creating multiple proteins from a single gene.

Unlike genes from plants, animals, and humans, bacterial genes usually do not contain introns and so they cannot be rearranged by spliceosomes. By inserting bacterial genes into plants, proponents argue that the transgene will not be alternatively spliced and will therefore produce only a single protein. But scientists almost always link introns to bacterial genes in order to enhance the production of the desired protein. (The introns facilitate the movement of messenger RNA from within the nucleus out to the cytoplasm.) These introns that are added to transgenes, however, are not located within the protein-creating portion of the gene. Rather, they are inserted next to it. Proponents assume that this placement of the introns will prevent alternative splicing from occurring within a GM plant, but this assumption has not been adequately researched.

Alternative splicing can theoretically create a protein that is toxic, allergenic, or the source of a new disease. But systematic analysis to verify the absence of unintended proteins is not required and is not done. Michael Antoniou says, "I think the possibility of a nearby intron within a transgene being involved in aberrant splicing is very low, but that doesn't mean that academia and industry shouldn't test for alternative or unexpected splicing events—it's very easy to do."

There is another way that an intron in a transgene can also generate an unintended proteins. As is observed in some plants, if the intron is not removed from the RNA, the intron sequence might contribute amino acids to the GM protein.

Altered reading produces new proteins

Specific sequences on the gene tell the transcription mechanism where to start reading and where to end. After the DNA is transcribed into RNA, every three bases are translated into a single amino acid. If the translation skips one base, than each subsequent group of three bases will be different. The reading frame will have shifted and the amino acids would be different. This can be illustrated using the alphabet. If groups of three letters formed the code, each amino acid would normally be created by the following groups: ABC DEF GHI. If the letter A was skipped, the code would change to BCD EFG HIJ. Hence, the amino acids would be different. Similarly, if the translation skips two bases, amino acids will also change. If it skips three bases, then it will simply leave out the first amino acid, but the rest will be the same. (In the alphabet example, shifting three means starting with DEF, then GHI, etc.) By shifting reading frames, the same gene can have different starting and ending points and produce completely different proteins. It is another method by which a transgene can produce unintended and potentially hazardous proteins. Frame shifts can be created by mutations that delete or add bases, which can occur through tissue culture or insertion mutations described in section 2.

Some genes naturally create more than one protein by having alternative start positions or end positions when DNA is transcribed to RNA. Although genetic engineers will likely avoid inclusion of such alternative signals within their transgene, mutation of the transgenes during or after insertion may create one of these alternate stopping or starting points.

Although assessments don't usually involve rigorous analysis of the protein profile of GM crops, the Canadian Food Inspection Agency reported that the *Bt*-11 corn produced four separate *Bt* proteins, each of different sizes. This was confirmed by a crude measure of weight, not sequence. The explanation put forward by some scientists was that the *Bt* toxic protein may be "processed or degraded in *Bt* 11."[44] However, it is also possible that the transgene produced more than one protein through the mechanisms described above.

4.5

Weather, environmental stress, and genetic disposition can significantly change gene expression

"*Living organisms interact with the environment, they behave quite differently under differing weather and soil conditions, they cross-pollinate, and they have a large range of natural genetic variability. . . . Genetically engineered plants are alive, and cannot be regulated with a system developed for inert chemicals.*"[45]

—William Freese, testimony before the EPA's Scientific Advisory Panel

1. Environmental factors, natural and man-made substances, and genetic disposition of a particular plant can influence levels of transgene expression and cause unique health effects.

2. These factors are not adequately accounted for in assessments.

Just as humans have genetic differences that make individuals and sub-groups unique, so do plants. Inserting the same gene into different varieties of the same plant species can have widely varying results. While this difference may be due to insert location and unique disruptions of the DNA, it may also be associated with innate differences from one plant to the next caused by slight variations of genes and overall patterns of gene expression.

Once the transgene is integrated into the genome, its expression may also differ from plant to plant and even within different parts of the same plant. This is due to individual genetic disposition and unique environmental influences. It is well-known that variations in water, soil nutrients, sunlight, temperature, and stress can alter nutritional value and health-related properties of plants. Transgene expression may be affected as well.

According to the Royal Society of Canada, "The nature of any such transgene-related changes is likely to be conditioned by the genetic background within which the new gene is being expressed; the developmental and physiological status of the transgenic organism; and the environmental pressures impinging upon it."[46] They say unanticipated changes "may only appear at a particular growth stage, or in response to specific environmental conditions."[47]

Bt-toxin levels vary in the same GM crop

The levels of Bt-toxin produced from GM crops, for example, can vary significantly. William Freese says, "You simply cannot do a study on a Bt corn plant and say that the results represent all other plants in the field—much less all plants of its variety. . . . we are dealing with living things here, not inert chemicals."[48]

Consider the experience of Filipinos described in section 1.7, where during the time of corn pollination, nearby residents reported severe skin, intestinal and respiratory reactions and fever. It is possible that the Bt expression of the corn was significantly elevated. When researchers tested the corn, amounts varied greatly, even between kernels from the same plant. Levels varied at least sixty-fourfold (from 0.014 ug to 0.9 ug) with other kernels expressing both above and below the limits of detection of the test equipment.[49]

It is unknown what caused this huge difference in Bt expression, but it is likely to be alterations in the molecular mechanisms that control overall patterns of gene function known as "epigenetics." These can change in response to environmental influences either natural or man-made.

Environment silences genes, boosts toxins

Scientists inserted a foreign gene into petunias, designed to turn petals red. Instead, flowers varied in both color and pattern. The variation was thought to be due to gene silencing brought about by a "position effect," i.e., changes based on where the transgene was inserted in the genome.[50] As the season progressed, however, the red in some plants disappeared as more transgenes switched off. This unexpected change in gene expression was apparently due to environmental changes and according to Michael Antoniou, probably working through an epigenetic mechanism.

Natural or man-made substances might also dictate how GM crops impact health. University of Wisconsin scientists, for example, accidentally discovered that Bt-toxin becomes more deadly to insects when mixed with very small amounts of a naturally occurring antibiotic (zwittermicin A—a byproduct of bacteria).[51] Tests have not been conducted to determine if the enhanced toxicity is also more dangerous to animals or humans.

Regulators overlook environmental effects

Several experts agree that "environmental influences" on GM crops "need more attention."[52] Codex, for example, "has pointed to the need for evaluation of stress in the approval of GM crops."[53] The Royal Society says that potential changes in the GM crop "need to be assessed empirically across time and environments."[54] Others ask "that every application for commercial release should include data from diverse climatic and ecological conditions and from several years." Overall gene expression will vary markedly from season to season and location to location as the plant tries to adapt to different environments.

According to Florianne Koechlin, "Monsanto tests its new Bt-maize in Missouri and claims validity of the results in Sweden or Kenya."[55] Cummins and Ho write, "It is certainly clear that GM crops approved under optimum environmental conditions cannot presume to be substantially equivalent to GM crops produced under conditions of extreme stress."[56]

By not evaluating the health impacts of GM crops under a wide variety of conditions, dangerous side effects due to variations within a species may be missed.

According to Freese, the natural variability of transgene expressions "is especially worrisome when we consider children eating pesticidal plant products. We know that children are especially prone to allergies, as reflected in their much higher incidence of allergic conditions."[56]

4.6

Genetic engineering ignores and disrupts complex relationships in the DNA

> "*Biology is so much more complex than technology.*"
> —Robert Mann, biochemist, University of Auckland

1. The GM transformation process can disrupt networks of genes that function together.

---

2. Synthetic transgenes may act different than natural ones.

---

3. Multiple transgenes may interact in unpredicted ways.

---

4. Genetic engineering may disrupt a newly discovered second code in the DNA.

Molecular geneticist Michael Antoniou told New Zealand's Royal Commission of Inquiry on Genetic Modification in 2001, "Genetic engineering technology, as it's being applied in agriculture now, [is] based on the understanding of genetics we had 15 years ago, about genes being isolated little units that work independently of each other." He explained that genes actually "work as an integrated whole of families." Two years after his testimony, he discovered that the biotech industry still espoused the outdated theory of gene independence. As a member of the UK's GM Science Review Panel in 2003, he sat with 11 other scientists who represented either the biotech industry or were appointed by the pro-biotech UK government. The 11 summarily dismissed the body of studies demonstrating coordination between genes and even claimed that the order of genes in the genome was entirely irrelevant.

A year later, a paper in *Nature Reviews Genetics* further validated Antoniou's position. It acknowledged that "gene order has typically been assumed to be random. However, the first statistically rigorous analyses of complete genomes, together with the availability of abundant gene-expression data, have forced a paradigm shift." It concludes, "Gene order is not random. It seems that genes that have similar and/or coordinated expression are often clustered."[57]

Researchers have also identified unusual genes, such as one that is nestled within a portion (intron) of another. In a second unusual variety, "protein is assembled when four different RNA molecules, made from DNA scattered over 40,000 base pairs, are assembled into one transcript."[58]

All this new information about genes was not considered when gene insertion technology was developed. A random insertion with its associated mutations and deletions might wreak havoc throughout a network of finely tuned and coordinated genes.

There are also other principles and properties of gene expression that are not accounted for in the simplistic model of gene insertion and its accompanying safety assessments. For example:

1. **Certain proteins are gene regulators.** They can switch genes on or off. If genetic engineering changes the amount of such proteins, that can disrupt other genes.
2. **Inserted genes are synthetic.** Since plant and bacteria genes use different sequences to code for certain amino acids, part of bacterial genes have to be altered so they will be read efficiently in the plant. Crop developers and regulators have made the assumption that synthetic and natural genes are equivalent, but there is insufficient research to verify this assumption.
3. **Some crops stack multiple transgenes on a single DNA.** One version of Monsanto's New Leaf potato, for example, was stacked with eight different traits—it created its own pesticide, resisted diseases, was tolerant to herbicide, gained more weight and reduced bruising.[59] Some GM crops also acquire additional foreign transgenes accidentally—through cross-pollination. Canola plants in Canada, for example, ended up with foreign genes from two different varieties, each conferring tolerance to a different brand of herbicide. Multiple transgenes increase the potential for unpredicted interactions. Regulatory agencies ignore this risk and have approved stacked varieties without additional evaluation.
4. **Scientists have discovered a new code in the genome (in addition to the genetic code) that is now known to be a major factor in determining which genes are turned on or off.**[60] This "epigenetic" code determines "the placement of the nucleosomes, miniature protein spools around which the DNA is looped"[61] and has a significant influence on the overall pattern of gene expression.

As our understanding of the complexity of DNA increases, it reveals how primitive genetic engineering is and how many subtleties and principles are not taken into account. While it is beyond our current understanding to identify the various effects from the GM transformation process, there are tools to help evaluate the results. Gene chips can be used to monitor gene expression from the entire DNA in a given part of the plant and proteomics measures proteins created. It seems an obvious choice to employ these techniques in safety assessments, but thus far, producers of GM crops have not generally used them.

"There is something profoundly amiss in our stampede down the biotech path for every trivial application. The level of the change now possible, the speed at which we can make these dramatic alterations and the potential consequences for animals, the environment and ourselves—for the world as we know it— ought to give us great pause. It is naive to think that this research, unbridled, will have only a trivial impact."[1]

—Autumn Fiester, bioethicist,
  University of Pennsylvania School of
  Medicine

SECTION 5:

Transfer of genes to gut bacteria, internal organs, or viruses

Genes transfer readily between bacteria and fungi. "This form of horizontal gene transfer (HGT) is part of an ongoing evolutionary process."[2] Since it had been assumed that HGT is rare in other kingdoms or between kingdoms, its consequences were not considered as part of GMO risk assessments. New information shows that not only do transgenes jump from GM crops to gut and soil bacteria, but the way they are constructed might actually facilitate gene transfer. Had this been known before, the current generation of GM crops might never have been approved. Nonetheless, assessments and regulations have still not been updated to adequately deal with this confirmed risk.

5 . 1

In spite of industry claims, transgenes survive the digestive system and can wander

> "There is evidence that relatively long fragments of DNA survive for extended periods after ingestion. DNA may be detected in the feces, the intestinal wall, peripheral white blood cells, liver, spleen and kidney, and the foreign DNA may be found integrated in the recipient genome. When pregnant animals are fed foreign DNA, fragments may be traced to small cell clusters in fetuses and newborns."[3]
>
> — Terje Traavik and Jack Heinemann

1. Industry advocates claimed that genes were destroyed during the digestion of food and therefore gene transfer to gut bacteria or organs was extremely unlikely.

2. Studies now verify that genes can survive digestion, both in humans and animals.

3. Animal studies on non-GM DNA also verify that it can pass through the placenta into the fetus, from the digestive channels into the blood and organs, and even penetrate the blood brain barrier.

In the 1970s[4] and 1980s,[5] researchers were unable to find any DNA that survived digestion in mammals. It was therefore commonly assumed that DNA was fully destroyed in the gut. According to Steinbrecher and Latham, "This understanding was largely responsible for the omission of [horizontal gene transfer] from risk assessment of GM plants and foods."[6] They did not explore the possibility that transgenes might transfer into gut bacteria or human DNA. In the mid-1990s, scientists used much more sensitive detection techniques (hybridization methods and polymerase chain reaction) and discovered that a significant percentage of DNA can survive the digestive system.

According to Traavik and Heinemann, "A restricted number of recent publications have demonstrated that foreign DNA and also proteins may escape degradation, to persist in the [gastro-intestinal tract] and even to be taken up from the intestines and transported by the blood to internal organs in biologically meaningful versions."[7]

DNA fed to mice was found to "persist in fragmented form in the gastrointestinal tract, penetrate the intestinal wall, and reach the nuclei of leukocytes, spleen, and liver cells."[8] When pregnant mice were fed DNA, it was also found in several organs of the offspring, including their brains.

In pigs fed GM and non-GM corn, transgene and gene fragments were detected in the lower gastrointestinal tract (rectal and cecal).[9] In chicks fed GM corn, antibiotic resistance marker genes were found in their stomachs.[10] The transgene for a *Bt* corn line (the full length of the coding portion for cry1AB) was found in-tact in sheep rumen (the first compartment of a ruminant animal's stomach). The authors concluded, "DNA in maize grains persists for a significant time and may, therefore, provide a source of transforming DNA [i.e., horizontal gene transfer] in the rumen."[11]

Short DNA fragments from plant chloroplasts were found in the lymphocytes of cows, and possibly in their milk. And gene fragments from feed were also found in muscle, liver, spleen, and kidney tissues in chickens.[12] And when humans were fed rabbit meat, fragments of rabbit DNA were found in the bloodstream.[13]

A test tube simulation of human digestion indicated that transgenes may survive in the stomach and small intestine for up to four hours.[14] A human feeding study was conducted on seven subjects who used ileostomy bags—their lower intestines had been removed and digestive material passed from the small intestine into an attached bag. They were fed a meal of GM soy burgers and a soy milkshake. In six of the seven, small but measurable amounts of the full length transgene from the soybean was present in the bag—it had survived digestion through the stomach and small intestine.

According to Steinbrecher and Latham, "The old assumption of risk analysis of [horizontal gene transfer] was that it was essentially impossible and that the consequences need not be considered. Now that evidence is steadily accumulating that HGT is likely to occur the onus must shift to an examination of the likely consequences."[15] It raises the risk that transgenes and/or promoters might transfer to gut bacteria and integrate into our own cell's DNA. Traavik and Heinemann say that uptake of transgenes could "ultimately lead to development of chronic disease conditions."[16] GM material may even pass into the unborn fetus through the placenta or integrate into adult sex cells, altering the genetics of future generations. The long-term impact of any of these possibilities, however remote, demands that they be evaluated carefully *before* GM crops are released.

5.2

Transgene design facilitates transfer into gut bacteria

*"*B*ecause small gene sequences and genes driven by the CaMV 35S promoter . . . are introduced into plants the opportunity for selective forces to operate on HGT [horizontal gene transfer] is significantly enhanced."[17]*

—Ricarda A. Steinbrecher and Jonathan R. Latham

1. Genes can naturally transfer between species and even kingdoms, but it is uncommon.

2. GM crops may be especially suited to overcome the natural barriers of this transfer.

3. Short bacterial sequences and higher herbicide residues, for example, may significantly increase the transfer rate.

4. Transgenes may therefore readily travel from GM food into the DNA of gut bacteria.

There is limited understanding about natural horizontal gene transfer (HGT) between species, genera, and even kingdoms,[18] but it is believed to be an uncommon occurrence. Certain environments are more conducive to HGT than others since they have the nutrients available to support a high density of bacteria. The gut of humans and mammals in particular is one such "hot spot" for gene transfer. Studies have confirmed that antibiotic resistance genes from soil organisms have transferred into the human and animal intestinal tracts, as well as the human mouth.[19] Several characteristics of GM crops, however, may overcome the natural barriers to transfer, making gene exchanges between GM foods and gut bacteria much more frequent.

1. Antibiotics: Gene transfer among certain bacteria increases one-hundredfold in the presence of the antibiotic tetracycline. Some herbicides used on herbicide-tolerant GM plants, such as glufosinate ammonium, "exhibit antibiotic activity[20] or are thought to do so."[21] The increased herbicide residues on these crops may stimulate transfer.

2. Similarity of genetic sequence (homology): For some types of bacteria, the critical factor allowing transfer is the presence of genetic sequences that are similar (homologous) to the bacteria's DNA. In *E.coli*, for example, "a minimal length of a 20 [base pair] homology is required[22] for recombination."[23] In many cases, as the similarity between the genetic sequences declines, there is an exponential decrease in the integration of the foreign gene.

Gene sequences *normally* found in plants are not similar to those in bacteria. GM crops, however, contain bacterial sequences. *Bt* and herbicide tolerant transgenes, for example, come from bacteria. Also, prior to insertion, transgenes are usually incorporated into circular DNA (plasmids) in order to generate multiple copies. The plasmids are made from bacteria, including *E. coli*—common gut bacteria—and are often inserted into the crop along with the transgene. Bacterial sequences from either the transgene or the flanking plasmids may therefore be similar to the DNA in gut bacteria and facilitate gene transfer.

Although scientists almost always alter some of the genetic sequences in bacteria-derived transgenes (so that they work properly in a plant cell), the changes may not be substantial enough to prevent gene transfer. Studies have verified that genetic material that is non-homologous can still become integrated into bacteria if the regions on either side of that material *are* homologous. In addition, analysis of plant DNA that had been integrated into bacteria showed that some sequences that had originally been deleted were actually restored.

A number of GM plants have sufficient similarities in their genetic structure to facilitate transfer into gut (or soil) bacteria. Chardon LL corn by Bayer, for example, contains most parts of a bacteria-derived ampicillin resistance gene, a modified bacterial sequence that is 70% homologous to the original, and most of a plasmid made from *E. coli*.

3. Self-replicating bacteria: The plasmids used to multiply transgenes contain a piece of DNA called an "origin of replication." This sequence causes the plasmid to replicate itself over and over again. Since the whole plasmid was often inserted with the transgene, many GM crops (e.g. GM papaya and potatoes) contain this origin of replication sequence. If activated, it might multiply the bacterial sequences, increasing the likelihood of horizontal gene transfer.[24]

4. Gene length and introns: Genes in plants normally have sections that do not code for proteins (introns) inserted between sections that do (exons). Plants cells have mechanisms that remove these non-coding sections from the RNA transcripts. The presence of introns in plant genes may inhibit gene transfer to bacteria in two ways. First, shorter genes may transfer more easily. Introns increase the length of the gene and may make it more difficult for bacterial DNA to take it up. Second, if plant genes do end up in bacteria, they may not function. That's because bacteria do not have a mechanism to remove the introns. This reduces its potential for harm and its chances for survival in a colony of bacteria. GM crops, however, do not have introns within the coding regions of the transgene. This may facilitate transfer and enable the gene to be expressed in bacteria.

GM crops may vastly increase the rate of gene transfer

Transgenes are present in every cell of a GM plant. By stripping them of natural barriers to horizontal gene transfer, they could, "in principle, transfer into any organism that ingests these materials or comes into contact with DNA released from that plant, including microorganisms (bacteria, fungi, protozoa, and viruses) of soil, of sewage, and of the digestive tract, including those of humans, cows, bees, slugs, or earthworms."[25] The potential for unprecedented cross kingdom gene transfers carries a significant element of risk.

5 . 3

Transgenes may proliferate in gut bacteria over the long-term

"There is horizontal gene transfer from plant material to gut bacteria and if for some reason there is a selective advantage for those bacteria expressing the gene (for example, during a course of antibiotics), they could become the dominant population within the gut."[26]

— David Schubert, molecular biologist and protein chemist, Salk Institute for Biological Studies

1. Once transferred into gut bacteria, transgenes may confer survival advantages, allowing them to endure and spread.

2. These advantages may be due to antibiotic or herbicide resistance, promoters that function in bacteria and genetic mechanisms that promote uncontrolled replication.

3. Having "infected" our gut bacteria, the foreign genes and the proteins they create may be harmful.

If transgenes end up in gut bacteria, will they live long and proliferate? If the transgenes give the new host organism some survival advantage, the answer is probably *yes*. There are several characteristics of transgenes that might facilitate this "selection pressure," allowing them to survive in the gut over the long-term.

Transgenes are more likely than natural plant genes to function in bacterial DNA. This is due in part to their shorter length and lack of introns described in the previous page. In addition, most transgenes are switched on with the cauliflower mosaic virus promoter (CaMV 35S), which *does* function in bacteria.[27] Plant genes, on the other hand, often use promoters that only function in plants and not in bacteria. Thus, if a transgene becomes integrated into bacterial DNA, it carries with it a functioning "on switch."

[For years, the biotech industry relied on the incorrect assumption that the CaMV 35S promoter does not function in bacteria. In a February 20, 2002 submission for their GM corn, for example, Aventis CropScience wrote: "The cauliflower mosaic promoter, associated with the pat gene is only active in plants, not in bacteria, thus even if horizontal gene transfer did take place, the PAT protein would not be expressed in the soil bacteria without the presence of a suitable promoter." In spite of several studies that had already proven this assertion false, the UK regulatory committee (ACRE) repeated the company's claim that the promoter does not function in bacteria.[28]]

Herbicide tolerant (HT) transgenes allow crops to survive herbicide applications. The most popular herbicides used with HT crops, glyphosate and glufosinate ammonium, can kill bacteria[29] and might be toxic to gut bacteria. HT transgenes may therefore allow gut bacteria to survive herbicide that enters the gut from crop residues.

In fact, HT crops typically have higher levels of herbicide residues. Thus, they provide a greater threat to gut bacteria (through their residues) and a key for the bacteria's survival (through their HT transgene). It appears to be a diabolical combination, uniquely designed to promote transgene survival in the gut.

Scientists from the Institute for Bee Research at the University of Jena in Germany reported that "the herbicide-resistant genes in . . . rapeseed transferred across to the bacteria and yeast inside the intestines of young bees." Professor HH Kaatz said, "This happened rarely, but it did happen."[30]

The gene that transferred inside the bees was the "PAT gene," used in Liberty Link crops. The gene produces an enzyme called the PAT protein, which converts the toxic Liberty herbicide into a supposedly non-toxic substance called NAG. NAG accumulates and is eaten as part of the crop. As described in section 6.1, certain gut microorganisms in mammals may re-toxify NAG, re-converting it back into herbicide inside our intestines. Since some enzymes facilitate chemical transformations in both directions, it raises a critical question of whether the PAT protein has this ability. If so—if it also re-toxifies NAG into herbicide—then pat genes in gut bacteria might create a dangerous feedback loop: we eat Liberty Link corn, for example. Our gut bacteria, equipped with the PAT protein, turns some of the NAG in the corn back into herbicide. The release of herbicide kills gut bacteria. Those bacteria with the pat gene have a survival advantage in the presence of the herbicide. The survival advantage creates selection pressure, prompting the transgene to further proliferate in the bacteria population. With this, *more* PAT protein is produced, which converts *more* NAG into herbicide, which threatens more bacteria, which creates more selection pressure, and so on. Since studies have not been done to see if such a cycle is occurring, we can only speculate.

Antibiotic resistant marker genes, used in most GM crops, could allow gut bacteria to survive in the presence of antibiotics. This would be particularly dangerous if disease-creating bacteria obtained the transgene, allowing it to withstand antibiotic medicine. (See page 132–133.)

Another way in which transgenes may proliferate in gut bacteria is via "origin of replication" sequences that were described on the previous page. They are part of the plasmids used to multiply copies of the transgene prior to insertion. Some GM crops contain this sequence, which, if transferred with the transgene into gut bacteria, may cause the transgene to rapidly multiply.

Some people argue that only one bacterium in a billion would take up a transgene. If this were true, with 10^{15} bacteria in the human gut and 10^{17} in a cow's gut, that works out to 1 million transformed bacteria in the former and 100 million in the latter. This may provide an ample start for selective pressure to expand the population.

5 . 4

Transgene transfer to human gut bacteria is confirmed

"Contrary to the views expressed by plant biologists, it has clearly been shown that a transgene from GE soya can survive passage through the small intestine and can transfer its DNA to the microflora of the small intestine. Although the gene was a fragment of the glyphosate resistance gene from soybeans, there is no reason why other genes could not also transfer."[31]

— David Schubert, molecular biologist and protein chemist, Salk Institute for Biological Studies

1. The only human feeding trial ever published confirmed that genetic material from Roundup Ready soy transferred into the gut bacteria in three of seven human volunteers.

2. The transferred portion of the transgene was stable inside the bacteria and appeared to produce herbicide-tolerant protein.

3. There is no known way to treat such a condition, which may be long-term.

In the only human feeding study ever conducted on GM foods, in three out of seven human volunteers, genes were found to have transferred from GM soy into the DNA of gut bacteria. Sequences from the herbicide tolerant bacterial gene, the CaMV promoter and a petunia plant, which are all part of the Roundup Ready soybean gene cassette, were confirmed as present in the bacteria (using PCR analysis).[32]

The bacteria were cultured in a medium containing glyphosate, the active ingredient of Roundup herbicide. The survival of the bacteria suggests that it had become "Roundup Ready," i.e, that the CaMV promoter was functioning in the bacteria and that the transgene was switched on, actively producing herbicide-tolerant protein within the human gut.

This UK government-funded research used seven volunteers who were ileostomy patients, i.e., they had their lower intestines removed and their food, after passing through the stomach and small intestine, was collected in a bag. Researchers identified the soy transgenes in the gut bacteria of three subjects, indicating that the transfer had occurred from previous ingestion of soy products and that the transgene was stably integrated. Harry Gilbert, one of the authors, said, "The thing I worry about in our work is that we have failed to identify the bacteria or bacterium that contains the transgene. We want to identify the microorganism and we want to know where in the genome it is integrated."[33]

All seven subjects were also fed a single meal consisting of a GM soy burger and a soy milk shake. Although GM DNA was found among the digestive material, there was no indication that any of the soy contained in the single meal had transferred into bacterial DNA. It was not clear why three of the seven subjects had integrated soy transgenes into their gut microflora in the past and why no subjects showed an increase in transferred transgenes after the single meal. The authors guessed that transfer might require long-term exposure to GM soy, but there was no data to support this. If degree of exposure were a factor, then the amount of transgenes in gut bacteria would presumably be much larger for subjects tested from the United States, where GM consumption is considerably more than in the United Kingdom.

The researchers also fed 12 healthy volunteers the same soy-based meal. In contrast to rat studies, in which GM DNA was found in feces for up to 79 hours after feeding,[34] analysis of the feces from the 12 human subjects showed no intact transgenic DNA. The detection method used in the study, however, was sharply criticized as not sensitive enough. Nonetheless, a lack of DNA in feces would simply indicate that the DNA had either been destroyed during passage through the digestive tract or transferred to microflora along the way. "Another interpretation," says epidemiologist Judy Carman "is that the transgenic DNA may have entered intestinal cells and/or passed into the bloodstream.[35] This went unassessed, even though several bacteria can invade intestinal cells and transfer genes into mammalian cells.[36]"

Health concerns dismissed without data or follow-up

Based on the detection methods used in the study, the researchers said, "The bacteria containing the transgene represented a very small proportion of the microbial population." On this basis, and without conducting any tests measuring possible health impacts of the gene transfer, they claimed, "It is highly unlikely that the gene transfer events seen would alter gastrointestinal function or pose a risk to human health." Many scientists were critical of this unsupported conclusion, which appeared more to echo attitudes of the pro-GM lobby rather than prudent scientific reasoning. The researchers, for example, did not address possible allergenic properties of the GM protein, the potential for spontaneous rearrangement of the transgene and resulting changes in protein structure and effect, selective pressure that might cause the transgenes to proliferate and the potential for the CaMV promoter to switch on other genes in the bacteria.

A more accurate conclusion might be the following: In the only human feeding study ever conducted on GM crops, long-standing assumptions that genes would not transfer to human gut bacteria were overturned. The findings should prompt immediate comprehensive follow-up tests to determine the implications for health among both the general population and at-risk subgroups. Additional tests should also look for genes from other GM crops, including antibiotic resistant markers, *Bt* genes, and viral transgenes.

5.5

GM foods might create antibiotic-resistant diseases

*"*I*T WOULD BE A SERIOUS HEALTH HAZARD TO INTRO-DUCE A GENE THAT CODES FOR ANTI-BIOTIC RESISTANCE INTO THE NORMAL FLORA OF THE GENER-AL POPULATION."[37]*

*"*T*he benefit to be gained by the use of the kanamycin resistance marker in transgenic plants is outweighed by the risk."[38]*

—Internal memos from FDA's Division of Anti-Infective Drug Products

1. Antibiotic resistant marker (ARM) genes have been inserted into most GM foods on the market.

2. If ARM genes were to transfer to pathogenic bacteria inside the gut or mouth, they might create super diseases, untreatable with one or more types of antibiotics.

3. GM crops may therefore accelerate the rise of antibiotic-resistant illnesses, which are already responsible for death and disease.

Antibiotic Resistant Marker (ARM) genes allow cells to survive applications of an antibiotic. They are attached to transgenes prior to insertion. After insertion, cells are doused with antibiotics. Only those whose DNA has integrated and activated the ARM gene survive. ARM genes remain in every cell of GM crops and are consumed by humans and animals.

Medical organizations worldwide[39] have expressed concern that ARM genes may transfer into bacteria in the digestive tract or environment, spread to pathogenic bacteria, and create antibiotic-resistant diseases. Such "super" diseases are prevalent due to overuse of antibiotics in food and feed. According to the FDA, they "increase risk of death, and are often associated with prolonged hospital stays."[40]

In the FDA's first GM crop review in 1992 (FlavrSavr tomatoes), the director of the Division of Anti-Infective Drug Products wrote, "The Division comes down fairly squarely against the [antibiotic resistant] gene marker in the genetically engineered tomatoes. I know this could have serious ramifications."[41] Political appointees approved ARM genes and a 1998 FDA document states, "It is highly unlikely that antibiotic resistance genes could be transferred from plant genomes to gut microorganisms."[42] This assumption has yet to be tested in humans, although antibiotic resistant genes can transfer into bacteria typically found in the human mouth (see section 5.8) as well as into soil microorganisms.[43] If transfer does occur, the presence of antibiotics might offer survival advantages to the antibiotic resistant bacteria and might also increase the rate of gene transfer (in one study, gene transfer increased one-hundredfold in the presence of tetracycline).[44]

Ampicillin resistant markers

Ampicillin is a widely used antibiotic and the drug of choice for several types of human and animal infections.[45] According to the UK's Department of Environment Antimicrobial Resistance Coordination Group, in some important animal pathogens there is "extremely low or no detected resistance (to ampicillin) in certain bacterial species," so that "any occasional transfer of resistance genes to these organisms would be a very significant event." If transfer occurred and other antibiotics were needed for the animals, "then there could be significant consequences for the consumer through the food chain."[46] by increasing disease resistance to other antibiotics.

The Bt-176 corn variety by Syngenta, which uses an ampicillin resistant marker, carries an additional risk—a genetic sequence that, "if it were transferred from the GM corn to a bacterium . . . could allow many copies of the gene to be generated in a cell." The UK Advisory Committee on Novel Foods and Processes (ACNFP) concluded in 1995 that the risk of transfer, "however remote, was unacceptable."[47] They therefore did not approve the use of the raw corn variety in animal feed. The committee was under the mistaken impression that transgenes and ARM genes would be destroyed when the corn was cooked. They therefore approved the use of Bt-176 for processed human food and animal feed.

In April 2004, the European Food Safety Authority declared that ampicillin resistant marker genes "should be restricted to field trials and not be present in genetically modified plants placed on the market." Spain promptly banned Bt-176 corn, which was growing there.[48] In March 2005, the US government revealed that an unapproved corn variety with ampicillin resistant genes (Bt-10) was accidentally mixed into the food chain by its producer Syngenta. The US government, which has not banned ampicillin resistant markers, insists that Bt-10 is safe.

Kanamycin resistant markers

Most GM crops on the market use kanamycin resistant genes. Regulators insist that the antibiotic is not used much anymore, so kanamycin-resistant bacteria would not be too dangerous. "There is evidence that the antibiotic is used extensively for some applications."[49] Geneticist Joe Cummins says,[50] "Kanamycin is used prior to endoscopy of colon and rectum[51] and to treat ocular infections.[52] It is used in blunt trauma emergency treatment[53] and has been found to be effective against E coli 0157 without causing release of the deadly verotoxin.[54]" It is also used often in veterinary medicine.

In addition, kanamycin-resistant bacteria may mutate and develop resistance to members of the same family of antibiotics.[55] That family (aminoglycoside antibiotics) includes streptomycin, gentamycin, tobramycin, and neomycin, all currently used on humans.[56] The bacteria may also cross-react with the other antibiotics. According to biochemist and nutritionist Susan Bardocz, after bacteria acquire one ARM gene, it is easier and quicker for them to take up additional antibiotic resistant genes. Cummins says, "the kanamycin-resistant gene" might "start a resistance chain reaction leading to the accumulation of multiple resistance on a plasmid"[57] in pathogenic bacteria.

In addition, the loss of effectiveness of animal antibiotics will increase the rate of infections. There is a possibility that animals with infectious diseases may have toxins that will impact those who eat the meat of the animals.

5.6

The promoter can also transfer and may switch on random genes or viruses

"*It is no longer acceptable to have bland assurances, such as that CaMV 35S promoter is specific to plants and will not work in animal cells, when indeed this is against the observed biological wisdom.*"[58]

—Arpad Pusztai and Susan Bardocz

"*To ignore [the CaMV promoter's] capacity to be universally active in almost any organism is irresponsible and careless and shows a serious lack of scientific rigor and commitment to safety.*"[59]

—Ricarda A. Steinbrecher, molecular geneticist, *Econexus*

1. Contrary to prior assumptions, the CaMV promoter does function in human, animal, and bacteria DNA.

2. This promoter does transfer into the DNA of human gut bacteria and might also transfer into human DNA.

3. Once transferred, it may switch on genes that produce toxins, allergens, or carcinogens, create genetic instability and, in higher organisms, switch on dormant viruses.

Critics of GM crops have been concerned that the CaMV promoter, used in nearly all GM crops, might transfer into gut bacteria or human DNA. If it does, it may permanently turn on native genes to produce toxins, allergens, carcinogens, or antinutrients. It may turn on genes that regulate cell division, causing cancer. In addition, the recombinant hotspot believed to be located in the promoter might lead to instability (additional recombinations) in the DNA, with unpredicted consequences. Since the DNA of higher organisms such as humans, animals, and plants contains dormant viruses, the transfer of promoters between species may also increase the likelihood that such a virus would be activated (see section 2.5).

Defenders of the promoter contend that humans are exposed to the cauliflower mosaic virus promoter all the time when eating vegetables infected with the virus. Thus, if there were a risk of transfer, we would find it commonplace. This position has three flaws.

1. By eating GM crops, humans are exposed to far greater quantities of the CaMV promoter than normal. The promoter is found in every cell of GM crops whereas the actual virus is limited to a small percentage of a few vegetables. Moreover, when the vegetable becomes infected, it typically looks or tastes[60] bad, inspiring avoidance rather than consumption.

2. The CaMV promoter operates differently in GM crops than in packaged viruses. As a packaged virus, it won't infect bacteria and may have a very low likelihood of integrating into the DNA of mammals. The promoter in GM crops, however, is without its normal protein coat. Studies have verified that naked viral DNA can infect species that are not susceptible to the intact virus.[61] The CaMV (a pararetrovirus) operates in the cytoplasm of the cell and does not integrate into the hosts' genome.[62] The promoter in GM crops, on the other hand, is placed into plant DNA and is more likely to transfer and integrate into foreign DNA.

3. Whereas CaMV will be killed when the vegetable is cooked, heating fragments of the CaMV promoter in GM crops may make it easier for the bacteria to take it up.

Proponents of the CaMV promoter have also claimed that it is plant-specific and will not function in bacteria or mammals if transferred. This assumption ignores research as far back as 1990, which verified that the promoter is active in bacteria,[63] fungi, and yeast.[64] Evidence that CaMV works in human cells dates back to 1982.[65] More recent research also demonstrates that it functions in bacteria,[66] mammalian,[67] and human cells.[68] A 2006 study, for example, showed that the promoter works in human enterocyte-like cells, similar to those found in the small and large intestines that would come in contact with GM food.[69] The authors wrote, "Taking the published studies together, it may now be concluded that the CaMV 35S promoter is capable of initiating gene expression in some mammalian cell lines under a range of different conditions and circumstances."[70]

Promoters may transfer

In the study published in 2004 in which GM soy transgenes were found to be stably incorporated in human gut bacteria (see section 5.4), possibly all (but at least part) of the CaMV promoter had transferred with the transgene. Furthermore, the bacteria survived in the presence of glyphosate, suggesting that the promoter had activated the herbicide-tolerant transgene. The same study was unable to simulate a transfer of the promoter into human enterocyte-like cells in test tubes, although the authors cautioned that conditions inside humans may differ from laboratory simulations.

An unpublished study presented at a conference in 2004[71] also reported that the full 1,100 base pairs of the CaMV promoter were found intact in rat tissues after a single meal. The promoter was found

- In stomach cells and in intestinal (mesenteric) lymph nodes two hours after eating;
- In intestinal lymph nodes, kidney, and liver cells six hours after eating; and
- In intestinal lymph nodes, spleen, and liver cells three full days after eating.

It was not clear if the promoter had integrated into the DNA or not.

[Study specifics: Groups of six rats were fed a balanced diet (through a tube), to which was added artificial DNA sequences similar to those used in GM crops. The genetic material, which was in both circular and linear forms, contained a CaMV promoter attached to a gene that codes for green fluorescent protein. Other groups were given genes without a promoter, with a promoter known to be active in all mammalian cells (human cytomegalovirus promoter) or no DNA at all. About half of the CaMV-fed rats in each of the circular and linear DNA groups were found to contain intact CaMV promoters.]

The evidence that the ingested CaMV promoter traveled to rat organs and integrated into human gut bacteria suggests that this powerful gene regulator could have random, unpredictable, and dangerous consequences.

5.7

If *Bt* genes transfer, they could turn our gut bacteria into living pesticide factories

"As shown in the human feeding experiment, a fully functional transgenic construct rendering Roundup Ready soya resistant to glyphosate can partially survive in the human gut, it is possible that funtional Bt-toxin transgenes can also survive, be taken up by bacteria resident in alimentary tract and convert us and our animals into pesticide factories."

—Susan Bardocz,
Biochemist and nutritionist,
University of Debrecen

1. Transfer of the *Bt* transgene could cause our intestinal flora to produce *Bt*-toxin.

2. With increased exposure to *Bt* crops and through selective pressure, the number of gut bacteria producing *Bt* may increase over time.

3. Since *Bt*-toxin has been associated with immune responses and damaged cells in animal intestines, long-term exposure may cause significant health problems.

Although much of the concern expressed about horizontal gene transfer has focused on antibiotic resistance, the impact of *Bt* gene transfer may be more dangerous. Earlier sections have revealed biological effects and apparent allergic or toxic reactions traced to *Bt* spray and *Bt* crops. The gene that codes for *Bt* has proven stable in the presence of saliva and within the digestive tract of animals.[72] The CaMV promoter, which drives the expression of *Bt* genes, is active in bacteria. There may be little standing in the way of *Bt* gene transfer.

If the gene transfers to gut bacteria, it is unknown whether there will be a selection pressure that enhances the trait's survival and replication. According to Steinbrecher and Latham, "For those traits/genes for which selection pressure is not known it does not follow that none exist. Too little is known about microbial communities in gut, soil or rhizosphere to make confident predictions."[73] In fact the purpose of the *Bt* gene in its original form in a soil bacterium (*Bacillus thuringiensis*) is not known.

Bt genes are used in GM corn. For the people of Mexico, Southern Africa, and elsewhere, corn is a food staple, eaten as much as three times per day. With greater exposure comes greater risk of gene transfer. If *Bt* genes become stably incorporated into gut bacteria and continue to produce the *Bt*-toxin, the impact of those infected might range from chronic low-level toxicity to life-threatening allergic reactions. The problems may be difficult to trace back to the *Bt* corn and the condition may be difficult to treat.

5 . 8

Genes may transfer to bacteria in the mouth or throat

Microbiologist John Heritage "said the risk of spreading antibiotic resistance occurred when cells were broken open during the processing of the food, releasing the modified DNA into the environment. The risk was magnified when the processing created dust, Dr. Heritage said, because the dust would be breathed in."[74]

—BBC

1. Bacteria in the mouth can take up free DNA.

2. GM DNA might similarly transfer from food.

3. Breathing dust or pollen from GM crops might cause genes to transfer to microorganisms in the respiratory tract.

4. These might impact health and possibly pass from person to person.

The argument that GM DNA is destroyed during digestion had been used to claim that antibiotic resistant marker genes would not transfer to gut bacteria. It is odd, however, that this line of reasoning completely overlooked the possibility of gene transfer in the mouth. Several studies now confirm that such transfers are possible.

Bt genes (in plasmid form) were placed in a sheep's mouth for eight minutes in order to evaluate how thoroughly they were broken down by the saliva. The authors concluded that there was still sufficient genetic material to allow for the possible transfer of antibiotic resistance genes into *E-coli*. They said that this implies "that DNA released from the diet within the mouth may retain sufficient biological activity" to transfer into "oral bacteria."[75]

In another study, an oral bacterium was able to take-up and express foreign genes within a minute.[76] And in a third study, 40%–65% of a GM plasmid survived after 10 minutes in human saliva and 6%–25% remained after a full hour. The authors also verified that partially degraded plasmids were able to transfer antibiotic resistance to bacteria (*Streptococcus gordonii*) that normally live in the mouth. Their data also "suggest that human saliva may itself contain factors that promote" the receptivity of the bacteria to gene transfer.[77]

The study concludes that there is no reason to assume that transgenes would not transfer to bacteria in the mouth. "It should be clear that even very infrequent transformation events can be highly significant if the transforming DNA bestows a selective advantage on the recipient."[78]

Thus, the bacteria within our mouth may already be transformed by the GM crops we eat. The antibiotic resistant markers, for example, may transfer to oral bacteria and contribute to antibiotic resistant infections of the mouth. *Bt*, Roundup Ready, or viral transgenes might similarly become expressed in our mouth and throat. Moreover, the bacteria might also pass to others via salvia.

Breathing GM dust may transfer genes

In a report sent to the FDA by experts on the UK Government's Advisory Committee on Novel Foods, scientists warned US regulators that antibiotic resistant genes may transfer into bacteria in the respiratory system from dust breathed in from GM crops. They said that when GM food is processed, dust containing DNA can become airborne and be inhaled.

One of the UK committee members, microbiologist John Heritage, expressed particular concern about meningitis bacteria becoming resistant to antibiotics. Approximately one person in five is a carrier of the bacteria, even though carriers do not necessarily contract the disease. Heritage says, "It's a huge concern to me. While the risk is small, the consequences of an untreatable, life-threatening infection spreading within the population are enormous."[79]

5 . 9

Transfer of viral genes into gut microorganisms may create toxins and weaken viral defenses

"*Some plant viral proteins may be harmful to humans. Therefore the transfer of viral genes from GM crops to gut bacteria could have very serious consequences.*"

—Jonathan Latham, molecular biologist and plant virologist, Bioscience Resource Project

1. As discussed earlier, proteins produced from viruses can be toxic and disable viral defenses.

2. If viral genes from GM crops transferred to gut microorganisms, they might produce large quantities of potentially harmful proteins.

3. Viral transgene characteristics make transfer to gut microorganisms much more likely.

Section 3.9 described how viral transgenes are inserted into crops to create resistance to infection from a specific virus. These transgenes produce viral proteins, which may be toxic or suppress viral defenses in humans. If transferred into the DNA of gut microorganisms, they may produce viral proteins (and RNA) in the gut over the long-term.

Viral transgenes increase transfer risk

According to molecular biologist and plant virologist Jonathan Latham, creating and inserting viral transgenes carries a potential risk that is not generally acknowledged. When scientists create a viral transgene from an RNA virus (as is the case with all US-approved virus-resistant GM crops) they synthesize a DNA version of a viral gene that had previously existed only as an RNA molecule. Since DNA only recombines with DNA, and RNA only with RNA, this means that the viral sequence can now integrate (recombine) for the first time into the genome of DNA-based organisms. Latham says, "The virus is available for recombination with a totally new spectrum of organisms." He warns, "The danger would become especially important if the transgenic protein were useful to the organism that picked it up."

Transferred genes may increase proteins

One of the "selling points" of the plum pox-resistant GM plum developed by the USDA is that it produces little or no viral proteins. This is not a trait of its viral transgene per se. When that same gene was inserted into other cells from the same type of plum, the resulting line did produce viral proteins. It just so happened that in one of the insertion "events," due to the unique location and characteristics of the insertion, viral proteins were not produced. Developers chose that line to develop for commercialization.

There is a possibility that over time, however, the gene may become unstable and begin to produce proteins. Furthermore, if the transgene from this plum variety transfers to gut bacteria, it may start to produce viral proteins. The level of expression of a transgene is governed by local factors. Whatever silenced protein expression in the plum might not be functioning in gut bacteria. Similarly, viral transgenes from any virus-resistant GM plant that transfers into gut microorganisms may produce higher levels of proteins than was produced in the plant.

"The gene-manipulators claim they can foresee the evolutionary results of their artificial transposings of human genes into sheep, bovine genes into tomatoes, altered bacterial genes into eggplant, etc. But such claims are a reflection more of arrogance than of scientific analysis."

—Robert Mann, biochemist,
University of Auckland

SECTION 6:

GM crops may increase environmental toxins and bioaccumulate toxins in the food chain

GM crops do not exist in isolation. They are a component of industrial farming practices and part of a complex ecosystem and food web. This section looks at potential health problems that may arise from these relationships. Topics include the impact of toxic herbicides that are applied to herbicide tolerant crops, bioaccumulation of other toxins within GM crops, concentration of toxins in the milk or meat of animals, and the consequences if virus-resistant GM plants promote new plant viruses.

6.1

Glufosinate-tolerant crops may produce herbicide "inside" our intestines

"Some of the N-acetyl-L-glufosinate had been converted back to the toxic form L-glufosinate in the intestine of the animals, probably by the activity of microorganisms in the gut.... the data obtained strongly suggest that the balance of gut bacteria will be affected, that the wellbeing of the feeding host will be affected."[1]

—Ricarda A. Steinbrecher, molecular geneticist, *Econexus*

1. Some crops are engineered to withstand glufosinate-based herbicide.

2. The crops transform the herbicide into a compound regarded as nontoxic, called NAG, which remains in the plant.

3. Once humans or animals consume NAG, gut bacteria can revert some NAG back into toxic herbicide.

4. The herbicide has known toxic effects, acts as an antibiotic and may kill off or disturb gut micro-flora.

5. If the herbicide-tolerant gene transfers to gut bacteria, it could magnify the problems.

Liberty Link crops, marketed by Bayer Crop-Science, are tolerant to Liberty herbicide (glufosinate ammonium). Liberty kills a wide variety of plants and can also kill bacteria,[2] fungi,[3] and insects.[4] It is toxic to humans and animals.[5]

The herbicide is derived from a natural antibiotic produced by two strains of a soil bacterium. So that the bacteria are not killed by the antibiotic they create, the strains also produce specialized enzymes that transform the antibiotic to a form called NAG (N-acetyl-L-glufosinate), believed to be non-toxic. The enzymes are called the PAT and bar proteins, which are produced by the PAT and bar genes. These genes are inserted into the DNA of GM crops, where they produce the enzymes in every cell. When the plant is sprayed, Liberty's solvents and surfactants transport glufosinate ammonium throughout the plant, where the enzymes convert it primarily into NAG. Thus, the GM plant detoxifies the herbicide and lives, while the surrounding weeds die.

The problem is that the NAG, which is not naturally present in plants, remains there and accumulates with every subsequent spray. Thus, when we eat these GM crops, we consume NAG. Once the NAG is inside our digestive system, some of it may be re-transformed back into the toxic herbicide. In rats fed NAG, for example, 10% of it was converted back to glufosinate by the time it was excreted in the feces.[6] Another rat study found a 1% conversion.[7] And with goats, more than one-third of what was excreted had turned into glufosinate.[8]

It is believed that gut bacteria, primarily found in the colon or rectum, are responsible for this re-toxification.[9] Although these parts of the gut do not absorb as many nutrients as other sections, rats fed NAG did show toxic effects. This indicates that the herbicide had been regenerated, was biologically active and had been assimilated by the rats.[10] A goat study also confirmed that some of the herbicide regenerated from NAG ended up in the kidneys, liver, muscle, fat, and milk.[11] [More information about the impact of this conversion is probably in documentation submitted to European regulators by AgrEvo (now Bayer CropScience), but public access was blocked by the company's threats of legal action.[12]]

Toxic to children, fetuses, and gut bacteria

Glufosinate is structurally similar to a natural amino acid called glutamic acid, which can stimulate the central nervous system and, in excess levels, cause the death of nerve cells in the brain.[13] The common reactions to glufosinate poisoning in humans include unconsciousness, respiratory distress, and convulsions. One study also linked the herbicide with a kidney disorder.[14] These reactions typically involve large amounts of the herbicide. It is unclear if the amount converted from GM crops would accumulate to promote such responses or if there are low-dose chronic effects.

Infants or fetal development may be impacted with smaller doses. According to Yoichiro Kuroda, the principal investigator in the Japanese project entitled "Effects of Endocrine Disrupters on the Developing Brain," glufosinate is like a "mock neurotransmitter" and disturbs gene functions that regulate brain development.[15] Exposure of a baby or embryo to the chemical can affect behavior.[16]

When mouse embryos were exposed, it resulted in growth retardation, increased death rates, incomplete development of the forebrain, and cleft lips,[17] as well as death of brain cells.[18] After pregnant rats were injected with glufosinate, the number of glutamate receptors in the brains of the offspring appeared to be reduced.[19] When infant rats were exposed to low doses of glufosinate, some of their brain receptors seemed to change as well.[20]

Glufosinate might also influence behavior. According to Kuroda, "female rats born from mothers that were given high doses of glufosinate became aggressive and started to bite each other—in some cases until one died." He added, "That report sent a chill through me."[21]

If the herbicide is regenerated from NAG inside our gut, since it has antibacterial properties, it will likely kill gut bacteria. Gut microorganisms are crucial for health. They not only provide essential metabolites like certain vitamins and short fatty acids, but also help the breakdown and absorption of food and protect against pathogens. Disrupting the balance of gut bacteria can cause a wide range of problems. According to molecular geneticist Ricarda Steinbrecher, "the data obtained strongly suggest that the balance of gut bacteria will be affected"[22] by the conversion of NAG to glufosinate.

The way the PAT protein detoxifies Liberty is by adding an acetyl group to the compound. The Public Health Association of Australia raises another risk: "No information is given as to the enzyme's specificity to just this substance. . . . If this enzyme is not specific to this substrate, it may acetylate or deacetylate other proteins in humans and farm animals." The Australian authorities claim "that processing to produce processed corn products would inactivate the enzyme. However, this ignores the minimal cooking of corn kernels or whole corn cobs as a vegetable, and the use of raw corn kernels in salads."[23]

6 . 2

Herbicide-tolerant crops increase herbicide use and residues in food

"*HT [herbicide tolerant] crops have increased herbicide use 138 million pounds.*"[24]

—Based on first nine years of use in the United States, according to USDA data, Charles Benbrook

1. Herbicide-tolerant crops increase the use of their associated herbicides.

2. Increased herbicide residues in crops can promote the toxic effects of these chemicals on humans, animals, and their offspring.

3. Increased herbicide use can also alter nutrient content, such as flavonoids, making GM crops less nutritious.

4. The accelerated emergence of herbicide-resistant weeds has resulted in the increased use of even more toxic varieties of herbicides.

When herbicide tolerant (HT) GM crops came to market in 1996, the biotech industry claimed that they would need less herbicide. That was true for the first three years. The repeated use of Roundup, however, caused weeds to develop resistance to the herbicide's active ingredient glyphosate. Farmers used more Roundup or added more toxic herbicide varieties, such as Paraquat and 2,4-D. According to USDA data, the net effect of HT soybeans, cotton, and corn in the United States was a 138 million pound (5%) increase in herbicides from 1996–2004. That is accelerating. By 2004, Roundup Ready soybeans received an estimated 86% more herbicide than conventional beans.[25]

Increased herbicide use is bad for human health:

1. Herbicides can alter crop nutrient content. Flavonoids, an important family of nutrients, for example, are reduced in Roundup Ready soybeans due to Roundup.[26]
2. Farmers and their families, herbicide applicators, and workers at food processing facilities are all exposed to higher levels of herbicides.
3. Herbicides may accumulate in the water table. In Denmark, for example, glyphosate contaminated the drinking water supply at five times allowable levels, overturning the belief that the toxin was fully broken down by soil bacteria.[27]

   Use of Roundup increased the rate of fusarium head blight (fungal infection) in spring wheat.[28] According to New Scientist, "The fungi that cause the disease also produce toxins that can kill humans and animals."[29] A USDA researcher also showed "that Roundup Ready soybeans . . . have significantly greater colonization of fusarium on their roots than untreated soybeans."[30] The increase was between 50% and fivefold.[31] According to the European Commission, "Findings do rather point in the direction of a change in soil microbial activity towards favouring fungi over bacteria. . . . It would in fact be rather surprising if such intensive use of one chemical would NOT cause a change in the microbial communities." [32]
4. Because herbicides are applied directly onto HT crops, herbicide residues on GM food is significantly higher. In 1992, Monsanto successfully petitioned the EPA to increase allowable residue levels of glyphosate on soybeans more than threefold (from 6 to 20 ppm) in anticipation of their HT crops.[33] They also asked regulators in Australia and New Zealand for a two-hundredfold increase in allowable residues.[34] When the company performs tests on its Roundup Ready soybeans, however, they typically use beans that were never sprayed with Roundup.
5. Roundup Ready soybeans convert much of the applied glyphosate into a metabolite called AMPA (aminomethylphosphonic acid) with unknown health properties. In one study, the beans contained 3 mg/kg of glyphosate and up to 25 mg/kg of AMPA.[35] "The presence of high AMPA residues in Roundup Ready soybean was not anticipated and presents a new type of consumer exposure."[36]

Glyphosate is toxic

According to the Journal of Pesticide Reform, "Symptoms of exposure to glyphosate include eye irritation, burning eyes, blurred vision, skin rashes, burning or itchy skin, nausea, sore throat, asthma and difficulty breathing, headache, lethargy, nose bleeds, and dizziness. Glyphosate and glyphosate-containing herbicides caused genetic damage in laboratory tests with human cells, as well as in tests with laboratory animals. . . . Exposure is linked with increased risks of the cancer non-Hodgkin's lymphoma,[37] miscarriages, and attention deficit disorder," [38] as well as Parkinson's disease.[39]

Exposure to mouse testicular cells (Leydig cells) resulted in a 94% reduction in sex hormone production.[40] In a study on human cells, a non-toxic concentration of Roundup as small as "100 times lower than the recommended use in agriculture," significantly disrupted the activity of aromatase—an enzyme crucial to sex hormone production.[41] Roundup administered to pregnant rats induced inhibition of enzyme activity in the liver, heart, and brains, which might lead to abnormalities in functional development of offspring.[42]

Although glyphosate is the "active" ingredient, Roundup contains many so-called "inert" ingredients. In herbicides, inert ingredients can be more toxic than the active one, and the combination of active and inert ingredients may surpass the toxicity of the chemicals on their own. Several studies demonstrate that Roundup is far more toxic than glyphosate.[43] For example, while Roundup is toxic to human placental cells at levels 10 times lower than those found in agricultural use, the toxicity of glyphosate alone was measured at half or less.[44] In an animal cell study, Roundup—but not glyphosate alone—disrupted the cell cycle, "the universal process by which cells reproduce." This may be linked to human diseases, including cancer.[45] And Roundup caused significant changes in rat liver activity, while glyphosate alone had no effect.[46]

Roundup's higher toxicity is often attributed to the inert ingredient POEA (polyethoxylated tallowamine), which helps the herbicide penetrate into leaves. It appears to help the toxin penetrate into human cells as well.[47] In spite of conclusive evidence that inert ingredients increase toxicity, many of the safety assessments on herbicides conducted by manufacturers for the EPA test only the active ingredient.

6.3

Tiny amounts of herbicide may act as endocrine disruptors

"Endocrine and toxic effects of Roundup, not just glyphosate, can be observed in mammals."[48]

—Sofie Richard, et al, *Environmental Health Perspectives*

1. Certain chemicals may disrupt endocrine function at extremely low concentrations.

---

2. Research on Roundup suggests it may be such a chemical, disrupting endocrine activity related to human sex hormone production, but more research on this and other herbicides is needed.

---

3. The increased use of Liberty and Roundup, due to GM crops, may expose the population through food and water to these low-dose effects.

Endocrine-disrupting chemicals (EDCs) can have significant hormonal effects at doses far below those previously thought to be significant. The disruptive effects are often found *only* at minute levels, which are measured in parts per trillion or in the low parts per billion. This is seen, for example, in the way estrogen works in women. When the brain encounters a mere three parts per trillion, it shuts down production of key hormones. When estrogen concentration reaches 10 parts per trillion, however, there is a hormone surge, followed by ovulation.

Herbicides may act as EDCs and their increased use on herbicide tolerant crops may multiply their low-dose exposure via food, air, and water. Unfortunately, the regulation and testing of agricultural chemicals, including herbicides, has lagged behind the findings of extremely low-dose effects. The determination of legally acceptable levels of herbicide residues on food was based on a linear model, where the effect of toxic chemicals was thought to be consistent and proportional with its dosage. But as the paper *Large Effects from Small Exposures* shows, this model underestimates biological effects of EDCs as much as ten-thousandfold.[49]

The shortcomings of testing and regulation were highlighted in comments submitted to the EPA by the Sierra Club. They were in response to Bayer CropScience's 2003 petition to approve maximum threshold levels of glufosinate ammonium on rice, anticipating the marketing of their Liberty Link variety.

"We find EPA's statements on the potential of glufosinate to function as an endocrine-disrupting substance in humans and animals as not founded on logical information or peer-reviewed studies. In fact EPA states that no special studies have been conducted to investigate the potential of glufosinate ammonium to induce estrogenic or other endocrine effects. . . . We feel it's totally premature for EPA at this time to dismiss all concerns about glufosinate as an endocrine-disrupting substance. . . . Due to the millions of Americans and their children exposed to glufosinate and its metabolites, EPA needs to conclusively determine if this herbicide has endocrine-disrupting potential."

The EPA responded that "glufosinate ammonium may be subjected to additional screening and/or testing to better characterize effects related to endocrine disruption"[50] but this will only take place after these protocols are developed. In the mean time, the agency approved glufosinate ammonium residues on rice at one part per million. At this level, the dosage range normally associated with EDCs is considered acceptable. As mentioned in pages earlier in this section, gut bacteria may convert small amounts of NAG residues in Liberty Link crops into glufosinate ammonium inside our intestines. This may carry significant health risks for ourselves and our children.

Roundup shows endocrine disruption

A 2005 study on Roundup illustrated that it may disrupt endocrine functioning at low doses. As described in the previous page, at concentrations 100 times lower than concentrations recommended in agriculture, Roundup disrupted an enzyme crucial to sex hormone production (aromatase) in humans.[51] The authors concluded, "The dilution of glyphosate in Roundup formulation may multiply its endocrine effect. Roundup may be thus considered as a potential endocrine disruptor."[52]

The residues of Roundup in the water supply might be of the concentration range that has an endocrine disruptive effect. In Denmark, they found a concentration of 0.54 micrograms per liter.[53] In addition, Roundup residues on beans were found to be 3 mg/kg, and allowable levels in the United States are 20 ppm. The impacts of Roundup at these levels in water and GM crop residues needs to be studied.

6.4

GM crops may accumulate environmental toxins or concentrate toxins in milk and meat of GM-fed animals

> *"There are new pesticide residues and possibilities of accumulation of residues because of the pesticide tolerance."* [54]
>
> —Gilles-Eric Seralini, toxicologist, University of Caen

1. FDA scientists warned that GM crops may concentrate toxins, such as heavy metals and herbicides, from the environment.

2. There is evidence of heavy metals in GM soybean oil.

3. FDA scientists also said that toxins in GM feed might concentrate in milk or meat.

4. GM DNA fragments were found in milk.

5. While very little research has been done on this, small amounts of Roundup may be retained in the body of animals and affect sperm quality.

6. The overuse of Roundup and Liberty herbicides on GM crops magnifies these types of risks.

The Division of Food Chemistry and Technology of the FDA outlined four potential dangers of GM crops. In addition to a potential "increased levels of known naturally occurring toxins," the "appearance of new, not previously identified" toxins, and "undesirable alterations in the levels of nutrients," they said that GM crops might gather "toxic substances from the environment" such as "pesticides or heavy metals."[55] The FDA division warned, "unless genetically engineered plants are evaluated specifically for these changes," the four potential dangers "may escape breeders' attention." The division recommended testing every GM food "before it enters the marketplace."[56]

Although their recommendation was ignored by the US government, research presented in the preceding pages did reveal that herbicide residues and their metabolic byproducts (NAG and AMPA) do increase in GM crops. A 2006 study also "showed that transgenic soybean oil in Beijing was presumably polluted with zinc, chromium, and lead," and also with arsenic and titanium.[57] The levels were not above the Chinese allowable limits and the study did not present data from non-GM soy oil controls. Thus, we can only conclude that heavy metals can accumulate in GM soy oil. As the paper states, little attention has been given to "whether the accumulation pattern and levels of heavy metals could change after the insertion of foreign genes."[58]

The scientists at the FDA's Center for Veterinary Medicine (CVM) also concluded that there is "ample scientific justification" to require testing and review of each GM food before approval. Their concern, according to CVM's director, was that "residues of plant constituents or toxicants in meat and milk products may pose human food safety concerns."[59] Bioaccumulation of toxins in animals is a well-documented phenomenon—when an animal eats a plant, some fat-soluble plant toxins may "collect in animal tissues and pass to humans when we eat the animal—and can be secreted in human and animal milk (for example, *solanine* from potatoes)."[60]

Any of the toxins that may be taken in from the environment or produced due to the process of GM transformation might possibly build up in animals and be consumed in milk or meat. According to the European Commission, "The European Communities considers that it is now clear that *Bt*-toxin could accumulate in *Bt* resistant herbivores (e.g. caterpillars which are able to ingest the *Bt*-toxin and thus accumulate it and/or its metabolites without dying), and so pass the *Bt*-toxin and/or its metabolites to organisms higher up the food web (e.g. to predators and parasitoids which feed on *Bt*-resistant herbivores)."[61]

Fragments of GM DNA were also found in milk. A 2006 study of 60 samples of 12 brands of milk purchased in Italy "demonstrated the presence of GM corn sequences in 15 (25%) and of GM soybean sequences in seven samples (11.7%)." The researchers also "demonstrated that the pasteurization process is not able to degrade the DNA sequences in spiked milk samples."[62] (The presence of the DNA may have come from GM feed that was fed to the cows, or possibly through contamination of the milk after it was produced.)

The high levels of herbicides used to treat herbicide-tolerant crops may also bioaccumulate in animals or humans. The inert ingredients in particular are fat soluble (nonionic), so they may be stored in cell membranes and other lipids in the body. Tests for these residues are not generally done.

Roundup may accumulate

"Even though absorbed Roundup is excreted rapidly from the body, usually in feces,"[63] researchers suggest that "a part may be retained or conjugated with other compounds that can stimulate biochemical and physiologic responses."[64] Although in one study, glyphosate did not appear to accumulate in fish,[65] evidence of glyphosate retention was found in a study of rabbits. Six weeks after male rabbits were exposed, the glyphosate still had a harmful impact on semen quality.[66]

Toxicologist Gilles-Eric Seralini called for labeling of animal products from GMO-fed animals "because pesticide residues associated [with] GMOs may bioaccumulate in the food chain, especially Roundup residues and adjuvants, and because animals may have metabolic disorders when they eat GMOs."[67]

The European Commission acknowledges that, "indirect environmental or human health effects that may arise from direct impacts on animal health or GM plant-induced imbalance in the animal interactions with the ecosystem is still largely an unexplored area."[68]

6.5

Disease-resistant crops may promote new plant viruses, which carry risks for humans

"GM crops may be especially susceptible to new infectious viral diseases."

—Coalition report, *Comments on GM Science Review*

1. Virus-resistant transgenes protect crops from one target virus, but may increase susceptibility to other plant viruses.

2. Infected plants put humans at risk due to increased pesticide use.

3. They may also lead to increased consumption of potentially harmful viral proteins.

Virus-resistant GM crops are designed to bolster the plants' defenses against one single virus. While the plant may successfully ward off that target virus, the presence of the viral transgenes and proteins in the GM crop can actually increase the likelihood that other viruses infect the plant. There are at least three routes by which this can occur:

1. Viral proteins produced by the transgene may attack the host cell's defenses, making it more susceptible to other viruses. In one study, proteins from viral transgenes even allowed a plant to become infected with an insect virus, not normally found in plants.[69]

2. One type of viral protein is called a coat protein. It surrounds (encapsidates) the RNA, protecting it from threats such as ultraviolet light or enzymes that would normally break it down. This allows that new virus to be picked up by an insect and transported to other plants. In fact, the coat protein typically specifies which species of insect can take up the virus. Since it is possible for a coat protein from one virus to encapsidate another virus, this would allow the latter to be picked up by a new insect species and be transported to a new spectrum of host plants. The risk of encapsidating the wrong virus (transcapsidation) is not unique to GM plants, but the presence of viral coat protein in every plant cell can greatly increase the probability that it will occur.

3. Inserted viral genes that come into proximity with related and unrelated natural viruses may recombine (exchange RNA) to create new versions. These "offspring" viruses can be quite different from either "parent." Numerous scientists have expressed concerns that viral inserts in GM crops may recombine with other plant viruses.[70] Several experiments specifically demonstrate that this takes place[71] (including recombination with the transgene used in plums developed by the USDA[72]). According to a paper by Latham and Steinbrecher, "In some cases recombination occurred at very high rates—in up to 80% of all plants tested. [73] ... The published scientific data best supports the conclusion that GM crops containing virus-derived transgenes should not at present receive commercial approval. This is because recombination (HGT) leading to the creation of new viruses is inevitable, while the consequences of such recombination cannot at present be predicted."[74]

By recombining with a transgene, the new virus may gain an evolutionary advantage. For example, one particular concern is that the viral transgene will transfer to a virus that does not normally infect the plant.[75] The invading virus, which is *not* adapted to that plant, would acquire a transgene that *is* adapted, thereby increasing its ability to attack it.[76] It is ironic that GM crops designed to resist one virus "may be especially susceptible to new infectious viral diseases."[77]

Diseased plants may impact human health

Plants that develop novel viruses are also more likely to be treated with pesticides, which increase human health risks. In addition, some forms of plant viruses produce large quantities of viral proteins. As described in section 3.9, consumption of viral proteins may increase susceptibility to viral infection or be toxic.

It is important to note that this concern about creating new viruses is related to plant viruses, not human viruses. Natural barriers tend to block a virus in one kingdom from attacking organisms in another kingdom. Therefore, the tendency to create new viruses in plants *does not mean* that they will attack humans. (However, instances of viruses operating between kingdoms do occur on rare occasions. As mentioned above, when genes from two distinct viruses were inserted separately into a plant, the two viral proteins made the plant susceptible to infection by an animal (insect) virus. There are also other examples of cross kingdom viral adaptations.[78])

USDA ignores scientific opinion

According to Latham and Steinbrecher, [79] "The views of many scientists working in this area (as reflected in the scientific literature) are at odds with the policy of widespread commercialization of virus-containing GM crops being pursued by the USDA." Biotech companies and regulatory agencies have ignored the data and cling to unproven or obsolete safety assumptions. (For examples of these assumptions, see part 3.)

"*Next time you hear a scientist asserting that gene splicing is safe, remind yourself that there is no scientific evidence for that statement. We are profoundly ignorant about what we are doing to the code that generates all life. And unfortunately some scientists, including those entrusted with public safety, are willing to lie*".

—Donella H. Meadows, biophysicist and environmentalist, Dartmouth College

SECTION 7:

Other types of GM foods carry risks

GM crops are not the only food items that are altered through genetic engineering. The technology is used to insert transgenes into bacteria, fungi, and yeast, converting the microorganisms into living factories. This technique is used to produce certain enzymes and additives used in food preparation as well as a sweetener called aspartame. It is also used in the production of recombinant bovine growth hormone, which is injected into cows to increase milk supply. This section looks at health impacts associated with these products of genetic modification.

7.1

Milk from rbGH-treated cows may increase risk of cancer and other diseases

> *"We feel fairly confident in being able to demonstrate that the safety of European citizens who consume [rbGH] products cannot be guaranteed."[1]*
>
> —Fredrich-Wilhelm Graefe zu Baringdorf, former Vice President of the Agriculture Committee of the European Commission

1. Monsanto's genetically engineered bovine growth hormone is injected into dairy cows in the United States and elsewhere, to increase milk production.

2. Milk from treated cows has much higher levels of IGF-1, a hormone considered to be a high risk factor for breast, prostate, colon, lung, and other cancers.

3. The milk also has lowered nutritional value, increased antibiotics and more pus from infected udders.

Monsanto inserted cow genes into bacteria to produce recombinant bovine growth hormone (rbGH), a drug that increases milk production in cows.[2] Approved in the United States in 1993, by 2002 it was used on 22% of the nation's dairy cows.[3] It is also used in South Africa and Brazil, but is banned in the European Union, Canada, Australia, New Zealand, and Japan.

Dairy products from treated cows carry several health risks, the most serious of which is higher levels of the hormone insulin-like growth factor 1 (IGF-1). It is one of the most powerful growth hormones in the human body and is naturally present in cows' milk. One study showed a 10% increase in the free levels of IGF-1 in subjects that drank milk; the controls showed no change.[4] Analysis of the diets of more than 1,000 nurses revealed that the food most associated with high IGF-1 levels was milk.[5] Neither of these studies used milk from cows treated with rbGH. If they had, the results may have been considerably more significant, since levels of IGF-1 in milk from treated cows can be up to 10 times higher,[6] and detection methods may underestimate the amount and impact of this increase by up to fortyfold.[7]

High levels of IGF-1 raise cancer risk

IGF-1 causes cells to divide; more than three dozen studies unequivocally link high levels to increased cancer risk.[8] A Harvard study of 15,000 white males found those with elevated blood levels to be four times more likely to get prostate cancer than average men.[9] In a *Lancet* study, premenopausal US women below age 50 with high IGF-1 levels were seven times as likely to develop breast cancer. "With the exception of a strong family history of breast cancer," the authors warned, "the relation between IGF-1 and risk of breast cancer may be greater than that of other established breast-cancer risk factors."[10] The *International Journal of Cancer* described a "significant association between circulating IGF-1 concentrations and an increased risk of lung, colon, prostate, and pre-menopausal breast cancer." It concluded, "Lowering plasma IGF-1 may thus represent an attractive strategy to be pursued."[11] A 1999 European Commission report concluded: "Avoidance of rbGH dairy products in favor of natural products would appear to be the most practical and immediate dietary intervention to . . . (achieve) the goal of preventing cancer."[12]

One way that IGF-1 may promote cancer is by reducing programmed cell death (apoptosis) in tumor cells. IGF-1 also inhibits the ability of various anti-cancer drugs to kill cultured human breast cancer cells.[13]

Rat pups fed IGF-I in milk increased the growth of their brains and livers.[14] And IGF-1 boosted the expression of the prion protein gene in rat cells, raising "unresolved questions on the possible effects of increased IGF-1 levels on susceptibility to bovine (BSE) and human prion disease (CJD)."[15]

Increased antibiotics, reduced nutrition

There are more than 20 side effects to cows listed on Monsanto's rbGH label, including cystic ovaries, uterine disorders, decreased gestation period, decreased calf birth weight, and increased twinning rates.[16] Udder infection (mastitis) is the most widely reported. This painful disease increases the pus (somatic cells) in milk; milk from treated cows has 19% more.[17] To manage infections and pus levels, farmers using rbGH typically treat their herd with extra antibiotics, which increases antibiotic residues in milk.

Milk from cows treated with rbGH has higher levels of bovine growth hormone (methionyl-rBST),[18] a thyroid hormone (tri-iodothyronine),[19] lactose and long chain fatty acids (up to 27%),[20] and less casein and short and medium chain fatty acids.[21] One reviewer said that the composition changed "in directions detrimental to the nutritional quality of milk. Health risks to individual consumers . . . would thus depend on how much of the milk consumed was from cows treated with [rbGH]."[22]

Regulators pressured for drug approval

One FDA scientist said he was fired after expressing concerns about insufficient data in the rbGH analysis. Other FDA employees sent an anonymous letter complaining of "fraud" and "conflict of interest" in relation to the drug's approval. They claimed, for example, that a Monsanto-researcher-turned-FDA-employee raised allowable levels of antibiotics in milk one-hundredfold, to pave the way for rbGH approval.[23] And when Canadian government scientists analyzed how the FDA approved rbGH, they wrote that the "evaluation was largely a theoretical review taking the manufacturer's conclusions at face value. No details of the studies nor a critical analysis of the quality of the data was provided." Because critical studies were not conducted, "such possibilities and potential as sterility, infertility, birth defects, cancer, and immunological derangements were not addressed."[24]

The Canadian scientists also testified before the Senate that they were pressured to approve rbGH by their superiors, that documents were stolen from a locked file cabinet and that Monsanto offered them a bribe of $1–$2 million to approve the drug without further study.[25]

7 . 2

Milk from rbGH-treated cows likely increases the rate of twin births

> "*The more IGF, the more the ovary is stimulated to release additional eggs at ovulation.*"[26]
>
> —Gary Steinman, obstetrician, multiple birth expert, Albert Einstein College of Medicine

1. Higher IGF-1 levels increase the rate of twin births.

2. Since milk drinkers increase their IGF-1, correspondingly they have higher twinning rates.

3. Milk from cows injected with bovine growth hormone has higher IGF-1 levels.

4. Drinking milk from injected cows should increase the twinning rate even more.

5. The number of twins grew at twice the rate in the United States compared to the United Kingdom, where rbGH is banned.

Higher levels of blood IGF-1 increase the tendency to have fraternal twins. The hormone increases ovulation and appears to support embryo survival.[27] Cows with high twin rates have IGF-1 levels 1.5–2 times higher than normal.[28] It is also noteworthy that the gene in cows that produces IGF-1 is located in close proximity to the genes that control the rate of twinning.[29]

In human populations, African Americans have higher IGF-1 levels than Caucasians, who in turn have higher levels than Asians. Correspondingly, the twinning rates for African Americans are 30% higher than Caucasians and 83% higher than Asians.[30]

Milk consumption increases IGF-1 levels. As mentioned in the previous section, one study showed that a glass of milk each day for 12 weeks increased blood IGF-1 levels by 10%.[31] Vegan women who do not drink milk have 13% less IGF-1 levels.[32] Male vegans have 9% less.[33]

Since milk increases IGF-1 and IGF-1 increases twinning rates, one would expect that milk consumption increases twinning. This is confirmed by several studies. For example, twinning rates in 15 European countries correlated with average milk consumption.[34] The rate of twins in some countries also dropped when dairy consumption fell during World War II.[35] A study in the *Journal of Reproductive Medicine* reported that mothers who consumed milk were five times more likely to give birth to fraternal twins, compared to vegans (1.9% compared to .4%).[36]

Bovine growth hormone increases twinning rates

Cows injected with recombinant bovine growth hormone (rbGH) have elevated IGF-1, increased ovulation and more embryos available.[37] Monsanto lists on its rbGH label that increased twinning rates is one of the possible side effects of use. Gary Steinman, an expert on multiple births and assistant clinical professor of obstetrics at the Albert Einstein College of Medicine, contends that since dairy products from injected cows have higher IGF-1 levels, they should likewise increase twinning rates among milk drinkers.[38]

Twinning rates have tripled over the last 30 years, in part due to the increased amount of *in vitro* fertilization and the tendency for women to have children later in life. Between 1992 and 2001, however, the rate of twins born in the United Kingdom increased by 16% while the increase in the United States was 32%. A significant difference between the two populations is that a large number of dairy cows in the United States are treated with rbGH, whereas the drug is banned in the United Kingdom and throughout Europe.

Steinman says, "Because multiple gestations are more prone to complications such as premature delivery, congenital defects and pregnancy-induced hypertension in the mother than singleton pregnancies, the findings of this study suggest that women contemplating pregnancy might consider substituting meat and dairy products with other protein sources, especially in countries that allow growth hormone administration to cattle."[39]

7.3

Food additives created from GM microorganisms pose health risks

---

> **"T**his is a novel pro-
> tein manufactured
> by genetically modified organ-
> isms and its characteristics
> have never been fully evalu-
> ated. It needs to be checked out
> before it is widely introduced
> into the human diet."[40]
>
> —Malcolm Hooper, emeri-
> tus professor of Medical
> Chemistry at Sunderland
> University, regarding GM
> fish protein used in ice
> cream

1. Certain food ingredients and processing agents are derived from GM bacteria, fungus, or yeast.

---

2. Even if the transgene is not found in the food, the GM process still carries risks.

---

3. The GM protein may be unhealthy, have altered properties or react with other compounds in unpredictable ways.

---

4. The gene insertion process might also disrupt normal gene expression of the microorganisms.

Several enzymes, cooking agents, and other proteins used in food are created from genetically engineered bacteria, fungus, or yeast. The GM organism is not added to the food; rather, the inserted genes produce proteins that are used.

By using GM microorganisms, companies may have access to proteins that would be too expensive to use otherwise. Genetic engineering, therefore, allows new ingredients, or higher concentrations of existing ingredients, into the human diet. Not only does this carry risks, the process of genetic engineering can lead to unpredictable outcomes.

Since the genes are not ingested, there is no risk of horizontal gene transfer. GM microorganisms also do not undergo tissue culture, so they avoid the associated genome-wide mutations that can occur with GM crops. But microorganisms still undergo insertion mutation, and transgenes may be truncated, fragmented, scrambled, mixed with host DNA, or be unstable. Gene insertion might also alter expression levels of natural genes in host DNA. In addition, the GM protein may be misfolded or attached to molecular chains, making it harmful. And the protein may also interact with other compounds produced by the microorganism, leading to new or higher levels of toxins, allergens, or antinutrients. These risks provide possible explanations why L-tryptophan, produced by GM bacteria, contained contaminants that were responsible for a deadly epidemic in the 1980s (See section 1.20).

Unfortunately, there are no special precautions for ingredients produced through GMOs. And like GM crops, the safety testing does not adequately guard against unpredicted outcomes of the technology.

Case study: fish protein in ice cream

To improve the taste and texture of its lowfat ice cream, Unilever introduced GM ice-structuring protein (ISP), which lowers the temperature at which ice crystals grow. Although ISP is naturally found in an eel-like arctic fish called the ocean pout, isolating the protein from the fish is expensive. To make it affordable, the company inserted multiple copies of a fish gene into yeast DNA.

After it produces ISP, the yeast is removed using microfiltration. The resulting mixture contains ISP, proteins, and peptides made by the yeast, as well as sugars, acids, and salts.[41] If the GM transformation process resulted in unexpected contaminants, it is possible that they might remain in the mix as well.

Although GM ISP has the same 66 amino acid sequence as the natural version, it is unknown if the protein is folded the same. There are certainly some differences in the shape, since a sugar chain is added in the ISP produced by the yeast. Such additions (glycosylation) to protein produced in GM peas led to a dangerous inflammation response in mice (see section 1.18). Geneticist Joe Cummins and others said that the ISP could likewise "be letting off an immunological time bomb,"[42] and called for long-term safety tests. Unilever refused. They claim that since the glycosylation pattern in their ISP is typical of yeast, and because yeast does not cause immune problems in humans, the protein should be harmless. This assumption, however, fails to take into account that when GM yeast was used to create human pharmaceutical proteins, the glycosylation *did* cause problems related to immunity and enzyme functioning. Scientists had to change (humanize) the yeast's sugar patterns to solve the issue.[43]

ISP has a history of use in the diet. Ocean pout has been used as a food in North America, particularly during World War II. Its presence in ice cream, however, vastly increases its exposure. A 160-pound young man in the United States who consumes a lot of ice cream would eat as much as 23 milligrams of ISP per day.[44] That's certainly enough to warrant concerns about allergies. Unilever tested their protein with the stability and amino acid sequence evaluations that are used for GM crops (see part 3). They also went a step further and looked for reactions in the blood (sera) from 22 individuals known to be allergic to cod fish. But according to Cummins, "This experiment was deceptive because the cod allergy is caused by a cod blood protein unrelated to grouper ISP."[45] Similarly, pediatrician Jim Diamond of the Sierra Club points out that "if this particular fish antifreeze protein is allergenic apart from the usual fish allergy to parvalbumin, the test wouldn't pick that up."

Unilever also fed ISP to human volunteers, five days a week for eight weeks. Although this was certainly not the long-term study called for by Cummins, it is a protocol that has not been used for GM crops assessments; they do not test products on humans.

Unilever's ice cream is not labeled as derived from GM ingredients. If ISP or a GMO-related contaminant created health problems in some people, it may be quite difficult to identify the cause—especially if the reactions were a common disease or took years to develop. "If labels are not provided for foods manufactured with protein produced from recombinant organisms," says Cummins, "serious human injury from such foods may go undetected in a huge unsuspecting population."

"While we have mounting evidences for epigenetics the outdated central dogma of the gene still exists – mainly in the field of agro-biotechnology and commercial applications of GM crops. We seem to hang in a state of suspense. The stubborn perseverance with which some still cling to the old dogma might have to do with commercial pressures and with patents. It's easier to patent genes than to patent complex epigenetic networks."[1]

—Florianne Koechlin, biologist,
Blueridge Institute

SECTION 8:

Risks are greater for children and newborns

This section explores the special risks that GM crops pose for children and developing fetuses.

8.1

Pregnant mothers eating GM foods may endanger offspring

> "*Over the past 10,000 years, it is likely that plant varieties that have adverse reproductive effects have been eliminated from our food supply, but modern GE technology may accidentally activate dormant pathways that adversely affect development.*"[2]
>
> —William Freese and David Schubert, *Biotechnology and Genetic Engineering Reviews*

1. Embryo development can be adversely affected by tiny amounts of substances in the mother's diet.

2. A pregnant mother's diet may even alter gene expression in children and be passed on to future generations.

3. GM crops may contain substances that impact normal fetal development, but have never been adequately tested for these effects.

Embryo development may be highly sensitive to changes in the diet due to GM foods, but almost no intergenerational feeding studies have been conducted. According to an article in *Biotechnology and Genetic Engineering Reviews*, "Embryogenesis is an exquisitely fine-tuned process controlled by ultra-low levels of small molecules, such as steroids and retinoids. Plants can make related molecules that may interfere with normal development."[3] These molecules may have little or no effect on adult humans or animals, they may be most active at very low levels, and may not even be identified or classified. All this makes testing of the effects of GM on the embryo more difficult, but no less imperative.

The safety evaluation is complicated by the fact that embryos develop in stages; some substances may have a measurable impact only during specific time periods. According to a paper in *Diabetes*, both human and animal studies provide "considerable evidence to suggest that maternal nutritional imbalance and metabolic disturbances, during critical time windows of development, may have a persistent effect on the health of the offspring."[4]

Epigenetics

Recent breakthroughs in the field of epigenetics have revolutionized our understanding of gene expression and add an unprecedented risk of GM foods. Not only will nutritional imbalances and metabolic disturbances affect infant health, they can even influence gene expression "and may even be transmitted to the next generation."[5]

This concept was illustrated by a remarkable study, featured on the cover of a 2003 issue of *Molecular and Cellular Biology*. "Scientists showed they could change the coat color of baby mice simply by feeding their mothers four common nutritional supplements before and during pregnancy and lactation." The diet changed the gene expression of the offspring and also lowered their "susceptibility to obesity, diabetes, and cancer."[6] These epigenetic alterations, which cause permanent changes in gene expression, have been seen for some time in cancer research.[7]

Diet choices during pregnancy can make the offspring healthier or have the opposite effect, and the impact may not show up until years after birth. This casts a long shadow over the vast number of unpredicted compounds that may be produced as a result of the GM transformation process. Natural genes can be deleted, scrambled, turned off, permanently turned on, reversed, duplicated, or moved, and the expression levels of hundreds of genes can be altered (see section 2).[8]

Other factors

Other risks to offspring that have been cited in this book include:

- Fragments of DNA from the diet of pregnant mice ended up in the brains of their offspring.[9] The effect of migrating transgenes or of natural DNA in food that has been mutated by gene insertion is not known. (See section 5 and section 2.)
- If transgenes were to transfer into human sex cells, they might impact the genetic expression of offspring and future generations. (See section 5.)
- GM soy adversely affected the structure and function of testicle cells in mice, potentially influencing offspring health. (See section 1.12.)
- Gene expression in early mice embryos was temporarily inhibited in the group whose mothers were fed GM soy. (See section 1.12.)
- Increased herbicide residues associated with GM crops might cause endocrine disruption or toxic effects in fetal development. (See section 6.)
- One of the few intergenerational studies reported more than a sixfold increase (55.6% vs 9%) in offspring mortality within three weeks. (See section 1.14.)

The vulnerability of the unborn and the lack of regulatory safeguards were highlighted in a January 2006 report issued by the Environmental Protection Agency's (EPA) Office of Inspector General. According to the document, studies demonstrate that certain pesticides easily enter the brain of young children and fetuses, and can destroy cells. The report concluded that the EPA lacks standard evaluation protocols for measuring the toxicity of pesticides on developing nervous systems.[10] EPA scientists also charged that "risk assessments cannot state with confidence the degree to which any exposure of a fetus, infant, or child to a pesticide will or will not adversely affect their neurological development."[11] This is even truer with GM crops.

Furthermore, three trade unions representing 9,000 EPA workers claimed that the evaluation techniques used at the agency were highly politicized. According to a May 24, 2006 letter to the EPA's administrator, the unions cited "political pressure exerted by Agency officials perceived to be too closely aligned with the pesticide industry and former EPA officials now representing the pesticide and agricultural community."[12]

8.2

GM foods are more dangerous for children than adults

> "Swapping genes between organisms can produce unknown toxic effects and allergies that are most likely to affect children."[13]
>
> —Vyvyan Howard, expert in infant toxico-pathology at Liverpool University Hospital, United Kingdom

1. Children are generally more susceptible to toxins, allergens, and nutritional problems.

2. They consume more milk, which may be from cows treated with rbGH.

3. The emergence of antibiotic-resistant diseases may also significantly impact those children who are prone to recurring infections.

Changes in nutrition have a greater impact on the structure and functioning of young, fast-growing bodies. More of the food is converted to build organs and tissues, whereas adults convert more to energy and store this as fat.

The UK Royal Society said that genetic modification "could lead to unpredicted harmful changes in the nutritional state of foods" and recommended that potential health effects of GM foods be rigorously researched before being fed to pregnant or breast-feeding women and babies."[14] Epidemiologist Eric Brunner said that "small changes to the nutritional content might have effects on infant bowel function."[15]

Children are more susceptible to problems

Children are three to four times more prone to allergies than adults and "are at highest risk of death from food allergy."[16] Infants below two years old have the highest incidence of reactions, especially to new allergens encountered in the diet. Even tiny amounts of allergens can sometimes cause reactions. One reason for this sensitivity, according to the EPA, is that "An immature gut or permeable mucosal epithelium is more likely to allow a higher degree of macromolecular transport and access to the immune system than the intact barrier of a normal mature gut. . . . The immune system must also be of sufficient maturity. . . . Both systems appear to be functioning optimally by age three to five."[17]

According to the Royal Society of Canada, "The potentially widespread use of GM food products as food additives and staple foods, including use in baby foods, may lead to earlier introduction of these novel proteins to susceptible infants either directly or via the presence of the maternally ingested proteins in breast milk."[18]

The UK Royal Society suggested that "post-marketing surveillance should be part of the overall safety strategy for allergies, especially of high-risk groups such as infants," but acknowledged that it is not clear "whether such monitoring is feasible for GM food."[19]

Children can react to much smaller doses of toxins than adults. Exposure to hormones or endocrine disruptors may also severely affect normal development. And children who are prone to infections may be severely impacted if antibiotics lose their effectiveness due to antibiotic-resistant genes in GM food and the overuse of antibiotics in rbGH treated cows.

Children have a high exposure to GMOs

Children consume a large amount of products that may be genetically engineered. They eat a higher percentage of corn in their diet compared to adults, and allergic children often rely on corn as a source of protein. Mothers using cornstarch as a talc substitute on their children's skin might also expose them via inhalation. Infants are sometimes reared on soy infant formula. The Royal Society wrote, "Infant formulas, in particular, are "consumed as a single food over extended periods of time by those who are especially vulnerable" and "should be investigated most rigorously."[20] Among the potential side effects are changes in soy's natural estrogen mimickers, which may influence sexual development.

Children consume a disproportionately large amount of milk. In the United States and elsewhere, dairy products may come from cows treated with the genetically engineered bovine growth hormone (rbGH). The milk contains increased amounts of hormones and antibiotics and an altered nutritional content (see section 7.1). According to a discussion paper on the public health implications of rbGH, published in the *Journal of the Royal Society of Medicine*, an "infant would be exposed to a dose of IGF-1, which was 12.5 times the recommended minimum."[21] Samuel Epstein, chairman of the Cancer Prevention Coalition and an expert on the health effects of rbGH, says that risks of high exposure to IGF-1 are "of particular concern . . . to infants and children in view of their high susceptibility to cancer-causing products and chemicals."[22] He also suggests that regular exposure might promote "premature growth stimulation in infants, gynecomastia [development of abnormally large breasts on males] in young children."[23]

Safety assessments ignore children

An FAO/WHO task force on GM food said that "Attention should be paid to the particular physiological characteristics and metabolic requirements of specific population subgroups, such as infants [and] children."[24] In practice, GM safety assessments ignore them. In fact, industry-funded studies often use mature animals instead of the more sensitive young ones, in order to mask results (see part 3).

Biologist David Schubert warns, "Since children are the most likely to be adversely effected by toxins and other dietary problems, if the GM food is given to them without proper testing, they will be the experimental animals. If there are problems, we will probably never know because the cause will not be traceable and many diseases take a very long time to develop."[25]

Connecting the dots: looking for patterns and causes

Part 1 began with 20 reports of adverse effects from GM foods. These included lab animals with damage to virtually every system studied, thousands of sick, sterile, or dead livestock and people around the world who traced toxic or allergic reactions to eating GM products, breathing GM pollen, or touching GM crops at harvest. Then, 45 ways in which genetic engineering may be responsible for these and other health problems were presented. Here we review the findings, looking for patterns and discussing probable causes for some of the adverse reactions.

Gambling with the genome and our health

Inserting transgenes is like throwing darts that can land in more than a billion possible locations in a genome. At the insertion site, the host's natural genes may become mutated, deleted, altered, or permanently turned on or off. In addition, up to 5% of the active genes throughout the genome may change expression levels, and growing GM cells in tissue culture can cause hundreds or thousands of additional genome-wide mutations. All this can change RNA, proteins, and other substances, including the countless natural products in plants. Any one might be harmful.

The inserted transgene introduces a new protein into our diet, which may be allergenic, toxic, or antinutritional. The structure and function of the protein may change unpredictably when processed in the new organism. In addition, the transgene sequence may be altered, truncated, or mixed with other DNA during insertion, or it may rearrange spontaneously years later—creating proteins with amino acid sequences that were never intended.

The unpredictable nature of GM crops is compounded by influences from the plants' genetic dispositions, growing conditions, interactions between multiple gene inserts, and heavier applications of herbicides. Toxins produced or accumulated in GM crops may also be concentrated into meat or milk, or bioaccumulate in humans.

In addition, the transgene, antibiotic resistant marker gene, or promoter might transfer into the DNA of our gut bacteria or internal organs; genetic material may also pass through the placenta into the unborn or possibly influence sex cells prior to conception.

Each of these risks is unique to GM crops in character and scale, but because regulators accept producers' myths about the safety of their products, GMOs are approved without checking for *most* potential problems.

Allergies and immune responses

According to the Indian Council of Medical Research, "The allergenicity potential of GM food has often been difficult to establish with existing methods as the transgenes transferred are frequently from sources not eaten before, many have unknown allergenicity, or there may be a potential for the genetic modification process to result in increase of an allergen already present in the food."[1]

The threat is not trivial. In 2001, scientists estimated that about "150 people die each year in the United States of food-related allergic reactions and 29,000 have a severe anaphylactic episode,"[2] (The actual number may be significantly different due to unreported or misdiagnosed cases.) Allergic reactions are a defensive, often harmful immune system response to an external irritant. The body interprets something as foreign, different, and offensive, and reacts accordingly. All GM foods, by definition, have something foreign and different. Studies confirm immune responses to GM crops and several reveal probable causes.

Soybeans outfitted with a Brazil nut gene created allergic reactions in the blood of those allergic to the nuts[3] (section 3.1). The cause is almost certainly the fact that the GM protein was an allergen. It provoked allergic reactions in sensitive people when it was produced in Brazil nuts, and those same people showed reactions when the protein was expressed in soybeans.

A GM enzyme produced in peas triggered inflammatory responses in mice, suggesting that it would cause allergies in humans[4] (section 1.18). In this case, the protein in its natural state—produced in kidney beans—was not harmful. Only when expressed in GM peas did it provoke a response. The reason is likely due to unpredicted subtle changes in the attached sugar chain patterns (glycosylation).

Potatoes engineered with a snowdrop lectin caused immune damage to rats[5] (section 1.1). Here too, the protein in its natural state was found to be safe. (Rats fed potatoes spiked with the lectin showed no such immune dysfunction). The cause was therefore either a modification in the protein or some other change in the composition of the potato brought about by the GM transformation process.

Soy allergies jumped 50% in the United Kingdom just after GM soy was introduced[6] (section 1.15). If GM soy was the cause, it may be due to several things.

1. The GM protein that makes Roundup Ready soy resistant to herbicide does not have a history of safe use in the human diet and may be an allergen. In fact, sections of its amino acid sequence are identical with known allergens[7] (section 3.2).

2. A portion of the transgene from GM soybeans is transferred into human gut bacteria. The transferred genetic material included the promoter, which turns on the transgene. In addition, the gut bacteria survived doses of Roundup's active ingredient glyphosate. This suggests that the transgene continues to produce its Roundup Ready protein from within the intestinal bacteria.[8] If true, than long after people stop eating GM soy, they may be constantly exposed to its potentially allergenic protein (section 5.4).

3. The GM transformation process may have increased natural allergens in soybeans. The level of one known allergen, trypsin inhibitor, was 27% higher in raw GM soy varieties. More worrisome, it was as much as sevenfold higher in cooked GM soy compared to cooked non-GM soy (section 2.11). Not only is this higher amount potentially harmful, the findings also suggests that the trypsin inhibitor in GM soy might be more heat stable and therefore even more allergenic than the natural variety.[9] There are also one or more proteins in natural soybeans that show cross-reactivity with a peanut allergens.[10] Changes in GM soy DNA may increase the amount or potency of this potentially dangerous source of allergies, and may have contributed to the doubling of peanut allergies from 1997 to 2002 (see section 1.15).

4. Changes in GM soy DNA may produce new allergens. Although there has never been an exhaustive analysis of the proteins or natural products in GM soy, unpredicted changes in the DNA were discovered. A mutated section of soy DNA was found near the transgene. This may contribute to some unpredicted effect. Moreover, between this scrambled DNA and the transgene is an extra transgene fragment, not discovered until years after soy was on the market. The RNA produced is completely unexpected. It combines material from all three sections: the full length transgene, the transgene fragment, and the mutated DNA sequence. This RNA is then further processed into four different variations[11] (section 2.9). These might lead to the production of some unknown allergen.

5. Another study verified that GM soybeans contain an IgE-binding allergenic protein not found in non-GM soy controls[12] (section 1.15).

6. One of eight subjects that showed a skin prick allergic reaction to GM soy had no reaction to non-GM soy[13] (section 1.15). Although the sample size is small, the implication that certain people react only to GM soy is huge.

7. Increased residues of Roundup herbicide in GM soy might contribute to increased allergies. In fact, the symptoms identified in the UK soy allergy study are among those related to glyphosate exposure. The allergy study identified irritable bowel syndrome, digestion problems, chronic fatigue, headaches, lethargy, and skin complaints including acne and eczema (section 1.15). Symptoms of glyphosate exposure include nausea, headaches, lethargy, skin rashes, and burning or itchy skin[14] (section 6.2). It is also possible that glyphosate's breakdown product AMPA, which accumulates in GM soybeans, might contribute to allergies.

8. The GM protein in the soy may have changed due to misfolding, attached molecular chains, or rearrangements of unstable transgenes (section 4). There is insufficient data to support or rule out these possibilities.

9. Mice fed GM soy had reduced levels of pancreatic enzymes[15] (section 1.11). When protein digesting enzymes are suppressed, proteins may last longer in the gut, giving more time for an allergic reaction to take place. Any reduction in protein digestion could therefore promote allergic reactions to a wide range of proteins, not just to the GM soy.

Bt-toxin triggers immune responses

Bt-toxin is consistently associated with immune and allergic-type responses. Even if unpredicted consequences of the GM transformation process contribute to allergic reactions from *Bt* crops, the evidence suggests that the *Bt*-toxin itself is a major factor. The *Bt* proteins found in most currently registered *Bt* corn varieties would not pass the allergy test protocol described in the 2001 FAO/WHO report[16] (section 3.2). They have amino acid sections identical with known allergens and are too stable in simulated digestive solutions. Furthermore, immune responses are triggered by both the natural *Bt*-toxin in spray form and *Bt* crops. (The concentration of *Bt*-toxin in crops, however, can be thousands of times higher than in sprays; and changes in its protein structure make the crop version more likely to provoke reactions in humans (section 3.4).)

Here is additional evidence:

- When populations were exposed to *Bt* spray, hundreds complained of allergic reactions and some were hospitalized[17] (section 3.3).
- Farm workers also exhibited antibody responses to *Bt* spray[18] (section 3.3).
- *Bt*-toxin fed to mice induced a significant immune response and an increased reactivity to other substances (section 3.3).
- Male rats fed MON 863 *Bt* corn had a significant increase in three types of blood cells related to the immune system: basophils, lymphocytes (22%), and total white cell counts (20%)[19] (section 1.3).
- Thousands of consumers complained to food manufacturers about possible reactions to StarLink corn and an expert panel determined that its *Bt* protein had a "medium likelihood" of being a human allergen[20] (section 3.5).
- Filipinos from at least five villages developed severe symptoms when nearby *Bt* cornfields were pollinating[21] (section 1.7).
- Indian farm workers exposed to *Bt* cotton developed moderate or severe allergic reactions[22] (section 1.5).
- And large numbers of sheep suffered illness and death when grazing on post-harvest *Bt* cotton plants[23] (section 1.6).

The consistency between the reactions related to *Bt* sprays and those reported by *Bt* cotton workers is astounding. The *Bt* spray was associated with sneezing, runny nose, watery eyes, skin inflammation and irritation, rashes, itching and burning, swelling, red skin and red eyes, exacerbations of asthma, facial swelling, and fever. Some people required hospitalization. *Bt* cotton workers in India reported sneezing, runny nose, watery eyes, skin eruptions, itching and burning, red skin and red eyes, facial swelling, and fever. Some people required hospitalization. The two lists are nearly identical. Only "exacerbations of asthma" was in one list (spray) and not the other (cotton).

Asthma and breathing difficulties *were* reported by Filipinos who inhaled *Bt* corn pollen. They also described swollen faces, flu-like symptoms, fever, and sneezing—all symptoms listed above. Some individuals in both India and the Philippines reported long-term effects after exposure. The list of symptoms in the Philippines, however, did contain items not reported by the other two groups. These included coughs, headache, stomachache, dizziness, diarrhea, vomiting, weakness, and numbness.

For the sake of comparison, sheep that grazed on *Bt* cotton plants had nasal discharge, reddish and erosive mouth lesions, cough, bloat and diarrhea, and occasional red colored urine. They were also described as dull and depressed.

Allergies are on the rise

It is difficult to confirm that GM crops are contributing to allergies among the GMO-eating United Station population. Although many scientists and organizations have called for post-marketing surveillance to find out, scientists Terje Traavik and Jack Heinemann question "whether post-marketing surveillance can provide useful information about allergens in GE foods. For a number of reasons," they conclude, "this is not likely to happen. Treatment of allergy is symptomatic, whatever the cause may be. The allergic case is often isolated, and the potential allergen is rarely identified. The number of allergy-related medical visits is not tabulated. Even repeated visits due to well-known allergens are not counted as part of any established surveillance system."[24]

According to a 2002 report looking at allergy research in the United States in relation to GM foods, there is a lack of "robust and reliable data on the prevalence (total cases), incidence (new cases per year), and trends of food allergy."[25] Under such conditions, it would be difficult to identify anything less than a huge increase. But according to the June 2006 *Chicago Tribune* article entitled, "Scientists see spike in kids' food allergies," "Medical personnel, from school nurses to chiefs of hospital pediatric departments," are describing just that—among US children. Dr. Jacqueline Pongracic, head of the allergy department at Children's Memorial Hospital in Chicago said, "I've been treating children in the field of allergy immunology for 15 years, and in recent years I've really seen the rates of food allergy skyrocket."[26] Whether GM food is a factor remains to be seen, but the evidence suggests that it is likely.

Several signs of toxic reactions

The same mechanism for producing allergens in GM crops can also lead to toxins. The GM protein, alterations in that protein, mutations in the host DNA, transferred genes, and excess herbicide residues can all have toxic effects. To see if the foods are toxic, Arpad Pusztai suggests that analysis of the digestive tract should be the first target of GM food risk assessment. The gut is the initial and largest point of contact and can reveal reactions to various toxins.

In one of the first animal studies, female rats fed the FlavrSavr tomato developed lesions in the stomach.[27] Although the researchers never looked at the intestines, other studies that did look found effects. Mice fed *Bt*-toxin and *Bt* potatoes had cell damage in the lower part of the small intestines (ileum). There was also abnormal and proliferative cell growth.[28] Similarly, rats fed GM lectin potatoes showed significant proliferative cell growth in both stomach and intestines.[29] Although the guts of rats fed GM peas were not examined for cell growth, the intestines were heavier, which might result from such growth.[30] Since proliferation of cells may be a precursor to cancer, it is an area of special concern.

Another indication of toxins is the state of the liver—a main detoxifier for the body. Several studies showed adverse effects. Rats fed lectin potatoes had smaller and partially atrophied livers.[31] Rats fed Mon 863 had liver lesions.[32] Mice fed Roundup Ready soybeans had altered gene expression and structural and functional changes in their liver cells.[33] In particular, the livers may have exhibited higher metabolic activity in response to a toxic insult. Rabbits fed GM soy also showed higher metabolic activity and the enzyme production in their livers was altered.[34] The livers of rats fed Roundup Ready canola were 12%–16% heavier, possibly indicating liver disease or inflammation.[35]

Post mortems conducted on the Indian sheep that ate *Bt* cotton plants showed severe irritation and black patches in both intestines and liver (as well as enlarged bile ducts). Investigators said preliminary evidence "strongly suggests that the sheep mortality was due to a toxin. . . . most probably *Bt*-toxin."[36] It is noteworthy that these animals had higher exposure to GM crops than any of those used in GM lab studies. The sheep grazed continuously and exclusively on *Bt* cotton plants. The results were chilling. Seventy-one shepherds reported that 25% of their herds died within 5–7 days.

Another area to look for toxic effects is in fetuses and children, the most vulnerable populations. The findings and risks have already been summarized in the preceding sections.

Consistent avoidance of further investigations

In a 2006 paper, Traavik and Heinemann write, "Some of the most crucial scientific questions concerning the health effects of genetic engineering (GE) and genetically engineered organisms were raised up to 20 years ago. Most of them still have not been answered at all, or have found unsatisfactory answers."[37] The lack of rigorous follow-up has been a consistent theme in this book.

Consider the issue of horizontal gene transfer. Many organizations expressed concerns, for example, that antibiotic resistant marker genes might transfer from GM food to gut bacteria. The primary defense for using the genes was the assumption that it could not happen—genes were destroyed quickly during digestion of GM food. When the only human feeding study verified that transgenes *can* survive digestion and *do* transfer into gut bacteria, no follow-up studies were conducted. No one has yet studied the frequency and impact of transgenes (Roundup Ready, *Bt*, and viral), promoters, or antibiotic resistant markers transferring to gut bacteria or human DNA. Since such transfers carry the potential for long-term damage from short-term exposure to GM crops, the lack of investigation is appalling.

So too is the non-investigation of deaths among lab animals and offspring, livestock sterility, reports of illness by those exposed to GM crops and pollen, unidentified proteins, and the overwhelming evidence linking cancer with a hormone that is significantly elevated in milk from rbGH-treated cows. Even when StarLink—a potentially allergenic corn variety unapproved for human consumption—contaminated the US food supply, the response was feeble at best.

It is not as if science lacks the tools for proper investigations. Rather, it seems that those promoting GM crops prefer the "don't look, don't find" strategy of avoiding problems. They even forgo basic analyses of their transgene and protein sequences, when not required.

This reveals the predominance of corporate interests over science. Companies don't want to set precedents of having to perform expensive tests on GM crops—and not finding problems promotes commercialization and helps shield companies from legal liability.

Normally, strong, independent regulation would step in and force compliance with basic principles of safety, but as part 2 illustrates, corporate interests predominate there as well.

"*The fundamental problem of the way in which GM foods have been approved is that they haven't really been tested properly at all. All that has happened is something which I would characterize as an exercise in wishful thinking.*"

—Erik Millstone, professor of Science Policy at the University of Sussex

INTRODUCTION
to Parts 2 and 3

Having characterized extensive risks associated with GM crops in part 1, parts 2 and 3 explain that there is no competent mechanism in place to protect the public from these dangers. Specifically, part 2 describes how the requirements by government regulators worldwide are not sufficient to identify *most* of the health issues described in the book. Part 3 exposes how the industry's safety studies—which are relied upon by regulators for GM crop approvals—are rigged to avoid finding problems.

The text is organized so you can scan these parts quickly. Each heading or subhead provides conclusions, which are illustrated or elaborated in the text or excerpts that follow. Reading just the headings, therefore, provides an executive summary, similar to the left hand pages of part 1. The excerpts are largely taken from expert reviews that spell out the shortcomings of regulations and industry studies in great detail. The authors of these reports are among the handful of people who have combed through scores of documents, many of which are obscure and unseen by the general scientific community.

Former EPA scientist Doug Gurian-Sherman, for example, wrote a report "Holes in the Biotech Safety Net," for the Center for Science in the Public Interest. He relied on 14 applications for GM crops presented to the FDA, which were obtained only through official Freedom of Information Act requests. William Freese, former research analyst for Friends of the Earth, also pored through industry submissions and government documents that most scientists working in the field have never seen. Epidemiologist Judy Carman did the same with submissions to Australia and New Zealand regulators, publishing her own critiques and supporting the position of the Public Health Association of Australia (PHAA) through their Food Legislation and Regulation Advisory Group. The Centre for Integrated Research on Biosafety (INBI), including Jack Heinemann, did an exhaustive analysis of a submission for high lysine GM corn by Monsanto, also to Australia and New Zealand regulators. Crop physiologist E. Ann Clark evaluates the Canadian approval system for GM crops. Biologist Arpad Pusztai and biochemist and nutritionist Susan Bardocz regularly review both published and unpublished submissions worldwide, and toxicologist Giles-Eric Seralini officially reviews submissions to the European Union both for a French committee and for an EU panel convened to defend the World Trade Association legal dispute. Molecular biologist and protein chemist David Schubert of the Salk Institute for Biological Studies regularly publishes scholarly articles that reveal the contradictions in the statements and assumptions used by industry and regulators to claim that GM foods are safe. Biophysicist and geneticist Mae-Wan Ho, director of the Institute of Science in Society, has authored numerous evaluations, critiques and books on the science and risks related to GM crops. Ian Pryme and Rolf Lembcke reviewed all published, peer-reviewed animal feeding safety studies in their 2003 *Nutrition and Health* article. Excerpts are also used from previous works by this author.

Because several documents are used multiple times, the sources are organized as a reference list at the end of the book, rather than numbered endnotes.

"*We should not lull ourselves into a false sense of security: we should not think that by regulating something which is inherently unpredictable and uncontainable it automatically becomes safe!*"

—Michael Antoniou, molecular geneticist, King's College London

PART 2

The Regulation
of GM Foods
is Inadequate to Protect
Public Health

Regulators are often hijacked by the biotech industry

In Indonesia, Monsanto gave bribes or illegal payments to at least 140 officials, attempting to get their GM cotton approved.[1] In a district in India, an official tampered with the report on *Bt* cotton, increasing the yield figures to favor Monsanto.[2] In Mexico, a senior government official allegedly threatened a University of California professor, implying "We know where your children go to school," trying to get him not to publish incriminating evidence that would delay GM approvals.[3]* While most industry manipulation and political collusion is more subtle, none was more significant than that found at the US Food and Drug Administration (FDA).*

The FDA set the stage for "non-regulation" of GM foods

The country most supportive of GM foods and the first to approve them is the United States. According to US law, GM ingredients are considered food additives. Normally, additives must undergo extensive safety studies, including long-term animal feeding studies prior to approval.[4] If approved, the label of food products containing the additive must list it as an ingredient.

There is an exception, however, for substances that are deemed "generally recognized as safe" (GRAS). GRAS status allows a product to be commercialized without any additional testing. According to US law, to be considered GRAS an additive must be the subject of a substantial amount of peer-reviewed published studies (or equivalent) and there must be overwhelming consensus among the scientific community that the product is safe. GM foods had neither. Nonetheless, in a precedent-setting move that some experts contend was illegal, the FDA declared that GM crops are GRAS as long as their producers say they are (which they do). Thus, FDA has required no safety evaluations (or labels) whatsoever. A company can even introduce a GM food to the market without telling the FDA.

Political and industry pressure won out over science

Such a lenient approach to GM crops was largely the result of Monsanto's legendary influence over the US government. According to the *New York Times*:

"What Monsanto wished for from Washington, Monsanto and—by extension, the biotechnology industry—got. If the company's strategy demanded regulations, rules favored by the industry were adopted. When the company abruptly decided that it needed to throw off the regulations and speed its foods to market, the White House quickly ushered through an unusually generous policy of self-policing.

"Even longtime Washington hands said that the control this nascent industry exerted over its own regulatory destiny through the Environmental Protection Agency, the Agriculture Department and ultimately the Food and Drug Administration was astonishing.

"'In this area, the US government agencies have done exactly what big agribusiness has asked them to do and told them to do,' said Dr. Henry Miller . . . who was responsible for biotechnology issues at the Food and Drug Administration from 1979 to 1994."[5]

Following Monsanto's lead, in 1992 the Council on Competitiveness chaired by Vice President Dan Quayle identified GM crops as a promising industry that could increase US exports. On May 26, Quayle announced "reforms" to "speed up and simplify the process of bringing" GM products to market without "being hampered by unnecessary regulation."[6] Three days later, the FDA policy on non-regulation was unveiled.

The person who oversaw its development was the FDA's Deputy Commissioner for Policy Michael Taylor, whose position had been created especially for him in 1991. Prior to that, Taylor was an outside attorney for Monsanto and the Food Biotechnology Council. Afterwards he became Monsanto's vice president. Based on FDA documents that were later made public from a lawsuit, we can piece together the key role that Taylor played.

---

*For a more detailed discussion on hijacked regulatory agencies, see *Seeds of Deception*.

His policy needed to give the impression that unintended effects from GM crops were not an issue. Otherwise their GRAS status would be undermined. According to an article in *Biotechnology and Genetic Engineering Reviews,* "This blanket GRAS exemption is based on the notion of 'substantial equivalence'—the strong, *a priori* presumption that GE crops are largely the same as their conventional counterparts. This assumes not only the safety of the transgenic protein, but also the absence of any potentially harmful, unintended effects of transformation."[7]

But internal memos showed that the overwhelming consensus among the agency scientists was that GM crops can have unpredictable, hard-to-detect side effects. Various departments even spelled these out in detail, listing potential allergies, toxins, nutritional effects, and new diseases. They had urged their superiors to require long-term safety studies.[8]

Freese and Schubert

"When this policy was being formulated in the early 1990s, scientists at the FDA raised numerous objections to a working draft of the policy.[9] For instance, FDA scientists at the Division of Food Chemistry and Technology and the Division of Contaminants Chemistry called for mandatory review, stating that 'every transformant should be evaluated before it enters the marketplace.'[10] Dr. Samuel Shibko, Director of the Division of Toxicological Review and Evaluation, recommended 'a limited traditional toxicological study with the edible part of the plant,' as well as 'limited studies in humans' and *in vitro* genotoxicity tests.[11] The most commonly expressed concern was unintended effects associated with the random nature of transformation techniques. Dr. Louis J. Pribyl's comments are typical: 'When the introduction of genes into a plant's genome randomly occurs, as is the case with the current technology (but not traditional breeding), it seems apparent that many pleiotropic effects [unpredicted changed characteristics] will occur. Many of these effects might not be seen by the breeder because of the more or less similar growing conditions in the limited trials that are performed.' Pribyl also raised concerns about 'new, powerful regulatory elements being randomly inserted into the genome' that could cause 'cryptic pathway activation' that breeders might miss. 'This situation is different than that experienced by traditional breeding techniques [sic].'"[12,13]

In spite of the warning by agency scientists, according to public interest attorney Steven Druker who studied the FDA's internal files, "References to the unintended negative effects of bioengineering were progressively deleted from drafts of the policy statement (over the protests of agency scientists)."[14] In their place, the policy manufactured the notion that there were no meaningful differences in GM crops.

Linda Kahl, an FDA compliance officer who summarized the position of agency scientists on GMOs, insisted that "the processes of genetic engineering and traditional breeding are different, and according to the technical experts in the agency, they lead to different risks."[15] Gerald Guest, the director of FDA's Center for Veterinary Medicine wrote, "I would urge you to eliminate statements that suggest that the lack of information can be used as evidence for no regulatory concern."[16] FDA microbiologist Louis Pribyl challenged the policy, writing: "What has happened to the scientific elements of this document? Without a sound scientific base to rest on, this becomes a broad, general, 'What do I have to do to avoid trouble'-type document. . . . It will look like and probably be just a political document. . . . It reads very pro-industry, especially in the area of unintended effects."[17]

The scientists' concerns were not only ignored, their very existence was denied. The final policy contained the statement, "The agency is not aware of any information showing that foods derived by these new methods differ from other foods in any meaningful or uniform way."[18] On the basis of this deceptive statement, the FDA did not require the testing normally necessary for a new food additive.

William Freese

"Contrary to popular opinion, the Food and Drug Administration (FDA) does not regulate GE foods. Instead, the FDA has a 'voluntary consultation' process that allows biotechnology companies to make all of the important decisions related to bringing their novel GE crops to market. The company, not the FDA, decides which, if any, safety tests to conduct and how they will be performed. The company, not the FDA, determines which data, if any, are shared with regulators. In fact, the company even determines whether it will consult with the FDA at all. Because the process is voluntary, biotech companies sometimes refuse to supply additional data requested by the FDA. And at the end of the consultation, the FDA does NOT approve the GE food as safe, or even as similar enough to its conventional counterpart to exempt it from scrutiny. Instead, the pertinent biotech company makes these determinations on its own authority."[19]

Freese and Schubert   "Without test protocols or other important data, the FDA is unable to identify unintentional mistakes, errors in data interpretation or intentional deception, making it impossible to conduct a thorough and critical review. The review process . . . makes it clear that, contrary to popular belief, the FDA has not formally approved a single GE crop as safe for human consumption. Instead, at the end of the consultation, the FDA merely issues a short note summarizing the review process and a letter that conveys the crop developer's assurances that the GE crop is substantially equivalent to its conventional counterpart. The FDA's letter to Monsanto regarding its MON810 *Bt* corn is typical:

'Based on the safety and nutritional assessment you have conducted, it is our understanding that Monsanto has concluded that corn products derived from this new variety are not materially different in composition, safety, and other relevant parameters from corn currently on the market, and that the genetically modified corn does not raise issues that would require premarket review or approval by FDA. . . . as you are aware, it is Monsanto's responsibility to ensure that foods marketed by the firm are safe, wholesome and in compliance with all applicable legal and regulatory requirements.'"[20]

Doug Gurian-Sherman   "FDA did not generate its own safety assessment, but merely summarized for the public the developer's food-safety analysis . . . The letter concluding the consultation between FDA and the developer clearly places responsibility for the safety of the GE food with the developer."[21]

The bias of the FDA in favor of company wishes over science is not unprecedented at the agency. In July 2006, the Union of Concerned Scientists and Public Employees for Environmental Responsibility distributed a 38-question survey to nearly 6,000 FDA scientists. Nearly 1,000 scientists responded, disclosing that 61% knew of cases in which "Department of Health and Human Services or FDA political appointees have inappropriately injected themselves into FDA determinations or actions," and 60% knew of cases "where commercial interests have inappropriately induced or attempted to induce the reversal, withdrawal, or modification of FDA determinations or actions." About one in five said, "I have been asked, for non-scientific reasons, to inappropriately exclude or alter technical information or my conclusions in an FDA scientific document," or "have been asked explicitly by FDA decision makers to provide incomplete, inaccurate, or misleading information to the public, regulated industry, media, or elected/senior government officials." Nearly 70% do not believe the FDA has sufficient resources to effectively perform its mission of "protecting public health . . . and helping the public get the accurate, science-based information they need to use medicines and foods to improve their health." An excerpt from one of the essay answers said, "*Scientific discourse is strongly discouraged when it may jeopardize an approval. . . . Whenever safety or efficacy concerns are raised on scientific grounds . . . these concerns are not taken seriously.*"[22]

The FDA voluntary review process is not competent to identify *most* of the unintended hazards described in this book

Doug Gurian-Sherman	"It is clear that FDA's current voluntary notification process (even if made mandatory) is not up to the task of ensuring the safety of future GE crops."[23]
Lancet **editorial**	"It is astounding that the US Food and Drug Administration has not changed their stance on genetically modified food adopted in 1992. . . . The policy is that genetically modified crops will receive the same consideration for potential health risks as any other new crop plant. This stance is taken despite good reasons to believe that specific risks may exist. . . . Governments should never have allowed these products into the food chain without insisting on rigorous testing for effects on health."[24]
William Freese	"Even though it is well-known that the process of genetic engineering causes numerous, unpredictable changes in plant composition due to its haphazard nature, neither industry nor government conducts the sort of testing needed to detect them and determine whether they have human health or environmental impacts. . . . In addition, companies sometimes evaluate GE plants by looking for gross abnormalities through simple visual inspection rather than conducting specific laboratory tests to detect the presence of potentially harmful compounds."[25]
Biotechnology at the Dinner Table	"The first consultation for the delayed-ripening FlavrSavr tomato looked at intended as well as unintended effects. . . . For the unintended effects, the consultation considered any changes in toxicity for one known toxicant in the tomato."[26]
Judy Carman	"Such results [compositional changes in GM food] have led the Royal Society of Canada to describe the notion of substantial equivalence [which was used by US regulators] as 'scientifically unjustifiable and inconsistent with precautionary regulation of the technology,'[27] and the American National Academy of Sciences to describe human health safety testing procedures to be 'woefully inadequate.' The Royal Society in London has also weighed into the argument, describing the current system of safety screening, developed in the United States, as flawed, subjective and inadequate and that manufacturers' tests on such foods should be tightened and opened to independent scrutiny."[28,29]
Philip Regal	"Over the last fifteen years, I and other scientists have put the FDA on notice about the potential dangers of genetically engineered foods. Instead of responsible regulation we have seen bureaucratic bungling and obfuscation that have left public health and the environment at risk."[30]
Suzanne Wuerthele (US Environmental Protection Agency toxicologist)	"This technology is being promoted, in the face of concerns by respectable scientists and in the face of data to the contrary, by the very agencies which are supposed to be protecting human health and the environment. The bottom line in my view is that we are confronted with the most powerful technology the world has ever known, and it is being rapidly deployed with almost no thought whatsoever to its consequences."[31]

The FDA's pro-GM attitude and dismissal of concerns has been institutionalized throughout the US government

Dan Glickman
(US secretary of agriculture under President Clinton)

"What I saw generically on the pro-biotech side was the attitude that the technology was good, and that it was almost immoral to say that it wasn't good, because it was going to solve the problems of the human race and feed the hungry and clothe the naked. . . . And there was a lot of money that had been invested in this, and if you're against it, you're Luddites, you're stupid. That, frankly, was the side our government was on. Without thinking, we had basically taken this issue as a trade issue and they, whoever 'they' were, wanted to keep our product out of their market. And they were foolish, or stupid, and didn't have an effective regulatory system. There was rhetoric like that even here in this department. You felt like you were almost an alien, disloyal, by trying to present an open-minded view on some of the issues being raised. So I pretty much spouted the rhetoric that everybody else around here spouted; it was written into my speeches."[32]

Canadian regulators are "compromised" by their determination to appease and promote the biotech industry

Royal Society of Canada

"In meetings with senior managers from the various Canadian regulatory departments, the Expert Panel addressed questions related to their handling of the issues of transparency and confidentiality in dealing with applicants for licensing of new biotechnology. Their responses uniformly stressed the importance of maintaining a favorable climate for the biotechnology industry to develop new products and submit them for approval on the Canadian market. . . . Such concern with industry development, though understandable, highlights another aspect of the regulatory conflict. The conflict of interest involved in both promoting and regulating an industry or technology . . . is also a factor in the issue of maintaining the transparency, and therefore the scientific integrity, of the regulatory process. In effect, the public interest in a regulatory system that is 'science based' — that meets scientific standards of objectivity, a major aspect of which is full openness to scientific peer review — is significantly compromised when that openness is negotiated away by regulators in exchange for cordial and supportive relationships with the industries being regulated."[33]

Many European regulators promote GMOs, accept poor industry research, and disregard science-based concerns

Friends of the Earth Europe

Regarding the European Food Safety Authority (EFSA) GMO Panel: "One member has direct financial links with the biotech industry and others have indirect links, such as close involvement with major conferences organized by the biotech industry. Two members have even appeared in promotional videos produced by the biotech industry. . . . Several members of the panel, including the chair Professor Kuiper, have been involved with the EU-funded ENTRANSFOOD project. The aim of this project was to agree [to] safety assessment, risk management, and risk communication procedures that would 'facilitate market introduction of GMOs in Europe, and therefore bring the European industry in a competitive position.' Professor Kuiper, who coordinated the ENTRANSFOOD project, sat on a working group that also included staff from Monsanto, Bayer CropScience, and Syngenta. . . .

"The importance of the ENTRANSFOOD project can be seen from its influence: For example, the biotechnology industry has received criticism from scientists worldwide for using antibiotic resistance marker genes (ARMs) in their GM crops, as they could be picked up and used by bacteria. In April 2004, the EFSA GMO Panel published a scientific opinion on the use of ARMs. But the ENTRANSFOOD project had also looked at this issue, and a paper was submitted to a scientific journal in November 2003. Astonishingly, the assessments of antibiotic resistance markers by the two groups were virtually identical, in places even down to the wording. . .

"Researchers commissioned by EFSA into how stakeholders view the authority, interviewed the scientific Panels [of the EU member states] and reported that 'GMO was mentioned as one very complex issue and there was some concern that the isolation of the safety assessment from other debates (socio-economical, biodiversity . . .) was somewhat artificial and that the EFSA "safe" stamp could potentially be abused for political purposes to legalize GMO.'. . .

"The Commission does not appear to be using the EFSA as a means to further scientific debate about GMOs and the concerns raised by scientists from around Europe. Instead, they are being used to create a false impression of scientific agreement when the real situation is one of intense and continuing debate and uncertainty."[34]

Jeffrey M. Smith

Regarding the French evaluation of Mon 863: "Without disclosure, says Seralini, just a few toxicologists can make the decision without public evaluation. And too often, the decision-making body is heavily influenced by the applying company. This appears to be the case with his French Commission for Biomolecular Genetics (CBG), which originally refused to approve Mon 863 based on the evidence. The CBG's president, a geneticist who works very closely with industry, asked a consultant to re-evaluate just one significant difference and then forced a second vote without a quorum. With only 5 of 18 members present, Mon 863 passed 3 to 2. According to Seralini, one of the scientists who voted in favor is a toxicologist who, oddly enough, is 'always against long animal toxicity tests.' In fact, he had been part of the French committee that approved Novartis (now Syngenta) E 176 corn after it had been tested for only two weeks with three cows. Actually, there were four cows at the start of the study, but one died and was removed. That toxicologist is also on EFSA [the European Food Safety Authority], which has come under attack for including primarily pro-GM scientists. . . . It is no surprise, therefore, that EFSA endorsed and even repeated each of Monsanto's excuses why the statistically significant health effects of rats fed Mon 863 were not relevant."[35]

Friends of the Earth Europe

Regarding the EFSA evaluation of Mon 863: "In fact, member states raised a large number of concerns about the quality of the assessment of MON 863. But the GMO Panel dismissed every one of the concerns and questions about MON 863 listed in its opinion as having been raised by scientific committees of the member states. This seems astonishing as it is hard to credit that so many scientists across Europe could be wrong in their concerns. It appears that the GMO Panel takes a far less precautionary approach to food safety than many of the member states' own scientific bodies."[36]

The European Commission privately expresses concerns about EFSA and GMO assessments while publicly touting product safety

Friends of the Earth Europe and Greenpeace The WTO [World Trade Organization] documents obtained by Friends of the Earth, show that the commission fully appreciates the extent of the uncertainties and gaps in knowledge that exist in relation to the safety of GM crops. However, the commission normally keeps this uncertainty concealed from the public whilst presenting its decisions about the safety of GM crops and foods as being certain and scientifically based. . . . The commission has commercialized 31 varieties of GM maize since September 2004. In all cases the commission informed member states and the public that the GM foods or crops were "completely safe." These new documents however show a different picture; one of uncertainties, lack of data, and subjective judgments that have to be made about the safety GM crops and food. They reveal that at the same time as taking a pro-GM line with the public, the commission was presenting evidence behind closed doors in the dispute at the WTO, that:

- there are substantial scientific concerns about the safety of GM foods and crops;
- new and complex risks are emerging;
- the risks to human and animal health can not be excluded;
- serious concerns remain about the environmental safety of growing GM crops;
- the environmental risks of GM organisms (GMOs) will vary according to the region and its environment;
- biotechnology companies provided poor quality applications and research in their applications to market GMOs; . . .

"One of the most striking aspects of the EC submissions [to the World Trade Organization] is that they frequently criticize the European Food Safety Authority (EFSA) and its assessments of the safety of GM foods and crops, even though the commission relies on these evaluations to make recommendations to member states. The commission has also continually used EFSA opinions to justify its decisions to approve new GM foods and feeds for import following a lack of agreement between member states."[37]

Inadequate testing requirements are the norm among GM crop regulators worldwide

Genetics professor Marcello Buiatti points out that "present day genetically modified plants are the result of the obsolete technology of the time of their development, nearly 20 years ago, and that such technology has not yet been updated in coherence with the new knowledge gained in the last 10 years or so, for reasons not related to science but rather to complex market and commercial dynamics." He calls for not only a "coordinated effort to update the methods of control of the genetic structure and function" of GMOs, but also "to drastically change" the requirements by regulators before GMOs are released into the environment or become part of the food chain.[38] Not only have regulators been negligent in following the progression of the science, they have failed to demand adherence to even basic principles of good science and regulation.

Public Health Association of Australia	Regarding Australia New Zealand Food Authority (ANZFA): "Its methodological and statistical reporting of animal experimentation is now much worse than it even was before. Now, it is routine for ANZFA to give **no** actual data from these experiments, but to just assert that no differences were found. This is totally unacceptable and a most retrograde step, particularly as the data of animal experiments in previous draft risk analysis reports showed adverse effects in spite of the assertion that no differences were found. It would seem that ANZFA now does not want outside scrutiny of these experiments.... ANZFA claims that it takes a cautious approach to the introduction of GE foods. However, ANZFA's own document 'GM Foods and the consumer, ANZFA's safety assessment process for genetically modified foods' clearly states that ANZFA considers that GE food is safe until proven unsafe, the opposite of the precautionary principle."[39]
Indian Council of Medical Research (From *The Financial Express*)	The Indian Council of Medical Research (ICMR) has raised some concerns over the safety of genetically modified (GM) food and has urged for an overhaul of the existing regulatory mechanism.... "Specific safety issues associated with GM foods include direct or indirect consequences of new gene product or altered levels of existing gene product due to GM, possibility of gene transfer from ingested GM food and potential adverse effects like allergenicity and toxic effects."[40]
Nature Biotechnology	Regarding insertion-site mutations: "Detailed inspection has shown that mutations such as these would almost certainly pass unnoticed through both the molecular and phenotypic characterization stages of the regulatory systems of both the European Union and the United States."[41]

Regulators rely on untested assumptions, animal studies that don't actually feed the GM crop to animals, and absurd research designs

Judy Carman	Regarding Food Standards Australia New Zealand: "Whenever FSANZ reviews the safety of a GM food, it reviews the information presented to it and generates a report of about 70 pages per application. A review of 12 reports covering 28 GM crops—four soy, three corn, ten potatoes, eight canola, one sugar beet and two cotton—revealed no feeding trials on people. In addition, one of the GM corn varieties had gone untested on animals. Some 17 foods involved testing with only a single oral gavage (a type of forced-feeding), with

observation for 7–14 days, and only of the substance that had been genetically engineered to appear [the GM protein], not the whole food. Such testing assumes that the only new substance that will appear in the food is the one genetically engineered to appear, that the GM plant-produced substance will act in the same manner as the tested substance that was obtained from another source, and that the substance will create disease within a few days. All are untested hypotheses and make a mockery of GM proponents' claims that the risk assessment of GM foods is based on sound science. Furthermore, where the whole food was given to animals to eat, sample sizes were often very low—for example, five to six cows per group for Roundup Ready soy—and they were fed for only four weeks."[42]

Public Health Association of Australia	(Note: ANZFA was the precursor to FSANZ) "ANZFA argues that feeding the whole food to experimental animals is not appropriate as it is 'not possible to conduct dose-response experiments for foods in the same way that these experiments are conducted for chemicals. In addition, a key factor … is the need to maintain the nutritional value and balance of the diet.' Such a toxicological view of food ignores the whole body of literature associated with animal feeding studies for nutritional research. Even a brief view of this literature would make it clear to ANZFA that the type of studies that they view as inappropriate are in fact routinely done. Moreover, previous risk analysis reports of GE foods published by ANZFA have contained such studies. In fact, in the nutritional literature, the usual way of testing the health effects of a food is to feed the whole food to experimental animals first, and then follow-up any adverse effects with subsequent feeding and other studies of the components, a process that is the opposite of [that] accepted by ANZFA for these foods. ANZFA should also note that the acute toxicity testing proposed as adequate would simply not pick up cancer, teratology [birth defects] or the long-term effects of nutrient deficiencies or increases in anti-nutrients."[43]
Doug Gurian-Sherman	"Of the 14 BNF [FDA] submissions reviewed, six conducted whole-GE-plant animal-feeding studies."[44]
E. Ann Clark	"Evidence accepted by Health Canada for approval varies inconsistently among submissions, with 10 of 15 GM corn crops and one of four potato crops presenting lab and purified protein feeding trial evidence, while the other five corn and three potato crops did not. Actual livestock feeding trial evidence, however limited, is provided for only one of five cotton crops and for one soybean, but not for other crops destined largely for livestock feed. Doses, durations, and all other aspects of experimental design appear to vary at the discretion of the industry sponsor, rather than under the direction of the regulatory bodies… "Heuristic (assumptions-based) reasoning is widely used in place of actual experimentation. In virtually every case, it is reasoned that because the target proteins synthesized in response to the transgene insertions … either do not share characteristics commonly found in mammalian protein toxins, or do not show either amino acid and/or nucleotide homologies with known mammalian toxins, then the crops themselves are presumed to have no toxicity risk. And thus, there is no need for testing."[45]
European Commission	"The information requested and supplied from the company was mixed, scarce, delivered consecutively all over years, and not convincing. The quality of the dossier can therefore be considered as not sufficiently informative. … The major weaknesses of the dossier relate to: no sufficient experimental evidence to assess the safety; compositional data insufficient for a product directly consumed by human; no in vivo experiments conducted on laboratory or farm target animals with grain of the event "sweet maize"; field maize used as a

control—grain material was spiked with *Bt* proteins (resulting in poor and unsatisfactory experimental conditions); further experiments performed on ruminants using the whole plant silage or stalk have no meaning for the safety assessment.... These issues could be considered to have justified requests for further evidence on the safety of the product." [46]

Regulators ignore compositional changes in GM crops used for oil, as well as exposure to humans via animal feed

Public Health Association of Australia

"The document states in several places the point that: 'processing of canola seed to oil involves the removal of all DNA and protein, which effectively results in the removal of the CP4 EPSPS and GOX [GM] proteins from the food fraction.' Yet in other places, it is stated that protein (and presumably DNA) is present in canola oil. Moreover, a concentration is even given for protein in refined oil, at 0.290 ppm for GT73 and 0.327 for the parent line, Westar. This is clearly contradictory. Moreover, no allowance is given for cold-pressed oil which may contain a much higher proportion of protein and DNA, as it may not go through the extent of processing as described in the document."[47]

"Only the proteins expected to be produced by the plant were tested for. Moreover, it is assumed that any health problems would come from the production of proteins. The production of fat-soluble substances that may be present in the oil fraction is not considered.... Animal feeding studies using oil from these GE canola lines were not done, even though this fraction is consumed by people, because it may 'cause nutritional and biochemical imbalances.' Yet the scientific literature in nutrition contains thousands of these types of studies. So why does ANZFA insist that they are not viable?"[48]

E. Ann Clark

Regarding Canadian GMO approvals: "No laboratory or feeding trial measurement of toxicity is presented in 70% (28 of 40) of the available crop Decisions.... The issue of potential toxicity in all canola and cotton crops is dealt with by assuming that a) all human exposure to GM plant toxins will occur only through consumption of oil, b) toxicity risk derives solely from proteinaceous material, and because c) all proteinaceous material is removed in the process of refining the oil, therefore, d) there is no risk, and hence, no need for testing. The evidence upon which each of these assumptions is made is not presented. ... In sum, 70% of the currently available GM crops, including all of the canola and cotton crops approved for commerce in Canada, have not been subjected to any actual lab or animal toxicity testing, either as refined oils for direct human consumption or indirectly as feedstuffs for livestock. The same finding pertains to all three GM tomato Decisions, the only GM flax, and to five GM corn crops ... [For the 12 crops that are tested] all testing is limited to the purified target protein(s) only....

"For crops such as canola and cotton, extraction of the oil for human consumption leaves a protein-rich byproduct, which is commonly fed to livestock, which then feed into the human food chain. ... However, with two exceptions, no actual lab or feeding trial assessment of toxicity (or allergenicity) to livestock is referenced.... The logic is internally inconsistent for assessment of the potential toxicity (and allergenicity) of canola and cotton. If such toxins or allergens exist, and are in fact present in the protein-rich residue left after refining the oils, why is toxicity assessment not more rigorous prior to feeding the protein-rich meal to livestock? Where are the trials showing lack of harm to fed livestock, or that meat and milk from livestock fed on GM feedstuffs are safe?"[49]

Regulators lack meaningful standards

William Freese	"Another problematic area is the lack of standardized procedures for those few tests that are conducted. Without standardization, companies can and do design test procedures to get the results they want."[50]
Doug Gurian-Sherman	"Some submissions are hundreds of pages long while others are only 10 or 20."[51]
E. Ann Clark	"Inconsistent standards detract from the perception of a meaningful, enforceable risk assessment process."[52]
Arpad Pusztai	"Nutritional scientists and leading journals would not accept these blatant inadequacies and misinterpretations. How can regulators accept it for a novel genetically modified food?"[53]

While proclaiming adherence to international standards and legal requirements, regulators regularly ignore them

Centre for Integrated Research in Biosafety	"We agree that FSANZ should benchmark with international food safety recommendations, but notes that FSANZ has accepted lower standards from submitted studies than recommended by these same bodies at several stages in assessing the safety of [high lysine GM corn LY038] . . . For example, FSANZ has accepted a study on cDHDPS [the GM protein] digestion that is outside of UN FAO/WHO protocols. It has ignored Codex Alimentarius recommendations for testing using cooked and processed LY038 corn, and their recommendations that all novel proteins be isolated. . . . In each case, the authority has, in our view, relaxed adherence to international standards for safety testing when that better suited the Applicant's submitted work, and imposed international standards whenever that was a lower standard than we recommended. . . . FSANZ claimed that cost to government was not in its purview, so they could avoid looking at labeling, etc. but regularly used costs to government when it suited their arguments, and used it in other decisions."[54]
Friends of the Earth Europe	"According to EU Regulation 178/2002 (Article 30), when different scientific opinions emerge the EFSA and the member state(s) "are obliged to co-operate with a view to either resolving the divergence or preparing a joint document clarifying the contentious scientific issues and identifying the relevant uncertainties in the data. This document should be made public." The use of this regulation to deal with different opinions is also recognized by the commission. . . . Despite the substantive differences between some member states and the EFSA on virtually every opinion, there has been to date no evidence that there are attempts to resolve these differences and certainly no such joint documents have been made public. Considering the legal obligation the EFSA has this is quite astonishing. . . . In addition the panel ignores EU requirements to identify the level of uncertainty in its assumptions, and fails to take in legal requirements that regard is given to the long-term effects of eating or growing GM foods."[55]

Regulators make errors in their evaluations or overlook errors in submissions

Freese and Schubert	"The FDA . . . states in its consultation note that MON 810 contains one complete copy of the cry1Ab gene, a NOS termination sequence, and a "nature-identical" Cry1Ab protein, none of which is correct.[56] Apparently, either Monsanto submitted incomplete summary data to the FDA, or the FDA made serious errors in its consultation note. In either case, it is troubling that the US agency responsible for food safety has fundamentally flawed molecular characterization data on such a widely planted GE crop."[57]
Doug Gurian-Sherman	"In three of the 14 reviewed submissions, obvious errors were found that were not identified by FDA staff during their reviews of the submissions. Had FDA conducted thorough reviews, the errors would have been easily detected." <u>Regarding altered ripening tomato and cantaloupe</u>: "In both cases, the developer of those crops argued that natural exposure to SAMase in T3 [the GM protein] found in the human digestive tract and drinking water supported a determination that the protein is safe for humans. . . . FDA considers previous dietary exposure to GE protein as important support for the safety of the GE crop. While the submissions claim scientific support for prior dietary exposure to SAMase, the papers cited for that support (and included with the data summary) do not mention T3 or SAMase occurring in the gut or in drinking water. Another paper, included but not cited in the submission, states that 'Coliphages [bacterial viruses] were not detected in finished drinking quality water.' Therefore, contrary to the developer's conclusion, the cited papers do not support prior dietary exposure, and no other support for dietary exposure (such as detection of SAMase in the intestines) is provided. There is no indication in publicly available files that FDA recognized the errors in the . . . data summaries. Reading of the developer-supplied and cited papers should have revealed the errors."[58]
Centre for Integrated Research in Biosafety	<u>Regarding high-lysine corn LY038</u>: "In one section . . . the authority indicates that cadaverine levels are elevated in LY038 relative to controls, but in another section asserts that cadaverine levels could not be measured because they were below detection concentrations in both LY038 and the controls. . . . [The breeding history of the control corn] in the breeding schemes provided by the Applicant . . . remains confusing. . . . The Applicant replied to a similar question from the Authority with the text they claimed they had also provided to the US FDA, but which is significantly different from what they told the USDA. . . . We do not see how both of these histories can be correct. . . . The amino acid sequence of cDHDPS [the GM protein] available on SwissProt reports a leucine [amino acid] at position 266. The applicant reports a serine at position 266. . . . It appears that the applicant performed their bioinformatics [comparison with a data base of amino acid sequences from known allergens] using the Swissprot sequence with a leucine at position 268."[59]
Public Health Association of Australia	<u>Regarding Mon 810 *Bt* corn</u>: "The text associated with table 4 does not match the figures given in table 4. The text states that 'the values were within the values reported in the literature.' However, it is clear in table 4 that this is not the case for cysteine and histidine, which are both higher than the quoted literature range. . . . Moreover, it is stated in the caption of table 4 that the level of tryptophan was significantly different in line MON 810 compared to its control, yet both have a mean of 0.6 in the table. It is highly unlikely that

two samples with the same mean would be significantly different, particularly with such low sample sizes."

Regarding Roundup Ready canola: "The concentration of arachidic acid ... is given as 1.02 in table 6. However, in table 9.1, the range for this is given as 0.6–0.8 for 1992 and 0.6–0.7 for 1993. Clearly, the two tables contradict."[60]

Mae-Wan Ho	"The researchers made a big blunder. Two of the cows in the non-GM group were inadvertently fed on the GM-diet, so they ended up with 13 data points in the GM diet group and only 5 data points in the control non-GM diet group."[61]

Regulators have unrealistic confidence in their own assessment and in industry reporting

FSANZ	"GM food products are not permitted on the market if any question associated with negative health effects is left unanswered during the pre-market safety assessment. For this reason post-market monitoring is not considered necessary or useful as there is no potential adverse health outcome to monitor. In Australia and New Zealand, as in most other countries, the responsibility for post-market surveillance is covered by an ongoing duty of care on the part of the developer. The developer is expected to monitor for existing and emerging risks that may be associated with its product and notify regulatory authorities whenever new information is uncovered."[62]

Multiple flaws in GM crop regulations and industry's control of the process leave consumers unprotected

Doug Gurian-Sherman	"The FDA consultation process does not allow the agency to require submission of data, misses obvious errors in company-submitted data summaries, provides insufficient testing guidance, and does not require sufficiently detailed data to enable the FDA to assure that GE crops are safe to eat. Under the current process, FDA largely appears to rely on the developer's judgment about what data it should provide to the FDA. That results in a conflict between the developer's need to market the GE crop and the public's need for assurance of safety."[63]
William Freese	"The StarLink debacle is a case study in the near total dependence of our regulatory agencies on the 'regulated' biotech and food industries. If industry chooses to submit faulty, unpublishable studies, it does so without consequence. If it should respond to an agency request with deficient data, it does so without reprimand or follow-up (e.g., statistics on allergic reactions reported to food companies). If a company finds it disadvantageous to characterize its product, then its properties remain uncertain or unknown. If a corporation chooses to ignore scientifically sound testing standards (e.g., by using surrogate protein without first establishing test substance equivalence), then faulty tests are conducted instead, and the results are considered legitimate. In the area of genetically engineered food regulation, the 'competent' agencies rarely if ever (know how to) conduct independent research to verify or supplement industry findings."[64]

So-called "independent" scientific bodies are often heavily influenced by industry

William Freese

"The expert bodies are often comprised mainly of plant science specialists who themselves receive research funding from biotechnology companies, or whose institutions receive such funding. . . . [A] common thread in the numerous expert reviews is their reliance on the opinions of national regulatory agencies, particularly the FDA, which as noted above are themselves based on 'data summaries' from the financially interested biotech companies rather than the company's full, original studies. Even if members of such expert bodies want to examine the original studies, they often either cannot gain access to this sensitive material (considered proprietary) or simply do not have time to examine those studies that may be available, relying instead on selective summaries of these studies by the regulatory agencies (e.g. Scientific Advisory Panels to the EPA)."[65]

Jeffrey M. Smith

"Geneticist Michael Antoniou, who works on human gene therapy, told the New Zealand Commission, "genetic engineering technology, as it's being applied in agriculture now, [is] based on the understanding of genetics we had 15 years ago, about genes being isolated little units that work independently of each other." He explained that genes actually "work as an integrated whole of families." In 2003, Antoniou represented non-governmental organizations on the UK's supposedly balanced GM Science Review Panel that was part of the nationwide "GM Nation?" public debate. He was shocked to find scientists there still supporting obsolete theories of gene independence, even claiming that the order of genes in the DNA was entirely irrelevant. But Antoniou was outnumbered by 11 scientists representing either the biotech industry or appointed by the pro-biotech UK government. His well-supported arguments fell on deaf ears. Since the debate, new studies have further verified Antoniou's position by showing that genes are not randomly located along the DNA, but clustered into groups with related functions."[66]

Centre for Integrated Research in Biosafety

"In our view, FSANZ has provided the applicant and industry with an impressive and unacceptable level of involvement in the process, undermining our confidence in FSANZ's impartiality. For example, FSANZ decided not to review our submission itself, but engaged an "independent" expert from the Monash Molecular Plant Breeding CRC in Australia to review our submission on high lysine corn. There are two worrying aspects about this. The first is that FSANZ sent our work to an institution with a clear vested interest in GM crops. For example, this institution lists the GM giant BASF as a corporate partner and has a joint 17 million euro investment in GM wheat development with it. The second is that FSANZ sent our work on human health to someone with no obvious training or experience in human health."[67]

"A Citizen Response"

"Immediately after its formation, serious questions were raised about the composition of the Health Commission GMO Task Force. Calls by both those supporting and opposing Measure Q to create a task force with equal representation were ignored. Instead: The selection process excluded persons openly expressing concern with GMOs; the selection process seated three pro-GMO activists, these three took the lead in composing three of the four main sections of the HC GMO Task Force Report; two task force members have direct financial ties to the GMO industry; the criterion for member selection has never been revealed even though numerous requests for this information have been made. As feared by many members of the public, a task force led solely by people with vested interests in the success of GMOs proved incapable of generating a report that accurately represented the science, regulatory, and ethical facts surrounding GMOs."[68]

Scientific organizations raise concerns about GM crops and regulations are often heavily influenced by industry

William Freese

"One source of confusion on the potential health impacts of genetically engineered foods is the tendency of many expert scientific bodies to issue reports that are inherently contradictory. (Examples include committees of the National Academy of Sciences and the UK Royal Society.) That is, they often call for more stringent testing regimens *and* state (or imply) that currently marketed GE crops are safe—which of course begs the question of how inadequately tested crops can be judged safe. The purveyors of sound-bite science have made a cottage industry of publicizing the latter claims while ignoring the serious criticisms of current testing regimens made by the very same bodies. Often, the contradiction is only apparent. The expert body will say that there is no evidence that GE foods on the market are unsafe. Yet 'lack of evidence' often reflects the lack of adequate studies—absence of evidence rather than evidence of absence."[69]

Friends of the Earth Europe

"Syngenta's *Bt*-176 GM maize contains a gene for ampicillin resistance (ampR) that has raised serious concerns from the competent authorities of member states. When the UK authorities looked at the data on *Bt*-176, they realized that the gene is structured in such a way that it could be used immediately by any bacteria that picks it up and it is different to naturally occurring ampR genes because it would allow bacteria to be able to break down ampicillin antibiotics much more rapidly than they could otherwise. During the original approvals process, 12 out of 15 member states were against granting European marketing approval for *Bt*-176, but they were overruled by the commission. The GMO Panel appears to have ignored the unique properties of the ampR gene in *Bt*-176, but even so they classified this gene as being in a group for which use "should be restricted to field trial purposes and should not be present in GM plants to be placed on the market." However, when the GMO Panel was later asked by the commission to consider the ban on *Bt*-176 put in place by the Austrian government, it stated that it was "of the opinion that the use of these genes should be avoided **in future** GM plants to be placed on the market" /emphasis added/ and therefore that the Austrian Government did not have a good case for a ban. This is an odd interpretation of their own opinion on ARMs - it is unclear why the panel considers that one GM crop, which Syngenta is already selling to farmers, should be safe if it believes that in the future similar crops shouldn't be allowed on safety grounds."[70]

Lack of safeguards exposes the food supply to GM contamination

G M crops are a source of self-propagating genetic and environmental pollution. They contaminate non-GM crops and wild relatives and will persist in nature for generations to come. A decade of contamination from cross pollination, seed movement, "volunteer" crops from unharvested seeds, and accidents by seed companies and farmers has made it clear that the situation is out of control. Containment of GM crops is not practically achievable. And unlike traditional invasive plants or animals, GM crops do not look different than their natural counterparts. We have no technology to completely clean them up.

Not only is the gene pool at risk from commercialized GMOs, field trials of unapproved varieties can quietly spread genes into natural populations. In the United States alone, between 1986 and 2005 the USDA approved over 10,600 applications for more than 49,300 field sites. The government is supposed to make sure that these trials won't contaminate the surrounding environment, but a report by the USDA Office of Inspector General in 2005 harshly condemned the oversight of these trials by the USDA's Animal and Plant Health Inspection Service (APHIS).[71] The report said that "at various stages of the field test process—from approval of applications to inspection of fields—weaknesses in APHIS regulations and internal management controls increase the risk that regulated genetically engineered organisms will inadvertently persist in the environment before they are deemed safe to grow without regulation." APHIS lacked "basic information about the field test sites it approves and is responsible for monitoring, including where and how the crops are being grown, and what becomes of them at the end of the field test. . . . APHIS does not review notification applicants' containment protocols, which describe how the applicant plans to contain the GE crop within the field test site and prevent it from persisting in the environment." Even with crops engineered to produce pharmaceutical and industrial products, "which are modified for nonfood purposes and may pose a threat to the food supply if unintentionally released," APHIS "does not require permit holders to report on the final disposition." In fact, the inspector found "that two large harvests of GE pharmaceutical crops remained in storage at the field test sites for over a year without APHIS' knowledge or approval of the storage facility. . . .

"Approved applicants sometimes allow harvested crops to lie in the field test site for months at a time, their seeds exposed to animals and the elements. Also, because APHIS has not specifically addressed the need to physically restrict edible GE crops from public access," the report said, "we found a regulated edible GE crop . . . growing where they could easily be taken and eaten by passersby." The report "concluded that APHIS' current regulations, policies, and procedures do not go far enough to ensure the safe introduction of agricultural biotechnology."

There is no guarantee that this critical report will make things right. Consider that 10 years ago after another Office of Inspector General (OIG) audit, "APHIS agreed to improve its tracking of inspection reports." Ten years later, the OIG said that "the agency continued to lack an effective, comprehensive management information system." APHIS also failed to update "its regulations to reflect the Plant Protection Act of 2000."

"While the public was fed a steady barrage of revised, updated, and reworked regulatory guidelines, giving the appearance of rigorous scientific oversight, the insurance industry quietly let it be known that it would not insure the release of genetically engineered organisms into the environment against the possibility of catastrophic environmental damage."

—Jeremy Rifkin, president,
Foundation on Economic Trends

Quotes from insurance spokespeople: [1]

"The worry is that GM could be like Thalidomide— only after some time would the full extent of the problems be seen."

"Fifty years ago they were writing policies for asbestos without a care in the world. Now they are faced with bills of hundreds of millions. There is a feeling that GM could come back and bite you in five years' time."

"If a farmer approached us with any kind of insurance policy relating to a farm associated with GM we would have to refuse their application—whatever the kind of insurance applied for."

PART 3

Industry Studies are Not Competent to Identify Most of the Unpredicted Side Effects

The enormous pressure not to discover problems results in very few studies, most of which are poorly done

Since GM food is proclaimed by proponents and some regulators to be as safe as its non-GM counterpart, the pressure on researchers to not contradict this assumption is considerable. Moreover, if *any* GM food study raises a safety issue, it might indict *all* GM foods on the market. This helps explain the lack of serious studies on GM foods and the explosive condemnations and denials that accompany adverse findings.

The tiny number of published safety assessments breathtaking. In December 2004, for example, Christopher Preston used the science search engine PubMed to find all studies in which animals were given food or food products from GM crops. The list contained only 41 studies.[2] That number combined both safety assessments and commercial feeding studies. Without the commercial studies, there were only 18 left, including four in Russian or Chinese.[3]

Ann Clark divided up Preston's list another way. She found that 19 of the 41 (46%) were authored by one or more employees of the biotech industry. Of the remaining, 14 were in foreign journals, "not readily available in agricultural libraries." That left eight studies, three of which "reported substantive concerns about GM crops."[4]

Pryme and Lembcke	"Although very many have voiced their opinions both in the popular and scientific press there is only very limited data published in peer reviewed journals concerning the safety of GM food.[5] It would seem apparent that GM food regulation is currently based on a series of extremely insufficient guidelines. . . . We feel that much more scientific effort and investigation is necessary before we can be satisfied that eating foods containing GM material in the long term is not likely to provoke any form of health problems. It will be essential to adequately test in a transparent manner each individual GM product before its introduction into the market."[6]
Pusztai and Bardocz	"The biological testing of GM feeds, as presently carried out, is rather limited in scope and mainly aimed at finding the best conditions for commercial animal production. . . . The almost total absence of published data in peer-reviewed scientific literature indicates that the safety of GM foods rests more on trusting the assurances given by the biotechnology industry than on rigorous and independently verified risk assessment."[7]
Traavik and Heinemann	"Most of the animal feeding studies conducted so far have been designed exclusively to reveal husbandry production differences between GEOs and their unmodified counterparts. Studies designed to reveal physiological or pathological effects are extremely few, and they demonstrate a quite worrisome trend: Studies performed by the industry find no problems, while studies from independent research groups often reveal effects that should have merited immediate follow-up, confirmation and extension."[8]
William Freese	"'Don't look, don't find' is a common strategy in both industry and regulatory circles."[9]

Industry stifles scientific criticism and thwarts independent studies

William Freese	"Even when independent researchers are funded, a finding of potential harm requiring follow-up can effectively disqualify those scientists from additional funding. For instance, one scientist found suggestive evidence that the insecticidal proteins found in *Bt* spray and *Bt* crops could be allergenic in a study approvingly cited and reviewed by expert advisers to the Environmental Protection Agency (EPA). He has been unable to obtain funding

for further research in this area. Another scientist has done EPA-sponsored research on unintended effects in *Bt* corn, as well as the environmental impacts of *Bt* insecticidal proteins. He, too, has had difficulty obtaining funds to continue these lines of research."[10]

Sue Kedgley (New Zealand Member of Parliament)	<u>Testimony before the Royal Commission of Inquiry on Genetic Modification:</u> "Personally I have been contacted by telephone and e-mail by a number of scientists who have serious concerns about aspects of the research that is taking place . . . and the increasingly close ties that are developing between science and commerce, but who are convinced that if they express these fears publicly, even at such a Commission. . . or even if they asked the awkward and difficult questions, they will be eased out of their institution."[11]
Turkish Daily News	"A bio-engineering scientist in Turkey with five years of experience in DNA testing of transgenic crops said that she came to the subject with an open mind, 'neither for nor against, but now the risk side seems to outweigh the benefits for me.' She declined to reveal her name while pursuing a court case against her university for this month reassigning her to another department and taking her lab away. The researcher had raised funds from government and industry . . . to set up an independent laboratory. She was days away from final stage testing on seed samples gathered around Turkey when the news came from her rector. "The chairman of the Agricultural Engineers Association, Gökhan Günaydin, said they were aware of the woman's situation and were writing a formal letter of support. 'Where the pressure comes from is not clear, except that the same pressure is coming to our association.'"[12]
Anderson Valley Advertiser	"The Mexican government had learned of the impending *Nature* publication [by Ignacio Chapela regarding findings of GM contamination of indigenous corn varieties] and went ballistico. Under-secretary of Agriculture Victor Villalobos fired off a furious letter accusing the microbiologist of 'doing incalculable damage' to the nation's agriculture and economy. "We hold you personally responsible," Villalobos wrote. . . . The director of Mexico's bio-security commission, Dr. Fernando Ortiz Monasterio, summoned Ignacio to a meeting in an abandoned building in a wooded zone just outside Mexico City. . . .[Chapela said] He told me . . . 'you will not stop us—no one will stop us!' I had the impression he was threatening my life. . . .Big Biotech, alerted to the Mexican corn study in advance, sought to pre-empt publication by hiring a high-powered Washington PR firm, the Bivings Group, which specializes in Internet subterfuge. The Chapela-Quist study had barely touched down on the newsstands when an orchestrated barrage of letters decrying 'fundamental flaws' in the research began clogging up the list serve operated by AgBioWorld, a creature of the industry. Investigative reportage by the British *Guardian* failed to verify the existence of the authors but traced the computer used to generate the e-mail campaign to one operated by a Bivings front. . . . 'They have made an example of me,' [said Chapela]. 'Other scientists see this and decide that maybe they should go back to studying the bristles on the back of a bug.' That Ignacio Chapela would be denied tenure was a foregone conclusion."[13]

Research is stopped when companies refuse to provide GM seeds

Nature	"A team led by Allison Snow, a plant ecologist at Ohio State University in Columbus, has uncovered preliminary evidence that a transgene that confers insect resistance can increase the number of seeds produced by wild sunflowers. This could allow the wild plants to proliferate as weeds. But Pioneer Hi-Bred International of Des Moines, Iowa, and Indianapolis-based Dow AgroSciences have now blocked a follow-up study by refusing to allow the team access to either the transgene or the seeds from the earlier study. "*Nature* has identified at least one other recent case in which a plant geneticist at a leading US research university, who wanted to carry out an evolutionary study of Mexican maize, was denied access to transgenic material by two companies."[14]
William Freese	"Scientists have been unable to obtain the GE crop for independent animal feeding studies. One example is a Japanese scientist who was denied access to modest amounts of DuPont's high-oleic soybeans by both DuPont and the Japanese government when that crop was being reviewed by Japanese regulatory authorities.[15] A scientist studying the potential for a GE crop to spread beneficial traits to sexually compatible weeds (creating so-called 'superweeds') was denied access to the transgene by the GE crop developer."[16]
GM Free Cymru	"When Prof. Bela Darvas and his colleagues in the Hungarian Academy of Sciences revealed a massive buildup of toxins associated with plantings of a GM maize called MON 810, and indicated that they wanted to repeat and extend their research, Monsanto immediately shut off supplies of seeds and effectively killed off the research project. . . . In 2005, when Dr. Judy Carman asked Bayer CropScience for 100g of GM InVigor canola seeds for field tests in Australia, the company simply ignored her request and made the research impossible."[17]
Lappé and Bailey	"We were directly told by a Hartz seed company (a wholly-owned subsidiary of Monsanto) representative who graciously supplied us with seed for our initial study, that he was told he could no longer provide us with seed samples. Even if we were to obtain seeds the chances of finding isogenically matched varieties is becoming increasingly more difficult. When we contacted Hartz a few months ago, we were told there were 23 varieties of Roundup Ready soybeans and only 8 varieties of conventional."[18]
Sacramento Bee	"Is the genetic diversity of Mexican maize—a biological insurance policy against pests and disease—in danger? . . . Two years ago, Gepts received a $25,000 grant to look for answers. But when he asked three biotechnology companies for the seed samples he needed for his research, the trail went cold. Pioneer Hi-Bred International Inc. in Des Moines, Iowa, said no. Syngenta, of Switzerland, and St. Louis' Monsanto Co. also turned him down. 'I was not surprised,' Gepts said. 'If you want to study the effects of biotechnology, you come up against a wall.'"[19]
Traavik and Heinemann	"Follow-up studies have not been performed. There are two main factors accounting for this situation: The lack of funds for independent research, and the reluctance of producers to deliver GE materials for analysis."[20]

Case study: One scientist's shock with GM research

Years ago, a pro-GM scientist with a stellar reputation was awarded a £1.6 million UK government grant to design a rigorous safety assessment protocol for testing GM foods. The protocol was supposed to become a requirement for GM approvals in the United Kingdom and eventually in the European Union. The scientist led a 20-member research team from three prominent institutions to work on the design.

About two years into his research, he was asked to review several confidential industry studies that were used to get GM soy, corn and tomatoes approved in the United Kingdom. Reading those studies, he says, was one of the greatest shocks of his life. The studies were so superficial, so poorly done, he realized what *he* was doing and what *industry* was doing were diametrically opposed. "I was doing safety studies," he said. "They were doing as little as possible to get their foods on the market as quickly as possible."

A few weeks later, the scientist confirmed that a GM potato he was working on caused considerable health problems in rats, including damage to their organs and immune systems. He also realized that his dangerous potatoes could have sailed through industry 'safety' studies and onto plates around the world. He went public with his concerns. The scientist's name is Arpad Pusztai and he paid dearly for his integrity.

When Dr. Pusztai publicly expressed his concerns about GMOs, he was a hero at his institute. But this quickly became a serious problem for the biotech industry and the pro-GM Blair government. Dr. Pusztai was the world leader in his field; he worked at the country's most prestigious nutritional institute. Using cutting edge research funded by the government, he found problems; and now he claims that GM technology may be inherently unsafe. The press was ravenous. For two days, the institute's director led the publicity efforts, describing Pusztai's research as a huge advance in science. Then two phone calls were allegedly placed from the UK prime minister's office, forwarded through the receptionist, to the director. The next morning, Dr. Pusztai was released from the institute after 35 years and silenced with threats of a lawsuit. His research team was disbanded and the government never implemented any long-term testing protocol. Disinformation was widely circulated. The institute and pro-biotech members of the Royal Society staged so-called peer-reviews, but didn't use all the test data, had no nutritionists doing the critique of a nutritional study and made sweeping claims that contradicted the research. According to a leaked document obtained by the *Independent on Sunday*, even three government ministers prepared 'an astonishingly detailed strategy for spinning, and mobilizing support for' GM foods, including rubbishing Pusztai's research.[21]

When Pusztai's gag order was eventually lifted and he gained access to his data, 23 top scientists from around the world reviewed the research and came to his defense. The study was peer-reviewed and published in the prestigious *Lancet* (in spite of threats made to its editor by a Royal Society official).[22]

Case study: Spinning failure into proclamations of success

GM peas under development were evaluated by tests normally applied to medicine—not to GM food.[23] The peas created a dangerous immune response in mice which, if found in humans, might be life-threatening. The 10-year pea project, costing over $2 million, was abandoned. If those same peas had been evaluated with tests used for other GM crops, however, they could have sailed through the approval process anywhere in the world.

So how did the GM industry defend a regulatory system that clings to outdated science and could have approved those dangerous peas if advanced tests had not been conducted? Tony Combes, Monsanto's UK director of corporate affairs, said, "The CSIRO decision to halt research and destroy the GM pea that inflamed lung tissue in laboratory mice showed how the regulatory system was working exactly as intended."[24]

This carefully crafted PR spin appears logical only to those unfamiliar with GM safety assessments. In truth, very few people *are* familiar with exactly what goes on. Even many biotech researchers and crop developers make the assumption that companies will do what is necessary to protect the public. If they discover the truth, they are often shocked.

Higgins, the GM peas' crop developer, may be in for such a shock. He too claimed that his pea study 'shows that the regulatory system works.'[25] His explanation reveals what he doesn't know. He said, "I didn't feel that we were breaking particularly new ground... We were following basically the recommendations for a proper risk assessment and I feel it is typical of the kinds of assessments that have been done for other GM crops around the world."[26] Pea researcher Simon Hogan said the same thing. But neither scientist could name a single GM food on the market that has had the same level of testing. Experts who have studied GM safety assessments submitted around the world know that there *are* none.

Arpad Pusztai, for example, who had coauthored a paper with Higgins on GM peas in the 1990s, has studied nearly every industry submission to regulators. In fact, he recently published an analysis of all peer-reviewed safety assessments. He says that the GM pea study, does, in fact, break new ground. Professor G.E. Seralini, who has officially reviewed all the submissions to Europe as well as all the commentaries on the submissions, wrote, "To my knowledge, no GM plant on the market has undergone such detailed experiments to assess allergenicity."[27]

Likewise, Doug Gurian-Sherman and William Freese, both experts on submissions to US authorities, acknowledge that industry immune studies are considerably weaker than the pea study. Judy Carman, who has analyzed GM applications to Australia and New Zealand, concurs. In fact, Marc Rothenberg, who is a coauthor of the current pea study and was also on an expert panel assessing the allergenicity of a GM corn variety (StarLink), said of the pea research, "It was very unique. It was much more extensive and rigorous than what was previously done."

There are currently seven such crops being produced for consumption: soy, corn, cottonseed, canola, Hawaiian papaya, zucchini, and crook neck squash. None have been evaluated like the GM peas. None have been tested through long-term feeding studies. Any one of them might be creating serious health problems in the population.[28]

Industry studies are designed not to find problems; if they do arise, they are misrepresented or hidden

Company-funded research that benefits the company is not new. Research bias has been identified across several industries. In pharmaceuticals, for example, positive results are four times more likely if the drug's manufacturer funds the study.[29] When companies fund economic analyses of their own cancer drugs, the results are eight times more likely to be favorable.[30]

Compared to drug research, the potential for industry manipulation in GM crop studies is considerably higher.
- Drug studies generally follow standardized procedures dictated by regulators. The Ag biotech industry largely uses its own testing parameters.
- Drug studies are published in peer-reviewed journals, while most GM studies submitted to regulators are not published and are kept secret from the public.
- Regulators are often biotech proponents, willing to accept shoddy research.
- Most importantly, drugs *can* show serious side effects and still be approved (GM food can't). There is no tolerance for adverse reactions.

These conditions, combined with the lack of money available for rigorous independent research, provide ample motivation and opportunity for rigging studies to avoid finding problems.

William Freese	"Biotech companies are left to essentially regulate themselves. Without the discipline of regulatory standards, corporate testing practices are often 'engineered' to get the desired results."[31]
Jeffrey M. Smith	"In 1996, Monsanto scientists published a feeding study in the *Journal of Nutrition*[32] that purported to test their soybeans' effect on rats, catfish, chicken, and cows. It has been used by the biotech industry as their primary scientific validation for safety claims. According to Arpad Pusztai, however, 'It was obvious that the study had been designed to avoid finding any problems. Everybody in our consortium knew this.' Pusztai, who had published several studies in that same nutrition journal, said the Monsanto paper was 'not really up to the normal journal standards.' Pusztai says that if he had been asked to referee the paper for publication, 'it would never have passed.' He's confident that even his graduate assistants would have taken the study apart in short order."[33]

Doug Gurian-Sherman	"To determine the adequacy of FDA's current voluntary consultation process, we performed a detailed examination of more than a fourth of the data summaries (14 of 53) that FDA has reviewed. Our evaluation found that the biotechnology companies provide inadequate data to ensure their products are safe. In addition, it was clear from our review that FDA performs a less-than-thorough safety analysis."[34]
Pryme and Lembcke	"The work in five studies was regarded as having been performed more or less in collaboration with private companies. In none of these studies were effects related to GM-materials reported. On the other hand, adverse effects were reported (but not explained) in independent studies by Pusztai (1998, 2002), Fares and El-Sayed (1998), Ewen and Pusztai (1999), and Pusztai *et al.*, (1999). It is remarkable that these effects have all been observed after feeding for only 10–14 days."[35]

Sound statistical methods are ignored or key statistical data omitted

Unlike peer-reviewed publications, the scientists seem to consciously avoid using or reporting appropriate statistics, which obscure the results and make analysis by others impossible.

Doug Gurian-Sherman	"The data summaries reviewed by FDA often lacked sufficient detail, such as necessary statistical analyses needed for an adequate safety evaluation. . . . Seven of the submissions . . . did not present chi-square (or any other) statistical analyses to verify the expected ratio of plants carrying the gene. . . . FDA did not comment on the absence of statistical analyses in the [submissions] we reviewed."[36]
Public Health Association of Australia	"In the statistical analyses presented in the draft risk analysis reports, often only a mean and a range are given. Peer-reviewed scientific journals would require most or all of the number (n), mean, standard deviation, 95% confidence interval of the mean, the nature of the statistical test (e.g. t-test), and a p-value for each measurement, or the paper would be rejected for publication. Similar non-parametric statistics would be required if the data are not normally distributed. Why have these not been given? Their omission prevents a full assessment of the data by others. For example, as no standard deviations are given, sample size calculations cannot be done by others." Regarding Roundup Ready corn: "Please describe what the 'least squares mean' is as it does not seem to appear in statistics text books and a number of statisticians consulted were unaware of its existence, and please provide reasons why this type of mean was used rather than a standard measure of central tendency."[37]

Companies keep information secret and unpublished, claiming "Confidential Business Information"

Royal Society of Canada	"In the judgment of the Expert Panel, the more regulatory agencies limit free access to the data upon which their decisions are based, the more compromised becomes the claim that the regulatory process is 'science based.' This is due to a simple but well-understood requirement of the scientific method itself—that it be an open, completely transparent enterprise in which any and all aspects of scientific research are open to full review by scientific peers. Peer review and independent corroboration of research findings are axioms

of the scientific method, and part of the very meaning of the objectivity and neutrality of science."[38]

Public Health Association of Australia	"ANZFA has not released information relating to the exact combination of elements present in each of the plasmids involved in the genetic engineering as ANZFA regards them as 'commercial in confidence.' This has prevented health experts from fully assessing the potential health effects of these foods and therefore ANZFA has placed commercial considerations ahead of health."

Companies do not always comply with regulators' requests

Jeffrey M. Smith	Regarding StarLink: "Cry9C created from StarLink corn has an added sugar chain. . . . The EPA had asked Aventis in 1997, long before the StarLink crisis, to determine the composition of the sugar chain in order to assess its allergenicity. Aventis responded that research was underway, but they never reported the results to the agency. . . . Also, the company consistently failed to provide critical information about the allergenicity of the product. Even before the contamination was discovered, an EPA Scientific Advisory Panel had asked Aventis to provide blood from animals fed StarLink and from humans who might have been sensitized by inhaling its pollen. They also asked that Aventis monitor agricultural workers who had the greatest exposure to StarLink and were more likely to develop sensitivity. In spite of repeated requests, the data was not submitted. . . .

"What Aventis did present to a July 2001 meeting of the EPA's Scientific Advisory Panel was wholly inadequate. Mistakes in the document obscured the results, conclusions were at odds with the study's own data, and Aventis failed to update a five-year-old test with newer more reliable methods. Moreover, it took the company eight months to deliver it to the panel.

"One frustrated panel member, Dean Metcalfe, MD, who heads the National Institutes of Health Laboratory of Allergic Diseases and is the government's top allergist, made the comment, 'It is important, I think, for people listening to this to understand that the questions that we have are not really minor questions. To try to put this in perspective, most of us review for a lot of journals. And if this were presented for publication in the journals that I review for, it would be sent back to the authors with all of these questions. It would be rejected.'"[39,40] |
| **Doug Gurian-Sherman** | "Six of the 14 FDA consultation files contained requests by FDA for additional information needed to fully assess food safety. In three (50%) of those cases FDA's requests were either ignored by the developer or the developer affirmatively declined to provide the requested information. FDA had to complete those reviews with less-than-thorough data summaries. FDA has no authority to require the developers to submit the desired additional data unless it decided to evaluate the crop as a food additive. . . . It is worth noting that the data that FDA desired would not have been expensive or time consuming to obtain."[41] |
| **Friends of the Earth Europe** | "Two member states raised concerns about the impact of glyphosate residues in the GM oilseed rape and the fact that no information on this issue had been provided by Monsanto. Pesticide residues in food have the potential to cause health implications for consumers and so it is important to know what the likely level of these residues might be. However, the GMO Panel could not examine this issue because Monsanto simply refused to provide the data, stating that it had been provided under the 91/414 procedures for assessing pesticides."[42] |

Studies are rife with unsupported assumptions

E. Ann Clark	"Food safety assessment is largely an assumptions-based process. Most or all of the conclusions of food safety for individual GM crops are based on inferences and assumptions, rather than on actual testing. Evidence is needed to substantiate and validate these assumptions. . . . Many of the assumptions are, in turn, based on other assumptions, which do not appear to have been validated."[43]
Public Health Association of Australia	"On the basis of these very limited animal tests on two GE canola lines, all seven canola lines were considered to be safe for human consumption."[44]
Jeffrey M. Smith	"Regulatory agencies do not require companies to check the gene and amino acid sequences to see if unpredicted changes have occurred. According to William Freese, a research analyst at Friends of the Earth, 'At present, the standard practice is to sequence just 5 to 25 amino acids', even if the protein has more than 600 in total. If the short sample matches what is expected, they *assume* that the rest are also fine. If they are wrong, however, a rearranged protein could be quite dangerous."[45]
Centre for Integrated Research on Biosafety	Regarding Monsanto's high lysine corn: "The Authority must refrain from substituting unsupported speculation—such as 'expected to be,' 'not expected,' 'considered to be,' or 'not considered to be'—for hard scientific data. . . . "It is impossible without testing to conclude that cDHDPS [the GM protein], in corn cells and through processing of foods with corn content, is 'no more likely to form amyloid fibrils than any of the naturally occurring proteins in LY038.'. . . [see section 4.1.] Its tendency to form aggregates of potential cytotoxicity cannot be determined by argument or reliance on GRAS [generally recognized as safe]. . . "Structural comparisons between cDHDPS (recombinant protein) with the natural corn DHDPS (mDHDPS) demonstrate non-equivalence.[46] Therefore, the safety of cDHDPS in cooked human food cannot be extrapolated from the historical presence of mDHDPS in cooked human food. . . "There is also no evidence that we are aware of that humans have had a significant exposure to cDHDPS in their diets. *C. glutamicum* is a soil microorganism. . . . At average daily corn consumption rates . . . the amount of cDHDPS consumed daily [in the United States, if the corn was the high lysine GM variety] would be . . . a total of 1mg for males and 0.857mg for females each day. For equivalent exposure, people would have to eat between 80–800 million (males) or 60–700 million (females) kg of soil each day, or nearly as much as 10,000kg/second 24 hours a day seven days a week. At actual estimated maximum daily soil intakes . . . we estimate daily human exposure to cDHDPS from natural sources to be . . . about 30 billion–4 trillion times less than exposure through LY038 corn. . . . The authority should justify how it can assume the history of safe use of cDHDPS based on historical human consumption of natural cDHDPS."[47]
Mae-Wan Ho	"The authors are wrong to claim that the 211-bp sequence is 'very unlikely to transmit genetic information.' For such sequences could be promoters or enhancers containing numerous binding motifs for transcription factors, and capable of boosting the expression of genes inappropriately."[48]
Judy Carman	"For the amino acid analyses, they also stated that no difference would be expected between Roundup Ready soybeans sprayed and not sprayed with Roundup, without apparently

measuring whether this would be the case. Yet, Roundup is designed to interrupt the biochemical pathway that makes some amino acids."[49]

For a list of some of the key assumptions that have been overturned, see table at the end of part 3.

Animal feeding studies overlook
most potential problems

Although animal studies have been used for decades to assess the safety of drugs, pesticides and other materials, companies conducting GMO assessments seem to ignore the protocols used and lessons learned by the scientific community.

Judy Carman

"Some of these experiments used some very unusual animal models for human health, such as chickens, cows, and trout. Some of the measurements taken from these animals are also unusual measures of human health, such as abdominal fat pad weight, total deboned breast meat yield, and milk production. So it would appear that many of these tests have not been designed to measure human health at all, but rather to reassure primary producers that GM feed will permit farm animals to grow sufficiently to get a reasonable price at market. In its safety assessments, FSANZ uses these kinds of experiments as evidence that these foods are safe for human consumption. Even worse is that often the only results given from these experiments were the death of experimental animals. If other information was given, it was usually only body weights, with possibly some organ weights. If gross pathology was examined, there was no description of what was involved. Certainly, biochemistry, immunology, tissue pathology, and gut, liver and kidney function, and microscopy results were not given. . . . In addition, animals were not fed for long enough for cancer studies, or studies into the effect on offspring, to be done. Consequently, those experiments could be regarded as initial experiments in what should have been a long series, starting with several thorough animal experiments and finishing with several detailed human experiments, yet they remain the only ones done."[50]

Public Health Association of Australia

"Animal feeding studies using canola meal were undertaken but the results of these are not provided by ANZFA on the basis that this is not consumed by people, even though meal from a previous canola (GT73), when fed to animals, showed unexpected adverse results that were not predicted by the other safety testing. Instead, two feeding studies using the whole canola seed are given, when humans do not eat these either. One of these studies was on chickens and the other was on rabbits. The chicken study had good sample sizes (280 chickens in total), but only fed the birds one of the seven canola lines . . . and only measured body weight, feed intake, and mortality during the study. At the end of the study, only chilled carcass weight and yield of deboned breast meat as a percent of carcass weight was measured. No actual data were given, only a declaration that no significant difference was found for body weight, feed intake, or mortality. The statistical difference or otherwise of the other variables was not given. Results of post-mortem examinations were not given.

"In the rabbit study, 10 animals per group were fed only one of the GE canola lines... were only fed for four days and only fecal samples were measured for dry matter, ash, nitrogen, fat, crude fiber, and gross energy. . . . No actual data were given, only a declaration that seed from this canola exhibited 'at least similar zootechnical performance as seed from the original Drakkar variety.' . . . On the basis of these very limited animal tests on two GE canola lines, all seven canola lines were considered to be safe for human consumption."[51]

Mae-Wan Ho

"Only six cows were used, three fed the GM diet and the others non-GM. But a peculiar 'single reversal design with three four-week periods' was used, which I believe, meant that the groups of three cows alternated between GM and non-GM diets. Thus one group would spend the first four weeks on GM, the next four weeks on non-GM and then four weeks back on GM; while the feeding regime for the other group would be non-GM, GM, and non-GM. This design generates nine data points each for the GM diet and non-GM diet. But, it also guarantees to balance out the effects of GM versus non-GM diets and hence is utterly worthless as far as detecting difference in weight gain or any other developmental or physiological indicators between the diets."[52]

Testing the novel protein alone overlooks unpredicted changes in the crop

Most animal feeding studies that are conducted on GM foods do not use the whole food. Instead, they feed animals the isolated GM protein. These tests miss the unpredicted side effects that can occur due to changes in the genome and in the nutrients and other compounds resulting from the GM transformation process.

In a 2004 review of the submissions for 28 GM crops to Food Standards Australia New Zealand (FSANZ), for example, 18 had never been fed to animals.[53] Seventeen of these did use acute oral toxicity studies. Animals were force-fed a single high dose of only the protein, not the whole food, followed by observation for 7–14 days.

Public Health Association of Australia

"The ANZFA state in their draft risk analysis reports . . . that animal experimentation using the whole GE food will not yield accurate information compared to testing the 'test substance' directly in dose-response experiments. ANZFA's argument appears to [be] based on the assertion that the only new substance that can be found in GE foods is the new substance that has been genetically engineered to appear. This is an untested hypothesis for these foods and a core matter of disagreement. It should be noted that unexpected substances have previously been known to appear in GE plants. . . . ANZFA's own documents indicate that new, unexpected substances may be appearing in the GE food. For example, in Application A346 for insect-protected corn line MON 810, the amino acid profiles indicate that out of the 18 amino acids tested, 8 were significantly different from the control corn. . . . This indicates that the concentrations of one or more existing proteins may have significantly changed, and/or that one or more new proteins may be being produced."[54]

Testing protein surrogates from bacteria further ignores many dangers

For the acute toxicity study mentioned above, as well as for other tests of the GM protein, biotech companies almost never isolate and extract the protein from the GM plant. While this certainly *can* be done, what they do instead is insert their transgene into bacteria and let it produce the protein. It's cheaper and easier to extract protein from the bacteria than from the plant. "This bacterial-derived surrogate protein (or its derivative) is then employed for all subsequent testing: short-term animal feeding studies, allergenicity assessments, etc."[55] They *assume* that the protein will have the same structure and effect as the protein from GM plants. But that same protein, if produced in a plant, could have added molecules, be misfolded, or have a different amino acid sequence. None of these potentially harmful changes would be picked up in a test that uses protein from bacteria.

According to the European Commission Scientific Steering Committee, "Extrapolating from the tested behavior of an isolated protein produced in a bacterium to predicting the behavior of the same protein when it is an integral part of the transgenic plant can be accepted only if the chemical identity (including conformational identity) of the two proteins has been demonstrated."[56] Similarly, the US National Academy of Sciences says, "Tests should preferably be conducted with the protein as produced in the plant." If surrogates are used, they say that "The EPA should provide clear, scientifically justifiable criteria for establishing biochemical and functional equivalency when registrants request permission to test non plant-expressed proteins in lieu of plant-expressed proteins."[57] According to an article in *Biotechnology and Genetic Engineering Reviews*, the EPA has not followed this recommendation, "even though its scientific advisers have proposed such 'test substance equivalence' criteria.[58] In fact, the toxicity and allergenicity assessments of the major *Bt* corn and cotton events currently on the market employed surrogate proteins that did not meet these criteria.[59,60]

William Freese	"Several scientists to whom we described this practice expressed amazement. They take it for granted that plant and bacteria will generate different transgenic proteins from the same gene ... Given the use of bacterially produced surrogate proteins as the norm, one cannot avoid the conclusion that the plant-produced transgenic proteins we actually eat in our food are virtually untested."[61]

Harmful sugar chains can be overlooked

When sugar chains are added to proteins, this process, known as glycosylation, can influence allergic responses. When GM peas created immune responses in mice (see section 1.18), researchers blamed a subtle, hard-to-detect difference in glycosylation patterns between the GM version and the natural version in a closely related plant. This change was considered dangerous enough to cancel the 10-year, $2 million project. Since most assessments use surrogate proteins, however, this potentially deadly chnage in a plant-produced protein would not be identified.

Proteomics	"Protein glycosylation is generally species-, tissue- and cell-type specific. Therefore, from a biological point of view, it is highly desirable to study the naturally expressed protein rather than a recombinant version."[62]
Freese and Schubert	"Even if precisely the same foreign DNA is expressed in bacteria and plant, the two organisms—which are kingdoms apart in biological terms—process proteins differently. For instance, bacteria are not known to add sugar molecules to proteins, while plants do. Glycosylation patterns influence the immune response to proteins, and glycosylation is considered to be a characteristic of allergenic proteins.[63] Other secondary modifications will certainly occur when proteins are expressed in foreign organisms or different cell types.[64] As a result, animal feeding studies and allergenicity assessments that make use of bacterial surrogate proteins or their derivatives may not reflect the toxicity or allergenicity of the plant-produced transgenic protein to which people are actually exposed."[65]
Pryme and Lembcke	Regarding a *Bt* tomato: "It is evident that all acute toxicity and stability studies on *Bt*-toxin were performed using an *E. coli* recombinant and not that isolated from the GM tomato. It needs to be emphasized that the structure and stability of the *E. coli* recombinant *Bt*-toxin, which they tested is almost certainly different from that synthesized by the plant. Indeed, in a later communication from the European Union it was stated that the *Bt*-toxin in the plant was glycosylated while neither *B. thuringiensis* nor *E. coli* would be able to perform this type of post-translational modification of the recombinant protein."[66]

Other structural changes will also be overlooked

Proteins from plants may fold or combine differently than those produced in bacteria. An altered shape can, for example, change which amino acids are next to each other or alter protein stability, both of which may increase allergenicity.

Centre for Integrated Research on Biosafety	"The safe use of the plant enzyme does not extend to the recombinant bacterial enzyme because the cDHDPS differs structurally from the plant version. This difference in

molecular architecture means that different faces of the protein are presented to the solution, with different direct allergenic potential."[67]

Properties of animal feed can mask results

GM feeding studies have inappropriately diluted their GM feed, used too much overall protein, too little GM protein, or too little nutrition, all of which will make detection of adverse reactions difficult or impossible. Other studies failed to prepare their crops in ways that humans will be exposed to it. For example, they have used herbicide-tolerant crops that were never treated with herbicide or used only raw feed for crops that are also eaten cooked or processed.

Too much protein in the diet

Pryme and Lembcke	Regarding Roundup Ready soybeans: "From the (rather poor) bar diagrams in the paper there was a significant difference in the growth rate of rats and catfish with the two different GM lines, even at the dietary protein levels which were artificially too high (close to 25%).[68] This very high protein content of the diet would almost certainly mask, or at least effectively reduce, any possible effect of the transgene, particularly when the inclusion level of the GM soya in any case was low. It is therefore highly likely that all GM effects would have been diluted out." [The authors contrasted this with Pusztai's studies,[69] which they said] "are remarkable in that the experimental conditions were varied and several ways were found by which to demonstrate possible health effects of GM-foods." [In particular,] "low protein feed was tried (the idea being that health defects would show up earlier at low protein intakes)."[70]
Pusztai and Bardocz	Regarding Roundup Ready soybeans (as above): "The absence of pancreatic hypertrophy, however, was not surprising because the unusually high dietary protein concentration, as pointed out by the authors, masked and/or diluted the biological effect of the trypsin inhibitors. This is of particular concern because the trypsin inhibitor content of GTS lines in unprocessed soybean was significantly higher than in the control line."[71]

Too little of the GM crop in the diet

Pryme and Lembcke	Regarding Roundup Ready soybeans: "In the unprocessed soy study the inclusion level of the GM soy was too low and would probably ensure that any possible undesirable GM effects did not occur."[72]
Pusztai and Bardocz	Regarding Roundup Ready soybeans: "The raw unprocessed soybean diets in which the GM meals were incorporated were only at the level of 5% or 10% of the diet.[73] Thus, these meals only replaced 8.5% and 17%, respectively, of the total protein of 24.7 g/100 g diet. In other words, the GM protein was diluted by other dietary proteins by twelvefold and sixfold, respectively, producing another possible masking effect."[74]
Jeffrey M. Smith	Regarding Mon 863 *Bt* corn: "African aid recipients rely on maize for about 90% of their caloric intake. Rats are stand-ins for humans. According to Pusztai, researchers should have started with the maximum amount of corn possible (while maintaining a balanced diet), and then used lower concentrations to evaluate dose effects. The maximum amount of GM maize fed to the rats was 33% of their diet, constituting only about 15% of their protein."[75]
Mae-Wan Ho	"It was work done with a mixture of both Monsanto's Roundup Ready soya GTS 40-3-2

(as soya meal) and Mon 810 maize (as maize grain) at the same time, comprising only 13% and 18.5% respectively of the total diet. This inevitably decreases the chance of detecting the GM DNA belonging to the varieties."[76]

Mixing feed with other GM products

Centre for Integrated Research on Biosafety	"The authority, at the very least, should seek a feeding trial using LY038 rather than a mix of transgenic strains that dilutes LY038." (The feeding included 20.5% of another GM variety.)"[77]
Jeffrey M. Smith	Regarding Mon 863 *Bt* corn: "Researchers also supplemented the corn with a commercial animal feed. Although its composition wasn't reported, it may have contained GM soy, which could have skewed the results."[78]

Too little of the GM protein expressed

Pryme and Lembcke	Regarding experimental tomatoes: "It would seem likely that the inclusion of 10% freeze-dried tomatoes distorted the diets' amino acid pattern. Moreover, at this inclusion level the *Bt*-toxin (a GM tomato protein) intake of the rats was insignificant (the *Bt* expression level was one-twentieth of that which is found in other *Bt* crops).[79] Thus one could expect nothing significant to be found and this indeed was duly confirmed by the authors." Regarding experimental potato: "The glycinin expression level and its intake by the rats was far too low to make the studies of major interest.... Hopefully, no food or feed additive is so toxic as to give adverse effects with the small dose used by Hashimoto *et al.*"[80,81]

Poor nutritional value of the feed

Pusztai and Bardocz	"The results of a separate study[82] with toasted glyphosate-resistant GM soybean, in which rats and mice were fed with this GM soybean at 30% inclusion level in the diet for 15 weeks, could not be seriously considered because rat growth was minimal (less than 30 g over 105 days) and mice did not grow at all on either the test or control diets. This invalidates the authors' observations of finding no significant differences ... "The conclusion by Kramer et al.,[83] that the GM corn developed by transferring the gene of egg white avidin to make the seed resistant to storage insect pests was safe for mice because they suffered no ill effects, can at best be regarded as premature. As the authors fed mice solely on GM or non-GM corn instead of on a balanced diet, it is not surprising that the mice did not grow at all with either. The results of a study with GM corn (CBH351) expressing *Bt. thuringiensis* toxin Cry9C,[84] in which rats and mice were fed with this GM corn at 50% inclusion level in the diet for 13 weeks in similar manner to their GM soya feeding study (Teshima et al., 2000),[85] are open to the same criticisms as the latter study."[86]

Not cooked or processed

Centre for Integrated Research on Biosafety	Regarding high-lysine corn: "The very latest research indicates that some allergens are attenuated or removed by heat or during processing, but other allergens become more

potent as a result of heating and in the presence of carbohydrates.[87] These can only be identified using food prepared in a fashion representative of how people will consume it....Only feeding studies, using whole plant material in food that has been cooked and processed in ways that humans would consume it, can provide the proper basis for a safety review. No such studies were provided for public review . . . and from the [Draft Assessment Report] we have no reason to suspect that such studies were ever provided to the authority."[88]

Arpad Pusztai   "The GM crop should be fed both raw and after heat-treatment."[89]

Using unsprayed herbicide tolerant crops

Judy Carman   "The soybeans assessed in the application were not treated with Roundup. They are therefore not equivalent to the soybeans that will come out of paddocks for human consumption. Experiments should be repeated with soybeans harvested from farms."[90]

Using mature animals instead of young ones masks serious problems

Nutritional studies typically use young, fast-growing animals, because they are sensitive to toxic and nutritional effects. According to Pryme and Lembcke, "during development the organism is highly dependent on appropriate feed." Young animals use protein to build muscles, tissues, and organs. Problems with GM food could therefore show up in organ and body weight. Pryme and Lembcke applauded Pusztai's research, stating, "Importantly, young rats were used throughout."[91] According to *The Pusztais' Guide to GMOs and Regulation*, "The organ- and body weights of older animals are less sensitive to dietary changes."[92] Studies funded by the biotech industry, however, routinely use mature animals.

Pusztai and Bardocz   "In gavage [feeding tube] studies, unlike in the work described, young, rapidly growing animals must be used to establish whether the gene product has any toxic effect, affecting the growth of the animal. With older animals any effect on growth could only be shown if they were gavaged with potent toxins."[93]

Jeffrey M. Smith   "Researchers tested GM soy on mature animals, not young ones. . . . 'With a nutritional study on mature animals,' says Pusztai, 'you would never see any difference in organ weights even if the food turned out to be anti-nutritional.' . . . Even if there were an organ development problem, the study wouldn't have picked it up since the researchers didn't even weigh the organs."[94]

     Regarding Mon 863 corn: "Monsanto used a mix of young and old animals, which may have hidden serious problems."[95]

Using animals with a wide variation in weight hinders detection of food-related changes

---

Bardocz and Pusztai   Animal starting weights should be close ... or it will be difficult to detect statistically significant differences in their growth, particularly in the short-term and with small group sizes."[96]

Jeffrey M. Smith	Regarding Mon 863 corn: "They used rats with a huge range of starting weights. Male rats ranged from 198.4 to 259.8 grams (or 143 to 186 grams according to conflicting data in the study's appendix). According to Pusztai, starting weights should not vary more than 2% from average. The wide range 'can make it impossible to find significant differences . . . at the end of the experiment.'"[97]

Short duration feeding studies miss long-term impacts

To analyze "harmful outcomes" from GM food, the Royal Society of Canada says to test for "short-term and long-term human toxicity, allergenicity, or other health effects." Biotech companies, however, do not employ such tests. They often rely on an "acute oral toxicity study" in which a high dose of the GM protein is fed to mice, which are then observed over several days to see if there's a problem. In Europe, 90-day feeding experiments with the whole food are used. Both of these tests are woefully inadequate to detect a range of possible problems.

Public Health Association of Australia	"The effects of feeding people high concentrations of the new protein over tens of years cannot be determined by feeding 20 mice a single oral gavage of a given high concentration of the protein and taking very basic data for 13–14 days, particularly when the protein fed to the mice came from partially-purified mEPSPS protein [Roundup Ready GM protein] produced in *E. Coli* in a laboratory, rather than from corn in a field. . . . "The acute toxicity testing proposed as adequate would simply not pick up cancer, teratology [birth defects], or the long-tem effects of nutrient deficiencies or increases in anti-nutrients."[98]
Pusztai and Bardocz	"It is of particular importance to perform long-term nutritional experiments with GM feed components because small changes in the nutritional value of GM crops are more likely to show up with extended feeding. For example, the effect on the growth rate of rats fed GM potato-based diets was too small to be seen in the 10-day feeding experiments, but a GM potato-induced reduction in rat growth was readily demonstrated in 110-day feeding trials, even when the potatoes were fully cooked. . . . Even at these similar growth rates the weights of some of the rats' vital organs, such as the gut and particularly the small intestine, the liver, and kidneys were still significantly different."[99] "One has to agree with the views of some biotechnologists that relatively short-term animal feeding/production experiments, particularly as they are presently carried out, do not contribute much to GM safety."[100]
Gilles-Eric Seralini	"As for animal feeding tests, 54 references were available by the end of 2000. Thirty-one are abstracts, websites and unavailable meeting reports. Two references are in press and 21 have been published in peer-reviewed journals. There from seven used rats (maximum duration 28 days for four of them), nine have been performed on chickens that do not go over 42 days. Four used pigs but only one test was published, which had fed an experimental maize. Two references fed cows of more than 42 days with *Bt* 176 maize that is not used anymore. Today there are no sub-chronic toxicity tests on rats that are obligatory. For new or pending GMOs there are only chronic toxicity tests for 90 days and not more."[101]
Jeffrey M. Smith	Regarding Mon 863 corn: "According to [toxicologist G.E.] Seralini, Mon 863 is new and unique; it differs from natural *Bt*-toxin in seven ways. It should require at least the level of evaluation used for chemical pesticides. In the Eropean Union, that requires research on three types of mammals, with studies ranging from 90 days to two years. Mon 863, however, was approved after only a short 90-day rat study."[102]

Short duration studies are also used for environmental evaluations

Freese and Schubert	"Feeding studies designed to detect potential effects of GE pesticidal proteins on non-target insects such as honeybees are often too short to give meaningful results, for instance nine days.[103] However, the EPA often accepts such inadequate studies as substantiating the hypothesis that GE pesticidal proteins are not harmful to insects at the tested doses.[104] Hilbeck and Meier[105] recommend full life-cycle testing to detect sub-lethal and long-term effects."[106]

Using so few subjects makes statistical significance nearly unattainable

"If one were seeking to show no effect, one of the best methods to do this is would be to use insufficient replication, a small n."[107] This comment was made in expert testimony in response to the chicken feeding study on the GM corn Chardon LL. The number of replicates (in this case, chicken feeding pens) was so low [n=4] that even a doubling of the death rate was dismissed as statistically significant. (see section 1.17) Many GMO studies funded by industry suffer the same limitation.

Judy Carman	"Groups of 5–6 Holstein dairy cows were fed uncooked soybeans. This is a totally inadequate sample size and would not be expected to show any differences between the groups. Yet a difference was found."[108]

Even animal deaths and serious conditions are discounted

Gilles-Eric Seralini	"In tests performed by Monsanto, 50 significant differences were noticed in rats eating the GM maize NK603 during 90 days. These differences have been judged 'not important' with bizarre explanations by two scientists from a governmental commission. Other differences were found in similar experiments with GM oilseed rape GT73 on livers that showed an increase in weight up to 20% and kidneys of rats. These differences were kept confidential in the commercial files. We only got access after actions in court."[109]
Public Health Association of Australia	Regarding Roundup Ready corn: "Why the unilateral corneal opacity, noted in one male mouse at the high dose level of the test material was considered not to be treatment-related and why further experimentation was not undertaken to determine the proportion of treated mice afflicted."[110]
	Regarding Liberty Link corn (Chardon LL): "The toxicity of the PAT protein was assessed using a single oral gavage to mice (5/sex/group) of 51% PAT protein. . . . The PAT protein used did not come from the corn, but from bacteria and was purified before use. Mice were observed for 14 days before being sacrificed and body weight and 'gross pathology' were done. There was no description of what was actually done in the gross pathology. One treated male mouse died. His pathology results were not supplied, but it was declared that 'as no other clinical signs were observed in animals of any group, these signs are not considered to be treatment-related.' No biochemistry, immune function, neurology, liver function, kidney function, gut function, complete autopsy, cancer, or teratological measurements were taken."[111]
Jeffrey M. Smith	"When [a] lawsuit made Calgene's rat study available, Dr. Pusztai reviewed it for the attorneys. With respect to the rats' bleeding stomachs, he pointed out that if similar reac-

tions were to occur in humans, 'they could lead to life-endangering hemorrhage, particularly in the elderly who use aspirin to prevent thrombosis.'[112] Pusztai also discovered a paragraph in the appendix which said 7 out of 40 GM-fed rats died within two weeks and were replaced. The cause of death was obliquely described as 'husbandry error.' Pusztai was astounded. It is entirely unacceptable for such a study to leave out the data from rat autopsies and substitute only meaningless, unsupported opinions. Likewise, replacing dead animals in the middle of a feeding study is not scientifically justified."[113]

Using irrelevant control groups hides significant findings

Arpad Pusztai   Regarding Mon 863 corn (section 1.3): "The study's use of six irrelevant controls and reference to historical databases obscured the true findings.... Monsanto defended changes in kidney weights by comparing results from the test animals with rats used in a completely different study, conducted in a different laboratory, using Mon 863 hybrids with other GM maize samples. In this study the results of the original MON 863 study were quoted (but not actually re-done) for comparison. This inter-experimental comparison is entirely inappropriate for nutritional evaluation and should be disregarded."[114]

Jeffrey M. Smith   Regarding Mon 863 corn: "Many health effects nonetheless remained significant even compared to these 'artificial' controls. So Monsanto claimed that they were biologically irrelevant if they fell within a wide range considered 'normal' for rats.... Thus, Monsanto dismissed a 52% decrease in immature blood cells as 'attributable to normal biological variability.' According to Pusztai, an allowance of 5% variability is the norm in food experiments. Similarly, he says that the increase in blood sugar levels by 10% 'cannot be written off as biologically insignificant, given the epidemic of diabetes.'

"In spite of the statistical sleight-of-hand, several results were *still* outside Monsanto's 'normal' range. They offered another excuse. Since the reaction among the rats was not consistent between males and females, it was not significant. 'This is really ridiculous,' says Seralini, who points out that everyone studying cancer and endocrinology knows that there are reaction differences between genders.

"And when the gender defense did not apply, Monsanto dismissed results claiming the reactions were not dose-specific. Specifically, changes in rats whose diet was 11% Mon 863 were sometimes more pronounced than those fed a 33% diet. Here again, Seralini says Monsanto's claims conflict with scientific understanding. In endocrinology and toxicology research, differences are not always proportional to their effects. A small dose of a hormone, for example, can cause a woman to ovulate, while a larger dose can make her infertile.

"When all other excuses failed, Monsanto claimed that with such a large study, one would expect lots of results to fall in the statistically significant category purely by chance. Thus, no follow-up is required. Pusztai, who was commissioned by the German government to evaluate the study in 2004, wrote, 'It is almost impossible to imagine that major lesions in important organs (kidneys, liver, etc.) or changes in blood parameters (lymphocytes, granulocytes, glucose, etc.) that occurred in GM Maize-fed rats, is incidental and due to simple biological variability.'"[115]

Judy Carman   "In addition to their normal diet, one group of rats was fed control potatoes while another was fed GE potato line BT-06. After a month, 'a number of' abnormal findings were noted, such as enlarged lymph nodes, hydronephrosis, and enlarged adrenal glands.[116] However, because at least some of these results were also found in the control rats, no statistical difference was found between the two groups, and so the GE potatoes were regarded as safe for eating! However, control rats are supposed to remain healthy, indicating that either rats are an inappropriate animal model for safety testing of potatoes, or that something unusual was happening with the rats. For example, a virus may have infected all the rats, masking any effect of the GE food, or the controls may have been inadvertently fed the GE food. To put it into perspective, consider a hypothetical clinical trial to determine the effects of a new aspirin. In this situation, one group of people would take the new aspirin and another group would take a sugar pill placebo for comparison purposes. After several weeks in this hypothetical trial, the manufacturing company followed-up its trial volunteers and found a high proportion of those taking the new aspirin had been hospitalized. However, the manufacturing company argued that because some volunteers taking the sugar pill had also been hospitalized, the new aspirin was safe. The regulatory authority agreed and released it for sale, without anyone asking: how can a sugar pill hospitalize a high proportion of those who take it? Put quite simply, the experiment should have been repeated and expanded to determine what was occurring and why, before the food was considered to be safe." [117]

| **Pusztai and Bardocz** | "The composition of the control diets should be the same as the GM diet, but containing the parent line with or without supplementation with the isolated gene product at the same level as expressed in the GM line. Unfortunately, although the use of the gene product-spiked control diet ought to be mandatory in these nutritional tests, they have rarely been used." [118] |

Essential data are missing

Pryme and Lembcke	Regarding Roundup Ready soybeans: "No data were given for most of the parameters but the authors give a bland assurance that there were no differences. . . . Terminal body weights and relative organ weights (liver, kidneys, testes) did not show significant differences (no data given). There were no gross pathologic findings related to genetic modification (no information about which organs were examined)." [119]
E. Ann Clark	Regarding submissions to Canadian regulators: "Details of the mouse or rat feeding trials, such as number of animals and rate and duration of exposure, are sketchy to nonexistent, and vary widely among Decisions. . . . Insufficient information is given on which to assess the statistical rigor of the feeding trials." [120]
Pusztai and Bardocz	Regarding tomato and sweet pepper: "However, some of these sweeping claims are difficult to accept on the basis of the actual data in the published paper. Additionally, there is a lack of precision in defining some of the parameters measured in the work. Thus, one of the major omissions is that the coat protein [CP] expression level in the plants is not given and in the toxicity tests it is impossible to see what is measured without making comparisons with equivalent amounts of CP, particularly as no attempt has been made to isolate CP from the two GM plants. "The nutrition study has not been described adequately, no starting or during-the-experiment weights of the individual animals are given. Means are no substitute, particularly when as in figure 3 the standard deviations in the bar diagram are so big (e.g. in 3 A at 3 weeks the mean weight of the rats is about 150 ±50 g) that it makes the in-between group comparisons meaningless. No diet composition and no animal management data are described, even though without pair-feeding no valid conclusions

about weight gain, organ weights, biochemical blood indices, etc., can be arrived at. The graphs and data are uninformative. The size of the most important tissues, such as the small and large intestines, pancreas, etc., has not been recorded. The methods used for histological evaluation are not detailed and therefore it is impossible to see whether the authors used appropriate methods or not. In view of these deficiencies it is difficult to accept the authors' conclusions that these GM plants are as safe as their conventional counterparts."[121]

Mae-Wan Ho	"Even though they had taken apparently carefully timed samples from individual animals in each four-week period, they pooled all the samples from the same animal together, thus losing potentially valuable information regarding the time course of the clearing of GM DNA from the gut to the tissues and out of the body."[122]
Arpad Pusztai	"The Mon 863 feeding study was poorly designed and reported. It is doubtful whether any prominent nutritional journal would consider it. It is odd, therefore, that it remains the key document used by government regulators to protect the health of European citizens." "**Nutritional data missing:** Nutrition studies require measurement and disclosure of the nutritional composition of the feed and the demonstration that it remains stable for the duration of the 90-day experiment. This assurance backed up by actual chemical analysis is not provided. "**Methodology missing:** The study fails to describe most of the methods used in the study. When methods cannot be evaluated or repeated, they remain suspect. . . . "The growth rates reported were inexplicable. During the experiment, for example, one rat lost 53 g in one week and then gained 102 g the next. Rats with the highest starting weight sometimes ended up with the smallest final weight. In the last four weeks, rats hardly grew at all, in spite of the similar feed intake and even though rats typically continue to grow throughout their lives. There is too little information provided to judge whether these are the result of animal mismanagement, degradation of the feed stored at room temperature, or some other problem."[123]
Jeffrey M. Smith	Regarding Mon 863 corn: "Overall, the research paper was confusing, conflicting, poorly reported, and at a whopping 1,139 pages, seemed to try and hide results in a mountain of irrelevant material. It failed to disclose the methods used to measure changes and therefore the research cannot be repeated and the results remain suspect. . . . Referring to the study as a whole, Pusztai says, 'Nutritional scientists and leading journals would not accept these blatant inadequacies and misinterpretations.'"[124]
William Freese	Regarding StarLink corn: "The studies submitted by AgrEvo (Aventis' predecessor) purporting to show that Cry9C is not allergenic are deficient in a number of ways. EPA criticized AgrEvo's rat study as follows: "The brown Norway rat model is not a validated test for food allergy at this point and the study submitted is significantly flawed ..." These significant flaws include AgrEvo's failure to report crucial data, including the concentration of Cry9C in the extracts injected into the rats, the number of rats that were tested, and the time that elapsed between injections of serum and challenge antigens. These are not minor oversights, but rather serious breaches of basic scientific protocol; a high school biology student would be flunked for less. . . . Most of the registrant's studies were not conducted according to standards of good laboratory practice; test protocols and other crucial data are routinely missing. In one study on the stability of Cry9C, the supposedly non-StarLink controls were contaminated with the Cry9C protein! "In short, the EPA and the SAP based their evaluations of StarLink corn on shoddy

corporate science. Given AgrEvo's obvious interest in approval, we cannot help but wonder why it left out crucial data. What did the company have to hide if this corn were in fact safe for animals and people, as it claimed?"[125]

Compositional studies are not comprehensive enough to detect hazards

As described in part 1, there are numerous ways in which the composition of GM crops can be unpredictably altered. The specific types of compounds measured and the methods used for detection are inadequate to identify potential hazards.

Changes in know toxins and antinutrients are not measured

Doug Gurian-Sherman	"Our review of 14 reviewed submissions found that developers do not evaluate all the compounds they should, and when they do, the methods they use are not always comparable to the contemporaneous state-of-the-art testing regimes. . . . The submissions did not evaluate some potentially deleterious compounds, such as scientifically recognized toxicants in tomatoes or anti-nutrients in corn. . . . Several anti-nutrients including phytate and trypsin inhibitor have been identified in corn. [Phytate was reported in two out of four submissions and trypsin inhibitor was reported in one of four.] The fact that both of those antinutrients were not measured in all engineered corn plants indicates that known corn food-safety concerns were not thoroughly assessed."[126]
Food and Chemical Toxicology	"Data from US and EC documents were investigated with regard to inherent plant toxins and antinutrients. Analyzed were documents of rape (glucosinolates, phytate), maize (phytate), tomato (tomatine, solanine, chaconine, lectins, oxalate), potato (solanine, chaconine, protease-inhibitors, phenols) and soybean (protease-inhibitors, lectins, isoflavones, phytate). In several documents used for notifications no declarations even on essential inherent plant toxins and antinutrients could be found. . . . Consistent guidelines, specifying data of relevant compounds, which have to be provided for notification documents of specific organisms have to be established. Because of the importance of inherent plant toxins and antinutrients on nutritional safety, also coherent databases of standard parental lines and clear criteria for mandatory declarations are necessary."[127]

Basic tests are not done and methods are often insensitive or obsolete

Jeffrey M. Smith	"In July 1999, independent researchers published a study showing that GM soy contains 12%–14% less cancer-fighting phytoestrogens. Monsanto responded with its own study, concluding that soy's phytoestrogen levels vary too much to even carry out a statistical analysis. Researchers failed to disclose, however, that they had instructed the laboratory to use an obsolete method of detection—one that had been prone to highly variable results."[128,129]
Pusztai and Bardocz	"Even the results of the analytical work done to date, using mainly conventional methods, have left many uncertainties about the chemical equivalence of the GM and non-GM soybeans, particularly as the design of some of the comparative studies was seriously flawed. Even more seriously, judging from the published literature, no attempt was apparently made to establish the equivalence of the GM to the conventional lines by more modern and high-resolving power technologies, such as proteomics, DNA microarray

analysis using GM soybean RNA isolated from different tissues and plants grown under different but relevant conditions. No data could be found using NMR combined with chemometrics for the characterization of metabolite differences in the plants.[130] Moreover, analysis of the possible different glycoforms of the 5-enolpyruvylshikimate-3-phosphate synthase [Roundup Ready protein] and other proteins has not been attempted, although variability in glycosylation patterns can lead to different biochemical and antigenic properties. Furthermore, no comparison was made between the GM and non-GM forms in their contents of small RNA molecules that are emerging as very important and inheritable gene regulators. In view of these omissions no claims by the authors that the GM and non-GM soybeans are substantially equivalent can be accepted without carrying out further and more critical studies."[131]

Mae-Wan Ho	"Their PCR method for detecting GM DNA is neither validated nor standardized. Its sensitivity varied over one-thousandfold between different tissues and tissue contents. The limits of detection is such that in some samples, I calculate that more than 40,000 copies of the soya genome or 9,000 copies of the maize genome must be present in the sample before a positive result is obtained. The usual detection limit of PCR is 10 copies or less.... No wonder there is a rather large number of neither positives nor negatives, but 'inconclusives' in the data."[132]
Centre for Integrated Research on Biosafety	Regarding high-lysine corn: "An adequate molecular characterization of all novel RNA molecules, that may pose a risk to consumers, is missing along with microarray analysis of the transcriptome of the LY038 line."[133]
Bardocz and Pusztai	"SDS-gel electrophoresis is a crude method for the determination of the molecular weight; it is unsuitable to determine the structural, and even less the functional similarity of two proteins."[134]
Jeffrey M. Smith	"In order to evaluate the difference between the GM protein in the peas and its natural counterpart in the beans, the Australians used the sensitive MOLDI-TOF test, which is almost never used in GM safety assessments. According to Doug Gurian-Sherman, a senior scientist at the Center for Food Safety and formerly at the US Environmental Protection Agency, those subtle differences in glycosylation patterns found in the pea study 'would not be detected by the tests that are currently required by US regulatory agencies.' In fact, in the 1990s, when the GM peas were tested with an inferior 'gel test' method that is sometimes used in GM food assessments, Higgins [the pea developer] didn't see any difference between the GM and non-GM proteins. The peas had passed this test."[135]

Studies typically combine poor reporting with missing data

Doug Gurian-Sherman	Regarding Bt corn from Dow AgroSciences: "FDA determined that the data summary had incomplete information about nutritional composition. FDA recommended to the developer that its 'composition data could be improved by addition of min/max [minimum and maximum] values to each analysis.' In a letter dated January 10, 2001, the developer responded to FDA's request by stating, 'We believe the addition of minimum and maximum values for individual composition analysis will not significantly enhance the data set nor provide useful support for the safety conclusions in the current FDA notification' and suggested that it is more useful to compare average values from its GE variety to the 'expected range' for the conventional crop. In other words, the developer decided

to rely on its own judgment about what data were useful for risk assessment rather than FDA's and did not comply with FDA's suggestion."[136]

Bardocz and Pusztai	"In some submissions there are pages marked as page 1 of 22. This means that this page is from a longer report, but the other 21 pages are not given.... There are references in the text as (figure X) or (table X), but these are not given in the files. Where are these data? Why are they not given?"[137]
Centre for Integrated Research on Biosafety	Regarding high-lysine corn: "The Applicant has assured the Authority that corn derived from LY038 and hybrids will have total lysine in the range of 3500 to 5300 ppm, and free lysine in the range of 1000 to 2500 ppm.... The applicant already possesses hybrid lines of corn with total lysine levels reaching 6160 ppm and free lysine levels reaching 2908 ppm, but apparently did not include that fact in the application.... "The applicant reports amino acid levels as a proportion of amino acids. This can mask important changes in the amounts of amino acids, especially in distributions between protein incorporated and free amino acids."[138]
Public Health Association of Australia	Regarding Liberty Link corn (Chardon LL): "Although analyses were done comparing sprayed GE corn with non-sprayed GE corn, no data were given, just a statement that no significant differences were found."[139]

The sample sizes used for compositional comparison are way too small

Judy Carman	"They found no significant differences but the sample sizes used are not given in the ANZFA document. Nor are sample size calculations to justify the sample sizes that were used.... If too small a sample size is used, any differences that may exist between Round-up Ready soybeans and ordinary soybeans will not be found. This is ... a serious scientific fault."[140]
Public Health Association of Australia	Regarding Roundup Ready canola: "It is clear that the sample sizes are most inadequate to find statistical significance. For example, n=2 in the glyphosate-tolerant canola line.... With such low numbers it is almost a foregone conclusion that a statistically significant difference will NOT be found between the GE food and the non-GE food for most analyses, even if one exists in nature. In fact, if a statistically-significant difference is found with such small numbers it indicates that the difference may be substantial indeed. "In spite of the very small sample sizes, the percent fat content was found to be significantly higher in the GE canola compared to the control. It is noted that the fat content was also higher in the 1993 and 1994 field trials, but was not found to be significantly different, probably due to the very small sample sizes. Therefore, the mean fat values may not be due to 'the natural range of variation that occurs in canola,' as stated.... We contend that the experiment needs to be repeated with much larger sample sizes, such as n=50."[141] Regarding Roundup Ready corn: "We contend that the compositional analyses require much larger sample sizes than n=5."[142]

Compositional changes are obscured by pooling crop data from varied growing conditions or making comparisons with plants of diverse genetics

In order to properly identify the compositional differences that come about due to gene insertion and not from random genetic variation and environmental conditions, according to the Organization of Economic Cooperation and Development (OECD), "Measurement data from the new variety should ideally be compared to those obtained from the near isogenic [parent line or nearly genetically identical] non-GMO line grown under identical conditions."[143] Food Standards Australia New Zealand (FSANZ) specifies this as "grown in adjacent plots at the same site and at the same time."[144] Furthermore, "the pooling of data from different sites is acceptable provided data from the separate sites is also submitted and separately evaluated."[145] Otherwise, it may be quite difficult for compositional differences to reach statistical significance. The specifications notwithstanding, the biotech companies appear to regularly construct their research in the opposite manner, going out of their way to obscure the data with faulty controls and pooled data from varied conditions.

Monsanto's application for high lysine corn provides an example. According to the Centre for Integrated Research on Biosafety (INBI):

"The applicant changed both the environment and the composition of genotypes by planting four different non-GMO 'reference' varieties at each of the different sites. The combined data then produces an overwhelming variance range because it is a composite of a few replications of each genotype, each genotype grown in only one environment, and five different environments. It is improbable, if not impossible, with this type of experimental design to recognize and eliminate outliers or produce useful baseline data for hazard identification. . . . In the statistical analysis, the range of observed values for the reference substances was always a combined value across all sites. There was no reference range reported by site."

The high lysine GM corn turns out to have levels of certain nutritional components (protein content, total dietary fiber, acid detergent fiber and neutral detergent fiber) that lie far outside the range of normal corn, as determined by the OECD historical ranges. Conveniently, Monsanto selection of non-GM reference varieties used at each site included those that were also substantially outside the historical range for corn on precisely these values. For example, the OECD list says the value of TDF in corn is 11.1. The GM variety was nearly double that (20.77 ±2.48). The non-GM corn used for comparison, however, had a range from 12.58–35.31. Thus, the high level in the GM corn was not considered significantly different because the controls it was compared to were so unusual. INBI said, "This observation again leads us to question how the applicant came to choose specific lines for this study, and whether or not those reasons were consistent with a design to optimize the analysis of LY038 as a human food."[146]

To obtain these unusual reference numbers, Monsanto used rather non-traditional corn varieties as controls, including two that had undergone genetic mutation in order to become tolerant to the herbicide imidazoline and five that were designated as high extractable starch corn.

In addition, the primary control corn that Monsanto used to determine molecular and compositional equivalence was "a sibling of the modified corn line and itself a product of gene technology." INBI points out that the studies' conclusions "were flawed because the comparisons were to another GM plant" and would not "reveal unintended hazards." They wrote, "The 'control corn grain' for which a lysine level is reported ... is not a valid control. [The Codex Alimentarius Commission][147] does not allow another GM crop to serve as a control, because neither crop has a history of safe use."[148] FSANZ also specifies that controls have "a history of safe use for consumption as food,"[149] but accepted Monsanto's studies nonetheless. FSANZ had requested Monsanto to justify why it did not use a non-GMO parental variety as a control in its compositional analyses. According to INBI, "We could find no explanation of the applicant's response to FSANZ. We can only assume that the authority has chosen to exercise a standard that is lower than it could under [the Codex Alimentarius Commission]."[150]

It is a standard that the regulators may have gotten used to, as this critique by the Public Health Association of Australia on Monsanto's Roundup Ready corn demonstrates.

"The composition of the glyphosate-tolerant GE corn was compared to control plants that consisted of 'the population of non-transgenic negative segregants (that is, plants lacking the mEPSPS gene addition) present in untreated plots of transgenic GA21 corn.' It would therefore appear that the control plants were those plants that had undergone the 'particle acceleration transformation system' to try to make them into GA21 plants, but where the process appears to have failed. Can the ANZFA [Australia New Zealand Food Authority, the precursor to FSANZ] please provide details as to why these plants were chosen as controls as it is contended that a more suitable control would have been plants that had not been treated at all in this manner. This is because of the possibility that minor sequences of DNA may have been incorporated into parts of the genome of these plants which may not have been picked up, but which may nevertheless alter the concentrations of amino acids or fatty acids."[151]

Doug Gurian-Sherman   "Test-crop growth conditions . . . can have dramatic effects on crop composition values. . . . [Monsanto's study on a *Bt* corn] gathered composition data about corn grown in six geographic locations and provided statistical analyses, but it pooled data from the different locations, which could obscure possible growth-condition effects. [Another *Bt* corn submission] from the same company, did not disclose locations, pooled the composition data, and did not supply statistical analyses."[152]

Pusztai and Bardocz   "The parent and GM lines must be grown under identical conditions, treated, and harvested the same way. . . . Unfortunately, fulfilling this condition is the exception rather than the rule."

Regarding Roundup Ready corn:[153] [Researchers collected data] "from 16 field sites over two growing seasons," [concluding that the composition was] "comparable to the control line. The comparison however, was carried out by a statistical method similar to that for GTS soybean [below] which is scientifically flawed."

Regarding Roundup Ready soybeans: "The statistical method for comparing the GM and non-GM lines was flawed. Instead of comparing sufficiently large numbers of samples of each individual GTS with its appropriate individual parent line grown side-by-side at the same location and harvested at the same time to establish whether they were compositionally 'substantially equivalent,' what the authors compared was a large number of different samples from different locations and harvest times.[154] As growth conditions have a major influence on seed composition, the range of the amounts of constituents in the different samples was so great (±10% or more) that the chances of finding statistically significant differences were unreal. This is all the more curious, because in the authors' experiment 1 in Puerto Rico the conventional and the GTS lines were grown at the same site, but the results of their analyses on these soybean samples were not included in the publication."

[When an investigator recovered the missing Puerto Rico data from the archives of the *Journal of Nutrition*, it became obvious why keeping the data a secret was beneficial to the company.]

"The data showed that the GM soybean contained significantly less protein and the amino acid phenylalanine, amongst many other things, and therefore it could not have supported the growth of animals as well as the parent line. . . . In practically all heat-treated GM soybean samples from the Puerto Rico trial, the amounts of lectin and the trypsin inhibitors were significantly higher in the GM samples than in the isogenic line. Even more curiously, heat treatment appeared to have a far lesser denaturing effect on the trypsin inhibitor content of the GM lines than on the parent line samples. Although for some unexplained reason the values were from single assays on single samples (table 3), one of the GM lines (61-67-1) appeared to have almost seven times as much trypsin inhibitor per mg sample dry weight as the parent. Indeed, the values in this GM soybean approached that found in untoasted soybean seed samples. Even the other GM line (40-3-2) contained three times as much trypsin inhibitor as the non-GM line."[155]

Statistically significant findings are often dismissed (without evidence) as "not biologically significant" or "natural variation"

Pusztai and Bardocz	<u>Regarding Roundup Ready Soybeans</u>: "Although several significant differences between GM and control lines, such as in ash, fat and carbohydrate contents were found,[156] . . . these were not regarded to have biological significance by the authors."[157]
Bardocz and Pusztai	"Without actual work this [often-used phrase 'is unlikely to be biologically significant'] is only an opinion, and not a scientific statement."[158]
Public Health Association of Australia	<u>Regarding Roundup Ready canola</u>: "When statistically significant differences in compositional analyses were determined between the GE plant and its control, Monsanto did not follow-up these results with substantial further experimentation to determine why these differences occurred. Instead, such differences in composition tend to be dismissed as being within the natural variation of the plant. Such a statement ignores the evidence from the controls and the reason for having controls in the first place. Controls are used in order to provide a proper comparison with the experimental group under the conditions present at the time of the experiment. For example, the GE canola GT73 . . . was compared to a control that was its parental line in field trials, presumably so that any differences between these groups could be attributed to the genetic engineering, and not to differences in soil, air temperature, rainfall, fertilizer, etc. However, when this comparison yielded statistically significant differences, the GE canola was then compared to the 'Westar range,' a database housed in Canada, presumably from canola grown over a number of years from a number of sites. Doing this permits differences due to soil, climate, etc. to creep in again. Moreover, proof should be provided for the assertion that the differences were due to the natural variation of the plant. It is normally the role of such things as the statistical test, the standard error and the 95% confidence interval of the mean to provide a measure of this. It is also important that the sample size be big enough to obtain an accurate measure of these. "We therefore contend that it is unacceptable to dismiss significant differences between the GE plant and its control and instead to compare the GE results to a broader pool of data as if this pool is the new control. Similarly, we believe that it is unacceptable to compare the mean concentration of something (e.g. proline in GE canola GT73) with 'previously reported values' because the concentration of proline lies outside the ranges of both the control and the 'Westar range.' . . . In table 6, the document states that there is no nutritional or toxicological significance associated with these fatty acids. . . . The document also states that these raised levels are considered to 'reflect the natural variation within canola rather than any affect of the genetic modification on the canola line.' Please provide reasons for this assertion."[159]
Centre for Integrated Research on Biosafety	"Natural variability is not a baseline for analysis, despite what the applicant repeatedly claims.[160] Hazard identification is the baseline for analysis. Thus, minimizing non-specific variability should be the goal of a risk assessment. This is most reasonably done using the proper non-GMO parental lines as controls."[161]
Bardocz and Pusztai	"The only relevant scientific comparison is with the isogenic parent line!"[162]

Processing samples can rig the results

William Freese	<u>Regarding StarLink</u>: "Even the data that Aventis did submit are seriously flawed. For example, buried deep in its 170-page study on Cry9C protein levels in food products, one discovers a serious breach of standard operating procedure in the processing of Star-Link corn that was made into dry-milled corn products that were tested for their Cry9C content. Instead of the standard 30-minute heat treatment, this batch of StarLink was heated for two hours—four times as long—surely resulting in a much greater degree of Cry9C degradation than standard food processing procedures. Aventis does not explain this lapse, nor why the processing was not repeated with a new batch of corn heated for the proper period of time. Neither is any adequate explanation given for the two- to nine-fold differences between two similar assays used to measure levels of Cry9C in these same dry-milled food products."[163]
EPA Scientific Advisory Panel	<u>Regarding StarLink</u>: "The panel was concerned that the methodology used to determine the concentration of Cry9C protein may be an inadequate approach for estimating biologically active Cry9C protein in exposed humans. The extraction of Cry9C has not been optimized nor standardized, and the solubility of the protein has not been fully assessed. The extraction times reported in studies were of short duration, and may not reflect the total Cry9C protein content."[164]

Evaluating allergenicity is not guaranteed

Testing for allergens in GM crops is a problem. There are no tests to guarantee that a novel protein, introduced into the human diet for the first time, is not an allergen. You can't simply give the food to a large number of people as a test, because allergic responses typically develop after a person has had multiple exposures. The percentage of people who react may be quite small (but the impact may be life-threatening).

In 1992, the FDA policy stated, "At this time, FDA is unaware of any practical method to predict or assess the potential for new proteins in food to induce allergenicity and requests comments on this issue."[165] Seven years later, a *Washington Post* article observed that there was still "no widely accepted way to predict a new food's potential to cause an allergy. The FDA is now five years behind in its promise to develop guidelines for doing so. With no formal guidelines in place, it's largely up to the industry to decide whether and how to test for the allergy potential of new food."[166] But Carl B. Johnson, a scientist at the Additives Evaluation Branch of the FDA, had already dismissed this as a viable option. He wrote, "Are we asking the crop developer to prove that food from his crop is non-allergenic? This seems like an impossible task."[167] The US EPA Scientific Advisory Panel concluded that "Only surveillance and clinical assessment of exposed individuals will confirm the allergenicity."[168] Unfortunately, no such surveillance exists.

Washington Post   <u>Regarding StarLink corn contamination in the food chain</u>: "There is no surefire way of testing a new protein like Cry9C for its potential to cause allergies in people. . . . 'We all wish there was a test where you plug in a protein and out pops a "yes" or "no" answer,' said Sue MacIntosh, a protein chemist with AgrEvo. But there is no such test, short of giving it to a lot of people and seeing what happens.'"[169]

At best, current assessments only *reduce* the likelihood of reactions

While "proving" that a protein is not an allergen remains impossible, the FAO/WHO and others[170] recommend a decision-tree screening process to minimize the likelihood that an allergenic GM crop gets approved. The procedure involves examining the transgenic protein for physical characteristics that are common to known allergens. According to *Biotechnology and Genetic Engineering Reviews*, "Three of these characteristics are amino acid sequence homology [similarity] to a known allergen, digestive stability, and heat stability. While none of these features is *predictive* of allergenicity, their presence (especially in combination) is regarded as sufficient evidence to reject the pertinent GE crop, or at least trigger additional testing, depending on the protocol."[171] But there are many ways in which GM crops with an allergenic protein might pass these tests.

Evaluating only the GM protein misses other allergens in GM crops

Part 1 of this book described several ways in which natural genes in the host genome can be altered by the GM transformation process. Naturally occurring allergens might increase and new allergens may be produced. The decision-tree allergenicity screening, however, focuses solely on the transgenic protein; it does not even look for these other potential allergens.

Protein stability tests are not reliable indicators

Transgenic proteins are put into test tubes with simulated gastric fluid (SGF), including digestive enzymes (e.g. pepsin) and acid, to measure how quickly they are broken down. This test is based on the theory that allergenic proteins often—but not always—break down slowly in the stomach and intestines. Since a protein that is broken down quickly may still cause allergies, potentially harmful allergenic proteins *can* pass this test.

In addition, the simulated gastric fluid is supposed to combine acid and enzymes to approximate average adult stomach conditions during digestion. While the FAO/WHO recommends a pH of 2.0, a person's actual acid level varies with age, the type and quantity of food consumed, illness and medicine. Infants, for example, have a higher (less acidic) pH of 3–4. Millions of adults take antacids and acid inhibitors—and there is a medical condition (achlorhydria) where the pH won't go below 4.0. Thus, even if the test accurately predicted protein stability for the average adult, it would fail to do so for a significant percentage of the population.

Test tube studies do not accurately predict what happens in the human gut

| Pusztai and Bardocz | "The results of such *in vitro* digestion assays . . . can be misleading because the interactions between the digesta and the gut wall and its enzymes, which can greatly influence the stability or degradation of the components of the diet, are absent in the test tube."[172] |

These studies cannot accurately distinguish between known allergens and non-allergens

| Centre for Integrated Research on Biosafety | "The authority has argued that 'most food allergens tend to be stable to the peptic and acidic conditions of the digestive system if they are to reach and pass through the intestinal mucosa to elicit an allergic response,' citing dated literature on the topic (1996–1999). More recent studies have undermined the generality of the statement that allergens are more stable. 'Food allergens were not necessarily more resistant to SGF [simulated gastric fluid] and SIF [simulated intestinal fluid] digestion than nonallergenic proteins of similar cellular functions.'"[173,174] |

GM proteins that break down quickly in test tubes survive much longer in the digestive system, further invalidating test conclusions

| Pusztai and Bardocz | Regarding mice study with *Bt*-toxin and *Bt* potato (section 1.4): "This was an important study because once and for all it established that, in contrast to general belief, exposure of the mouse gut (ileum) to the CryI gene product caused profound hypertrophic and hyperplastic changes in the cells of the gut absorptive epithelium and these could lead to mucosal sensitization, as was later demonstrated.[175] These changes could only have occurred because, in contrast to the artificial stability shown in the *in vitro* simulated gut proteolysis tests, the *Bt*-toxin did in fact survive, in a biologically active form, the passage through the digestive tract."[176] |

| European Commission | "The 'sound scientific evidence'. . . consists only on checking protein homologies with existing allergens and a study of the isolated purified transgene product in a simulated gastric fluid. Based on this, *Bt* proteins are degraded within minutes. However, today we know that when embedded within transgenic plant material *Bt*-proteins can pass even through the intestinal tract of cows."[177] |

Scientists test proteins made from bacteria, not from actual GM crops

Bardocz and Pusztai	"Because recombinant proteins expressed in *E. coli* or in the GM plants can be different, the use of *E. coli* surrogates or other microbial recombinant protein in digestibility studies is scientifically invalid."[178]

Some tests use proteins with different amino acids

Doug Gurian-Sherman	"Safety tests, such as for allergencity, used forms of the protein that may differ from the GE protein found in the transgenic plant. . . . SGD assays should be performed using the form of the protein found in the transgenic plant, because even minor alterations may change one or more of the properties of the protein. In tests reported in [the submission], instead of testing SAMase [the GM protein] itself, a SAMase fusion protein was used in digestive and heat-stability assays. A fusion protein is a single protein produced from a hybrid gene that joins two otherwise separate proteins. [The GM crop submitted], however, does not contain the fusion protein. It is possible that the fusion could have reduced the stability of the SAMase portion of the protein by altering its structure in the combined protein. FDA did not comment on any aspect of the allergenicity assessment of [the submission]."[179]

Companies fail to test proteins after cooking and processing, which might *increase* allergenicity

Centre for Integrated Research on Biosafety	"The Applicant should report digestibility measurements after processing/cooking of material from whole food. . . . The very latest research indicates that some allergens are attenuated or removed by heat or during processing, but other allergens become more potent as a result of heating and in the presence of carbohydrates.[180] These can only be identified using food prepared in a fashion representative of how people will consume it."[181]
Journal of Agricultural and Food Chemistry	"In contrast to these so-called pollen-related allergens, roasting has been reported to increase the allergenicity of raw peanuts. For example, protein extracts of thermally treated peanuts have been shown to bind IgE antibodies from patients' sera at up to ninetyfold higher levels than extracts obtained from the corresponding nontreated peanuts. In addition, inhibitory ELISA experiments revealed a significant increase in the IgE binding activity of the purified major allergens Ara h 1 and Ara h 2 after thermal treatment in the presence of carbohydrates."[182]

Companies use stronger pH and more enzymes, to breakdown the GM protein more quickly

The speed of protein breakdown is largely influenced by how strong the acid is and how much digestive enzymes are present. One study demonstrated, for example, that, the stability of the major egg allergen ovalbumin changed from greater than 120 min to 0 min as the ratio of pepsin to test protein (by weight) increased from 0.1 to 100."[183] Doug Gurian-Sherman writes, "a common plant protein that was rapidly digested at one ratio was stable when the pepsin concentration was reduced one-hundredfold.[184] Several recent studies also show that the stability of some known allergens can be reduced or eliminated when the relative pepsin concentration is increased.[185] In particular, some GE proteins that would be stable, and would be considered potential allergens, if tested, according to Metcalfe et al., may be unstable at relatively high pepsin (or low GE protein) concentrations, and would pass the SGD assay. Therefore, using inappropriate concentrations of pepsin and the GE protein can potentially give misleading results."[186]

William Freese	"Monsanto's digestive stability test on Cry1Ab employed highly acidic conditions (pH 1.2) and a huge excess of pepsin relative to test protein—conditions that favor the most rapid possible digestion.[187] Thus, it's no surprise that Monsanto's results (over 90% degradation in just two minutes) vary by a factor of 60 from those of Hubert Noteborn.[188] Dr. Noteborn found that 10% of Cry1Ab survived for one to two hours, not two minutes. Under the authoritative allergenicity testing protocol recommended by international experts at FAO/WHO and accepted widely by national regulators outside the United States, Cry1Ab would show itself to be still more stable than in Noteborn's test."[189]
Freese and Schubert	**"Industry procedures used to measure digestive stability frequently employ highly acidic conditions and a very large excess of pepsin relative to test protein—conditions that favor the most rapid possible digestion.[190]** Under the authoritative allergenicity testing protocol recommended by international experts at FAO/WHO, digestive stability tests are to be carried out at a higher pH (2.0) and in SGF with a ratio of test protein to pepsin over three orders of magnitude greater than the conditions used by some.[191]"
Centre for Integrated Research on Biosafety	**"The applicant has used 2000 times the amount of pepsin by weight recommended in the FAO/WHO protocol."[192]**
Doug Gurian-Sherman	"Several papers examining food-protein digestibility that were published prior to [submission] BNF-01 and BNF-02 used pepsin-to-food-protein ratios thousands of times lower than in either FDA submission.[193] The basis for using the relative concentrations of pepsin to test proteins in BNF-01 and BNF-02 could not be evaluated by FDA because the methodology was not provided in the data summary. Had the relative concentrations of pepsin to CP4 EPSPS [Roundup Ready protein for soybeans] or ACCd [delayed ripening protein for tomatoes] been disclosed in BNF-01 or BNF-02, as would be the case in a full description of methodology, FDA may have had concerns about the allergenicity of the engineered proteins."[194]

Less sensitive measurement methods can lead to false conclusions

Doug Gurian-Sherman	"Antibodies are often used to detect digestion-resistant food-allergen proteins or fragments remaining after SGD, and several different types of antibodies that differ in their ability to detect the protein can be used. Polyclonal antibodies, which can typically detect several distinct sites, or epitopes, on a food-allergen protein are most appropriate because they may detect stable protein fragments that often result from the SGD tests. By contrast, monoclonal antibodies can detect only one type of epitope on the GE protein, and would not detect a digestion-resistant fragment that does not include that epitope. Monoclonal antibodies were used to detect SAMase during the SGD assays in [the submission]. Therefore, the detection method used in [the submission] could have missed a digestion-resistant SAMase fragment. . . . "Resistance to degradation in assays simulating the human stomach was the primary reason that the GE protein in StarLink corn was not approved for human consumption. Entire food allergen proteins, or large fragments of them, remained undigested in SGD

assays for at least two minutes.[195] In the . . . SAMase SGD assay, the first measurement was not made until five minutes, which would not have detected resistance to digestion at between two and five minutes."[196]

Comparing amino acid sequences to known allergens will not identify many potential allergens

Comparing the protein's sequence with amino acids from known allergens is done in two ways. The first, as recommended by FAO/WHO, is to look at the sequence of 80 or more amino acids and determine if "there is more than 35% identity."[197] The second method looks for an exact match of sequences of six or more contiguous amino acids. They specifically look at sections (epitopes) from known allergens, where the immune system's Immunoglobulin E (IgE) antibodies are known to attach. There are several shortcomings to this approach.

1. Not all epitopes have been identified.
2. The databases used by companies do not even encompass all the known epitopes.
3. Epitopes with less than six amino acids can bind with IgE, but biotech companies reject even the criteria of six as too likely to give false positive. Some use eight.
4. Epitopes are for allergic reactions which involve IgE. Not all allergies are IgE-related.
5. Since proteins fold, IgE usually attaches to amino acids that end up next to each other only after the fold. The database comparisons, however, identify only sequences that are contiguous *before* folding.
6. The criterion of 35% similarity over 80 amino acids is somewhat arbitrary.

Bardocz and Pusztai	"Using databases to establish the lack of allergenicity from the lack of sequence identity of eight consecutive amino acids in the GM protein and a known allergen is not sufficient. . . . Occasionally six or even less amino acid identity is enough to evoke allergic reactions. . . . Present databases are not sufficiently large or inclusive to contain all toxins and allergens. . . . Allergic reaction is to an epitope (a steric structure) on the allergen which, in most cases, is made up of non-consecutive amino acids."[198]
Centre for Integrated Research on Biosafety	"The FAO/WHO[199] suggests a procedure where: a complete set of 80 amino-acids derived from the expressed protein is prepared and then compared to the allergen or toxin database; a search for identity over six contiguous amino acids is performed. The applicant used a search over eight contiguous amino acids, saying that "the results demonstrated that searches with six or seven amino acid windows led to high rates of false positive matches."[200] . . . For allergen identification, we are more concerned with false negatives than false positives. Thus we ask the authority to review the bioinformatics data using the parameters set by FAO/WHO. The applicant has provided three references in defense of this claim, all produced by the applicant and Novartis, another GMO producer. However, six contiguous amino acids is the standard for the research on protein epitopes. If too many false positives are found, it is possible to apply "filters" (as explained in Kleter and Peijnenburg)[201] that will distinguish between false and true positives."[202]

Regulators have ignored evidence that some *Bt* crops fail the three allergenicity tests and may cause allergies

Freese and Schubert

"While the EPA [which regulates the pesticide portion of *Bt* crops] ostensibly 'requires' data on these three parameters [sequence homology to a known allergen, digestive stability, and heat stability] for all *Bt* crop proteins 'to provide a reasonable certainty that no harm will result from the aggregate exposure' to them,[203] in practice it has simply not collected pertinent studies, accepted substandard ones, or ignored relevant evidence.

"For instance, the EPA apparently did not make use of a study by FDA scientist Steven Gendel that demonstrated sequence homology between several Cry proteins and known food allergens. . . . Gendel found that Cry3A (*Bt* potatoes) and β-lactoglobulin, a milk allergen, shared sequences 7–10 amino acids in length. He also identified sequences of 9–12 amino acids shared by Cry1Ab (*Bt* corn) and vitellogenin, an egg yolk allergen. Gendel concluded that: '. . . the similarity between Cry1A(b) and vitellogenin might be sufficient to warrant additional evaluation.'[204] The EPA knew about this study because it had been discussed by its scientific advisers.[205] But the agency re-registered *Bt* corn for seven years in 2001 without discussing or even citing Gendel's study in its review document, with no corresponding study on file from Syngenta, and only incomplete data from Monsanto.[206]. . .

"Two digestive stability studies on Cry1Ab, the GE toxin found in *Bt* corn, by Hubert Noteborn established that: 1) After 30–180 minutes in simulated gastric fluid (SGF), 9–21% of Cry1Ab remains undigested; 2) After 2 hours in SGF, Cry1Ab degrades only to fragments of substantial size at the low end of the range considered typical of food allergens (15 kilodaltons); and 3) Cry1Ab is substantially more resistant to digestion than four other transgenic proteins tested, including one other Cry protein, Cry3A. Of the six proteins Noteborn tested, only StarLink corn's Cry9C exhibited greater digestive stability."[207] . . .

"Noteborn also found that Cry1Ab possessed 'relatively significant thermostability . . . comparable to that of the Lys mutant Cry9C protein' found in StarLink corn.[208] Noteborn found that Cry9C was stable for 120 minutes at 90° C, but gives no further information on Cry1Ab's heat stability. The EPA failed to collect any heat stability study from Monsanto on MON 810."[209,210]

William Freese

"Regulators have failed to collect *any* studies on some of these important [protein properties] parameters in the case of most *Bt* crops. . . . The EPA failed to collect any amino acid homology studies from Monsanto prior to the product's original registration in 1996, or even upon its re-registration in 2001."[211]

The most common varieties of *Bt* corn either raise red flags or have been inadequately evaluated

Summary of Available Data for Human Health Assessment

Company Crop *Bt* protein	Digestive Stability	Heat Stability	Amino Acid Sequence Homology
Monsanto Yieldgard Corn Cry1Ab	**RED FLAG** Digestive stability similar to (though lesser than) that of StarLink Cry9C (1)	**RED FLAG** Heat stability comparable to that of StarLink Cry9C (2)	**RED FLAG** Matches found with vitellogenin, an egg yolk allergen, over 9–12 amino acid-length subsequences (3)
Syngenta *Bt* 11 Corn Cry1Ab	**RED FLAG** Digestive stability similar to (though lesser than) that of StarLink Cry9C (1)	**RED FLAG** Heat stability comparable to that of StarLink Cry9C (2)	**RED FLAG** Matches found with vitellogenin, an egg yolk allergen, over 9–12 amino acid-length subsequences (3)
Monsanto BollGard Cotton Cry1Ab/Ac	**INADEQUATE** Flawed study shows degradation in 2–7 minutes (4)	**INADEQUATE** Only shown to be "inactive" in processing study (5)	**RED FLAG** Cry1Ab/Ac has the same vitellogenin-matching subsequences as Cry1Ab in the pertinent region (3, 6)
Mycogen & Pioneer Herculex Corn Cry1F	**INADEQUATE** Test conditions not specified by EPA (7)	**INADEQUATE** Only shown to be "inactive" in bioassay after 30 min. at 75° & 90°C (5)	**OK** Though more stringent test would be desirable (8)
Monsanto NewLeaf Potato Cry3A	**INADEQUATE** Test conditions not specified by EPA (7)	**NONE** (9)	**RED FLAG** Amino acid sequences found in which 7–10 matched β-lactoglobulin, a milk allergen (10)

This table is excerpted from a study by Friends of the Earth. Original citations and notes from this table are reproduced after the Endnotes.

Regulators do not acknowledge evidence that their test methods are faulty

Based on the test tube studies, the EPA operates on the assumption that *Bt*-toxin is destroyed in the stomach. In fact the primary reason that StarLink *Bt* corn was not approved for human consumption was that Cry9C might survive digestion in the stomach. When mice were fed *Bt* potatoes,[212] the study confirmed that a natural *Bt* variety *did* survive past the stomach and caused cell damage in the lower part of the small intestines. Even though this invalidated their test methods and showed that the risk of *Bt* causing allergic reactions was far greater than they believed, the EPA did not change the status of the approved *Bt*s, did not initiate additional studies and continues to rely on their test tube methods.

Regulators ignore recommendations for updating their methods

US National Research Council	"Priority should be given to the development of improved methods for identifying potential allergens in pest-protected plants, specifically, the development of tests with human immune-system endpoints and of more reliable animal models."[213]
Bardocz and Pusztai	"For allergenicity testing, in addition to the decision-tree approach, in vivo immune-tests are needed, such as anti-gene product antibody tests (humans and animals) and immunization model studies (Brown Norway rats, etc.)"[214]
EPA's Scientific Advisory Panel Report	"The importance of this [Bernstein's] report is that reagents are available that could be used for reliable skin testing and serological evaluation of *Bt* protein-exposed individuals."[215] (The EPA ignored this recommendation and has not used this method of evaluating potential allergenicity using human subjects.)
Pew Study	<u>Regarding allergy tests in the United States and their relevance for GM foods:</u> "A number of important areas of scientific investigation are either not being addressed or are receiving very limited federal attention. The authors conclude that current federal efforts are insufficient to provide the timely and comprehensive information needed by food safety regulators. . . . The majority of studies underway focus on foods that have traditionally caused food allergy (nuts and milk), while there is almost no work exploring the allergenicity of novel proteins in food. . . . No studies examine the dose response or exposure assessment information needed for setting 'safe' levels for new proteins produced by biotechnology. Efforts to develop animal models or in vitro tests for food allergy are extremely limited in this sample. Furthermore, the studies on identifying and characterizing susceptible subpopulations are insufficient, particularly as epidemiological studies are not well represented in this sample. Finally, there is little research on identification and characterization of new allergens or the molecular determinants of food allergy."[216]
Doug Gurian-Sherman	"Allergenicity testing was not always performed using the best tests available."[217]

Case Study: The blood test on StarLink's protein was flawed

Just five weeks after the FDA/CDC declared StarLink safe, based on the blood tests, advisers to the EPA—including some of the nation's leading food allergists—released a thorough critique of the FDA's allergy test and other aspects of the StarLink investigation. Their conclusion? "The test, as conducted, does not eliminate StarLink Cry9C as a potential cause of allergic symptoms."[218] They said the research had many shortcomings. For example, the test lacked adequate controls, was not sensitive enough and failed to follow standard protocols that helped prevent false interpretations.

The researchers used as their control group twenty-one blood samples that had been frozen since before 1996—before its donors could have been exposed to StarLink and developed an antibody reaction. This control blood served as the baseline; in order for StarLink to be considered allergenic, reactions to Cry9C by the blood of the 17 people who had suffered allergic responses to corn needed to be at least 2.5 times greater than the reactions by the control blood. But when tested, reactions in the previously frozen control blood varied widely and were not reproducible. Moreover, the control blood reacted far more to the Cry9C than did the blood from the allergic group. No one knew why this happened but, according to [biochemist Masaharu Kawata], the "CDC, after apparent brain racking, came up with an excuse that the blood serum, [which] had been freeze preserved . . . could be different from that of fresh blood samples."[219] Kawata says that this obviously should have disqualified the controls. But researchers stuck by their quirky frozen blood, and since it reacted more to Cry9C than the test groups, StarLink was off the hook. In the end, after careful analysis of all the available data, however, the EPA's Scientific Advisory Panel upheld their original assessment that there is a medium likelihood that StarLink was an allergen.[220]

Case Study: Irregularities marred evaluations of Monsanto's GM drug, recombinant bovine growth hormone (rbGH)

Several claims made by FDA scientists in defense of rbGH have not held up under scrutiny. For example, they said that bovine growth hormone does not increase substantially in milk from treated cows. The study they cited, however, shows a 26% increase in the hormone. Furthermore, those researchers injected cows with only a 10.6 mg daily dose of rbGH compared to the normal 500 mg bi-weekly dose used by farmers. In fact, they didn't even use Monsanto's rbGH, but rather another version that was never approved. They then pasteurized the milk 120 times longer than normal in an apparent attempt to show that the hormone was destroyed during the process. They only destroyed 19% of the hormone. They then spiked the milk with powdered hormone—146 times the naturally occurring levels—heated that 120 times longer than normal, and were then able to destroy 90% of the hormone.[221] FDA scientists reported that 90% of the hormone was destroyed during pasteurization.[222]

Documents revealed that in order to show that rbGH injections did not interfere with fertility, industry researchers allegedly added cows to the study that were pregnant prior to injection.[223]

FDA Veterinarian Richard Burroughs described how industry researchers would often drop sick cows from studies, to make the drug appear safer. When Burroughs ordered more tests than the industry wanted, he was told by superiors he was slowing down the approval and was fired. The remaining whistle-blowers in the FDA had to write an anonymous letter to Congress, complaining of fraud and conflict of interest in the agency. They described one FDA scientist, Margaret Miller, who arbitrarily increased the allowable levels of antibiotics in milk one-hundredfold. This was necessary before approving rbGH. Since the drug increases the chance of udder infections, farmers inject cows with more antibiotics. This leads to a higher risk of antibiotic resistant diseases in cows and humans. Miller had formerly conducted research on rbGH while with Monsanto and then moved into the FDA department that evaluated her own research.

In 1998, six Canadian government scientists testified before the Senate that they were being pressured by superiors to approve rbGH, even though they believed it was unsafe for the public. Their detailed critique of the FDA's evaluation of the drug showed how the US approval process was flawed and superficial. They also testified that documents were stolen from a locked file cabinet in a government office and that Monsanto offered them a bribe of $1–$2 million to approve the drug without further tests. (A Monsanto representative went on national Canadian television claiming that the scientists had obviously misunderstood an offer for research money.) The Canadian scientists later described how their superiors retaliated against them for testifying. They were passed over for promotions, given impossible tasks or no assignments at all, one was suspended without pay. Three of the whistleblowers, who also spoke out on such controversial topics as mad cow disease, were ultimately fired on July 14, 2004.[224]

Canadian GM food approvals are assumption-based

According to crop physiologist E. Ann Clark, "People who assume that there is actual testing, and more specifically, actual testing involving actual grain from transgenic crops, will be amazed to learn that risk assessment of GM crops is largely heuristic or assumptions-based, as is disturbingly clear from the summary statements that accompany Health Canada's assessment of GM submissions." The organization Common Ground says, "The Canadian GM regulatory process is a ruse, claiming to safeguard human and environmental health, but actually intended to facilitate commercialization of GM crops."[225] A review of some GM crop approvals demonstrates the dangers of assumption-based regulations.[226]

Monsanto Canada's insect resistant corn, MON 810

As part of this variety's 1997 approval, documents from Health Canada state:

1. "The human safety assessment of the CryIA(b) protein was confirmed in experiments, which included protein characterization, digestive fate in simulated gastric and intestinal fluids, and acute oral toxicity in mice. Data were generated that demonstrated that the active CryIA(b) protein product in MON 810 was equivalent to that produced in the naturally occurring B.T.K."

This statement is incorrect. In reality, the transgene was truncated during insertion and the final protein combines amino acids coded by the transgene and host DNA (see section 4.2).

2. "The CryIA(b) protein is rapidly degraded and its insecticidal activity lost under conditions that simulate mammalian digestion."

In reality, the stability of the protein is comparable to StarLink corn, banned for human use (see *Bt* protein chart, page 228). In addition, the loss of insecticidal activity is not necessarily a guarantee that the protein will not be allergenic, as demonstrated by GM peas (see section 1.18). And the test tube studies don't accurately simulate mammalian digestion (see part 3).

3. "There was no indication of toxicity as measured by treatment-related adverse effects in mice administered CryIA(b) protein by oral gavage."

Only a bacteria-derived protein was fed to mice. No studies fed the actual corn to animals.

4. "The introduced protein was compared to databases of known protein toxins and did not show any meaningful amino acid sequence similarity to known protein toxins, with the exception of other *Bacillus thuringiensis* (*Bt*) proteins. The studies support the safety of the CryIA(b) protein and are consistent with the history of safe use of *Bt* and CryIA(b), which has been demonstrated to be highly selective for insects, with no activity against other organisms such as mammals, fish, birds, or invertebrates (US EPA, 1988)."

In reality, mammal studies show *Bt* to be bioactive, and humans react to *Bt* spray (see section 3.3).

5. "The introduced CryIA(b) protein was compared to known allergens. Using sophisticated computerized search capabilities, the evidence showed that the CryIA(b) protein did not show meaningful amino acid sequence homology to known allergens."

In reality, matches were found in another study with vitellogenin, an egg yolk allergen, over 9-12 amino acid-length sequences (see *Bt* protein chart, page 228).

Monsanto Canada's Roundup Ready cotton (Line 1445)

This variety was approved without reference to any scientific analysis whatsoever. They wrote: "Health Canada's review of the information presented in support of the food use of refined oil from cotton line 1445 concluded that this refined oil does not raise concerns related to safety. Health Canada is of the opinion that refined oil from cotton line 1445 is as safe and nutritious as cottonseed oil from current commercial cotton varieties."

Monsanto Canada's Roundup Ready Canola (GT73)

This variety, as well as other canola and cotton crops, were approved without tests. Health Canada wrote: "Since only the processed oil from transgenic GT73, or lines derived therefrom, will be available for human consumption and the processing removes proteinaceous material, there are no additional toxicity or allergenicity concerns with this product."

In reality, some cold pressed oils may contain GM protein and a fat soluble toxin produced from the GM transformation process may be found in the oil. In addition, the non-oil portion is fed to animals and may influence human health through milk and meat.

Monsanto Canada's NewLeaf-Y potatoes (Shepody)

This variety was approved without any animal testing whatsoever. Health Canada offered the following assumptions instead. "Amino acid sequence of the CryIIIA protein . . . closely related to the sequence of the same proteins that are present in strains of *B. thuringiensis* . . . used for over 30 years . . . did not show homologies with known mammalian protein toxins...not judged to have any potential for human toxicity . . . history of known safe consumption." As for allergenicity, "The Cry3A protein and PLRV replicase do not possess characteristics typical of known protein allergens...no regions of homology to amino acid sequences of known protein allergens . . . the Cry3A protein is rapidly degraded by acid and/or enzymatic hydrolysis when exposed to simulated gastric or intestinal fluids . . . extremely unlikely to be allergenic."

In reality, another study identified 7–10 amino acid sequence matches with β-lactoglobulin, a milk allergen (see *Bt* protein chart, page 228).

Calgene's FlavrSavr tomato

Health Canada used just a few nutritional comparisons and assumption-bases assessments to declare that "this novel variety does not raise concerns related to human food safety."

They did not mention the feeding study submitted by Calgene to the FDA that described stomach lesions and deaths among the subjects (see section 1.2).

Chart of several safety-related assumptions that have been proven wrong

"The science upon which current GM experiments are based, as stated or assumed by the experimenters, is in many places wrong."[227] —Robert Mann, biochemist

Assumption	Actual Status	Quote
Inserted genes will produce a single protein.	Inserted foreign genes might create multiple proteins, with unpredictable consequences.	"The fact that one gene can give rise to multiple proteins…destroys the theoretical foundation of a multibillion-dollar industry, the genetic engineering of food crops." Barry Commoner, biologist, Center for the Biology of Natural Systems at Queens College
The proteins created by inserted genes will act exactly the same way in a new organism.	Foreign proteins may be folded improperly or become attached to other molecules, which could change their properties. Likewise, gene expression may be affected by the genetic disposition of a host organism, or even the environment.	"An incorrectly folded form of an ordinary cellular protein can under certain circumstances … [duplicate itself] and give rise to infectious neurological disease." Peter Wills of Auckland University [The effect of a protein on a plant or animal] "can be modified by the addition of molecules such as phosphate, sulfate, sugars, or lipids." David Schubert, molecular biologist and protein chemist, The Salk Institute for Biological Studies
Inserting foreign genes is precise and non-disruptive.	The process of inserting foreign genes can damage the structure and function of the host's DNA, switch genes on or off, create never-before-seen genetic sequences and render the genome unstable.	"Genetic engineering is generally a hit and miss affair. The genes may be inserted the wrong way round or multiple copies may be scattered throughout a plant's genome. They may be inserted inside other genes—destroying their activity or massively increasing it. More worryingly, a plant's genetic make-up may become unstable. . . . Rogue toxins may be produced or existing ones amplified massively. Such problems may only arise hundreds of generations after the crops are originally modified." BBC's *Tomorrow's World Magazine*
Foreign genes will not transfer to bacteria in the digestive system. Therefore, use of antibiotic resistant genes is safe.	Roundup Reaady transgenic sequences transferred into human gut bacteria and appeared stably integrated.	"British scientific researchers have demonstrated for the first time that genetically modified DNA material from crops is finding its way into human gut bacteria, raising potentially serious health questions." *The Guardian* "IT WOULD BE A SERIOUS HEALTH HAZARD TO INTRODUCE A GENE THAT CODES FOR ANTIBIOTIC RESISTANCE INTO THE NORMAL FLORA OF THE GENERAL POPULATION." Murray Lumpkin, former director the FDA's Division of Anti-infective Drug Products

Assumption	Actual Status	Quote
The promoter that keeps foreign genes switched on only influences that one gene.	The promoter may turn on native genes. This can create a flood of proteins with unpredictable consequences. Some scientists theorize that the promoter might even switch on dormant viruses that are deposited along the DNA.	"When inserted into another organism as part of a 'genetic construct,' it [the promoter] may also change the gene expression patterns in the recipient chromosome(s) over long distances up- and downstream from the insertion site." Michael Hansen, Consumers Union, publishers of Consumer Reports "Horizontal transfer of the CaMV promoter . . . has the potential to reactivate dormant viruses or [create] new viruses in all species to which it is transferred." Ho, Ryan, and Cummins in, "Cauliflower Mosaic Viral Promoter—A Recipe for Disaster"
The promoter is stable.	Studies indicate that the promoter may create a "hotspot" in the DNA, whereby the whole DNA section, or chromosome, can become unstable. This can cause breaks in the strand or exchanges of genes with other chromosomes.	[A promoter can have] "the same impact as a heavy dose of gamma radiation." Joe Cummins, geneticist
The promoter only works with plant organisms.[228]	Research indicates that the promoter can influence human and animal genes. Some scientists believe it can transfer to internal organs and accelerate cell growth, possibly leading to cancer.	"It is possible GM DNA could affect stomach and colonic lining by causing a growth factor effect with the unproven possibility of hastening cancer formation in those organs." Stanley Ewen, histopathologist
Nutritional properties are unaffected by genetic modification.	Significant differences in nutritional content between GM crops and their natural counterparts have been observed.	"Roundup Ready beans were significantly lower in protein and the amino acid phenylalanine. More disturbing were [increased] levels of the allergen trypsin inhibitor in toasted Roundup Ready meal. . . . Lectins in Roundup Ready beans almost doubled the levels in controls."[229] Barbara Keeler, on data that had been omitted from Monsanto's published study
Genes and their expression will act in isolation, not impacting other metabolic processes.	Insertion of foreign genes and their new proteins may create complex, unpredictable interactions, not well understood. Similarly, inserting two or more foreign genes into the same plant may also cause interactions that have not been studied.	"When you insert a foreign gene, you are changing the whole metabolic process . . . Each change is going to have an effect on other pathways. Will any one gene kick off a whole slew of changes? We don't know for sure."[230] Sharad Phatak, University of Georgia "Genetic engineering results in the formation of higher than normal concentrations of certain enzymes and products; these could provide the basis for the synthesis of higher levels of toxic substances."[231] Charles Yanofsky, Stanford

Assumption	Actual Status	Quote
There is no risk from breathing pollen from GM crops.	Inhalation of pollen may cause unpredicted health problems. Transfer of genes from inhaled pollen may also be possible.	"Experts on the Government's Advisory Committee on Novel Foods and Processes have issued a warning about plants being grown in the United States and parts of Europe which contain a gene resistant to antibiotics. They are concerned that, if workers breathe in dust as the crops are processed, the resistance could be transferred to bacteria in their throats."[232] *Daily Mail* "Many if not all of the villagers exposed to GM-maize pollen in 2003 have remained ill. . . . 31 signed a petition circulated by a member of the Parish Social Action Center, claiming they fell ill during the flowering period. . . . Around 20 children (aged 5–10 years) got sick during the flowering period."[233] Mae-Wan Ho, biophysicist and geneticist
The chances of GM crops being allergenic are minimal.	After GM soy was introduced into the UK, soy allergies sky-rocketed 50%. Current GM corn would not pass tests recommended by FAO/WHO for potential allergenicity. The EPA's Scientific Advisory Panel determined that GM protein in StarLink corn has a "medium likelihood" of being an allergen.	The FDA's 1992 policy states, "At this time, FDA is unaware of any practical method to predict or assess the potential for new proteins in food to induce allergenicity and requests comments on this issue." FDA scientist Carl Johnson wrote, "Are we asking the crop developer to prove that food from his crop is non-allergenic? This seems like an impossible task." According to FDA microbiologist Louis Pribyl, "the only definitive test for allergies is human consumption by affected peoples, which can have ethical considerations."
The same transgene produces the same protein whether in a GM plant or *E. coli*.	Different organisms process genetic information and synthesize proteins differently.	"DNA is only coding for the amino acid sequence but not necessarily for the conformation, function and biological activity of the protein."[234] Susan Bardocz and Arpad Pusztai, GMO safety assessment experts
If the amino acid sequences in the active (working) site of a GM protein is the same as those in a non-GM protein, that proves the two are the same.	There are proteins with identical (active site) sequences that differ in other amino acids, and as a result, function differently.	"The identity of a small part of the amino acid sequence of two proteins does not necessarily show the identity of the rest or that their conformation and stability are the same."[235] Susan Bardocz and Arpad Pusztai
Substitution of one amino acid by another does not alter the protein structure.	One amino acid can alter both the structure and the function of a protein, especially if the change occurs at the active site of an enzyme.	"Without stability and conformational studies this is just an unsupported opinion."[236] Susan Bardocz and Arpad Pusztai

Assumption	Actual Status	Quote
Transgenes are stable.	The actual transgene sequences of several GM crops differ from that which was registered by the company.	"In a recent study on five commercially approved transgenic lines carried out by two French laboratories, all five transgenic inserts were found to have rearranged, not just from the construct used in transformation, but also from the original structure reported by the company. This was clear evidence that all the lines were genetically unstable."[238] Mae-Wan Ho
Food processing destroys DNA.[237]	Several types of food processing leave substantial amounts of DNA intact.	"Food that comes from a GM crop, such as maize, can be processed, for example into flour, and the GM DNA is still present in the food and can be identified."[239] Food Standards Agency, UK
Since cooking denatures proteins, no additional allergy tests are necessary on cooked or processed proteins.	In some cases cooking does not destroy allergenicity but rather makes proteins more allergenic.	"The very latest research indicates that some allergens are attenuated or removed by heat or during processing, but other allergens become more potent as a result of heating and in the presence of carbohydrates.[240] These can only be identified using food prepared in a fashion representative of how people will consume it."[241] The Centre for Integrated Research on Biosafety
If cooked pesticidal proteins such as Bt no longer function as a pesticide, they no longer can cause allergic reactions.	The loss of pesticidal properties does not insure the loss of allergenic properties.	"The GM peas were boiled for 20 minutes. After cooking, the alpha-amylase inhibitor was denatured and was no longer effective in protecting against weevils. Industry assumptions notwithstanding, the cooked pea protein still caused an immune response in mice."[242] Jeffrey M. Smith
RNA is harmless.	RNA can impact gene expression, even in subsequent generations.	"Some small RNA molecules can be transmitted through food, causing lasting, sometimes heritable, effects on consumers and their children."[243] New Zealand Institute for Gene Ecology
The NOS terminator will end the "reading" of the transgene.	In Roundup Ready soybeans, the NOS terminator was ineffective in ending transcription, and may have helped process the RNA into four variants.	"The NOS terminator signal of transcription introduced into the genome in [Roundup Ready soy] is (at least in part) ignored, resulting in the production of an over-length transcript. Furthermore, this transcript was found to be processed . . . resulting in the production of different RNA variants. . . . Since the NOS terminator was introduced as regulatory region in several other GMOs, read-through products and RNA variants might be transcribed in these transgenic crops as well."[244] Andreas Rang, et al, *European Food Research and Technology*

False assumptions that viral genes in disease-resistant crops won't recombine to create new viruses

The insertion of viral transgenes into GM crops carries a significant risk. The transgenes may recombine with natural viruses in the same plant to create new "offspring" viruses. Many experts insist that this is inevitable and that the danger of such recombination outweighs the advantages of using viral transgenes. Crop developers and regulatory agencies, however, defend virus-resistant GM crops, using five common arguments. These are presented below, along with responses that are based on a paper by Latham and Steinbrecher.[245]

Argument: The likelihood of recombination is the same as that of natural plants that have two (or more) viral infections. Since that occurs naturally, we shouldn't consider GM plants as a special cause for concern.[246]

With GM crops, viruses will come into proximity with the transgene at a much higher rate. Most natural plants are *not* infected by viruses and *do not* have viral sequences available. When viruses do attack plants, they are often restricted to certain types of tissue[247] and will not readily encounter viruses present in other tissue. For those attacking the same tissue, some viruses have a mechanism (superinfection exclusion) to prohibit other viruses from infecting the same cell.[248] In other cases, viruses may occupy different compartments within the cell and thus be prevented from interacting. These natural barriers to viral recombination are largely dismantled in GM crops, which contain viral sequences in every cell.

Argument: The quantities of messenger RNA (mRNA) produced by some viral inserts are less than those found in natural viruses. Therefore, the rate of recombination (of the mRNA) will be lower.[249]

Naturally occurring viruses are usually surrounded (encapsidated) by a protective coat of protein and many also replicate in areas of the cell that are enclosed by membranes.[250] GM viral sequences are neither encapsidated nor enclosed. They therefore may come into contact with natural viruses more often, even if the total amount of mRNA is less. Furthermore, the level of transgenic mRNA may increase in those cells that are infected by a non-target virus,[251] because the introduced virus may disable the mechanism that keeps the transgene expression low.[252]

Argument: Recombinant viruses "are unlikely" to survive competition from pre-existing viruses or will not give rise to significant new strains.[253]

These assertions are not supported by data.[254] On the contrary, new and significant viruses do arise naturally by recombination[255] (as well as mutation) and some demonstrate superior fitness compared to their parents.[256] Also, some viruses don't compete with pre-existing ones, but rather move into a different niche.

Argument: Viral sequences are inserted into GM crops so that the plants resist viruses that carry that same sequence. When the USDA approved the first virus-resistant plant (the ZW-20 squash),[257] they argued that if the inserted viral sequence recombines with a natural virus, the new virus will be suppressed by the same mechanism.

This assumption has been overturned by the discovery that infecting viruses can disable gene silencing mechanisms.[258]

[All four of the arguments above appear in *every* application for new GM virus-resistant varieties and are the primary defense against the risk of recombination. A fifth rationale, which is sometimes used by advocates, is as follows.]

Argument: The widespread use of GM virus resistant plants will so effectively reduce the prevalence of viruses, that it will reduce the rate of recombination.[259]

No data is presented to support this position, which overstates a GM crop's ability to suppress viruses beyond one or a few targeted strains.

"Up till now all technologies were controllable. Electricity, even nuclear power can be turned off. GM is the first irreversible technology in human history. When a GMO is released it is out of our control; we have no means to call it back. We can insert a transgene, but we cannot take the released transgene out. Since GMOs are self-replicating, releasing them might have dire consequences for human and animal health and for the environment and can change evolution."

—Professor Susan Bardocz, biochemist and nutritionist

PART 4

Flaws
in the Arguments
Used to Justify
GM Crops

Why GM crops are not needed to feed the world

Hundreds of millions of dollars have been spent by biotech companies trying to convince the world that GM crops are needed to feed the world. Their message targets those in developed countries in order to create an impression that it is morally wrong to oppose the technology. This tactic is described by Prince Charles and others as "emotional blackmail."

If GM crops are truly the solution to hunger, all five of the following statements should be true. GM crops must:

1. Be safe;
2. Produce higher yields;
3. Have consistent and reliable yields; and
4. Be better than competing options;
5. World hunger must be solvable by increasing food productivity.

All five are false.

Food from GM crops is not safe

Perhaps sometime in the future scientists will be able to reliably and predictably manipulate genes for the betterment of health and the environment, but as this book demonstrates, that is not the case thus far.

GM crop acreage produces lower average yields

According to plant physiologist E. Ann Clark, "GM crops are not bred for higher yield, thus, any yield benefit can only occur when the target trait affords weed or pest control benefits more cost effectively than what is attainable through non-GM methods. Yield can be enhanced for *Bt*-corn when populations of the target European cornborer pest are high, but that occurs infrequently and unpredictably. . . . Yield of soybean actually appears to be constrained by the Roundup Ready (RR) trait, as inferred in a report presented at the 2004 Midwest Soybean Conference in Des Moines, Iowa.[1] Ron Eliason documented that US soybean yields peaked in 1994 and then flattened following release of RR cultivars, consistent with the conclusions of Fernandez-Cornejo and McBride,[2] Benbrook,[3] and Martinez-Ghersa et al.[4] Eliason[5] attempted to account for this pattern from severe weather events, but something more than weather appears to have been happening, leaving open the possible effect of the RR trait itself. A range of industry-, university-, and state-sponsored surveys summarized by Benbrook[6] and Martinez-Ghersa et al.[7] showed that RR soybean yields averaged 5%–10% less than conventional soybeans. The general absence of a yield benefit discounts the notion that biotech is necessary to 'feed the world,' or could somehow do better than conventional plant breeding is already doing."[8]

In addition, there are reports of lower yields from GM canola and cotton. These reports do not generally come from biotech companies themselves. Monsanto in particular has been accused of presenting yield figures in excess of actual performance. According to a report on *Bt* cotton grown in India, Monsanto commissioned studies to be done by market research agencies, not scientists. One, for example, claimed four times the actual reduction in pesticide use, 12 times the actual yield, and 100 times the actual profit.[9] Case studies presented in a poster series by the company were similarly skewed. The posters were called, "TRUE STORIES OF FARMERS WHO HAVE SOWN BT COTTON." But when investigators tracked down one featured farmer who had claimed great benefits, he turned out to be a cigarette salesman, not a farmer. Another poster gave yield figures of a farmer that were four times what he actually achieved. A third featured a photo of a farmer standing next to a tractor, suggesting that sales of *Bt* cotton allowed him to purchase it. But the farmer was never told what the photo was to be used for and said that with the yields from *Bt*, "I would not be able to buy even two tractor tires."[10]

Peter Rosset

"Some researchers have shown that none of the genetically engineered seeds significantly increase the yield of crops. Indeed, in more than 8,200 field trials, the Roundup Ready soybeans produced fewer bushels of soybeans than similar natural varieties, according to a study by Dr. Charles Benbrook, the former director of the Board on Agriculture at the National Academy of Sciences."[11]

GM crop yields can be dangerously inconsistent

Reliability of yields is essential in developing countries, where a loss of a single season's crop can spell starvation for some farmers. The severity of this became clear when farmers in India began planting *Bt* cotton. A 2005 study of 87 villages in the state of Andhra Pradesh over a period of three years[12] showed that non-GM cotton yielded about 10% more than the *Bt* variety. But the performance of *Bt* cotton was erratic and plagued by numerous problems, including increased pests and disease, brittle stems, failure to germinate, drought damage, smaller cotton bolls, increased labor requirements, poorer quality and a shorter harvest season. Some farmers complained "that they were not able to grow other crops after *Bt* because it had infected their soil."[13] Where farmers did not have access to irrigation, the yields from *Bt* were often a disaster. The overall average return to *Bt* cotton farmers over three years was 60% less, and 71% of farmers who used *Bt* cotton ended up with financial losses. (Similarly, about 70% of the 4,438 farmers growing *Bt* cotton in Indonesia were unable to repay their credit after the first year of planting.[14])

In the spring of 2005, the government of Andhra Pradesh acknowledged that the losses to *Bt* cotton farmers for the season totaled about $10 million.[15] Crop wilting in Madhya Pradesh cost an estimated $87.5 million.[16] And in parts of Tamil Nadu, "Up to 75% of the *Bt* cotton seeds failed to germinate."[17] The true cost of *Bt* cotton cannot be calculated in financial terms. Thousands of indebted *Bt* cotton farmers in India committed suicide.

Other methods are far better for improving yields and the life of farmers

A 2001 *New Scientist* article reported on the world's largest study on sustainable agriculture at the time. The story was called, "An Ordinary Miracle: Bigger harvests, without pesticides or genetically modified crops? Farmers can make it happen by letting weeds do the work." The research looked at more than 200 projects in 52 countries,[18] involving more than four million farms "covering an area the size of Italy—3% of fields in the Third World. And, most remarkably, average increases in crop yields were 73%." The study's author concluded that the sustainable agriculture methods are "cheap, use locally available technology and often improve the environment. Above all they most help the people who need help, the most-poor farmers and their families, who make up the majority of the world's hungry people."[19] *New Scientist* wrote, "This 'sustainable agriculture' just happens to be the biggest movement in Third World farming today, dwarfing the tentative forays in genetic manipulation. . . . And some experts think GM crops will pale by comparison with sustainable agriculture, at least for the time being."[20]

An even larger study in 2006 looked at 286 projects to introduce sustainable techniques "on more than 12 million farms in 57 countries, mostly in Africa." According to a report on SciDev.net, the research evaluated yield effects when farmers used "approaches such as less tilling to conserve soil, integrated pest management—which favors ecological pest control over pesticide spraying—and improved management of soil nutrients. According to the study, adopting such approaches meant yields increased by an average of 79% and harvests of some crops such as maize, potatoes and beans doubled."[21]

These sustainable solutions help people reclaim the ability to feed themselves by applying scientific rigor to make old-fashioned crop improvement methods more systematic and efficient using seed varieties that are well-suited to local conditions. The model for GM crops, however, concentrates ownership of agriculture into the hands of a few multinational corporations, forces farmers to buy seeds each year and reduces the diversity of seed genetics. In addition, in developing nations, people gain valuable nutrients by harvesting a diversity of wild plants that grow in the field with the crops. Herbicide-tolerant GM crops bundled with their herbicide applications, however, would kill off this important food source. The overuse of *Bt* crops also hasten insect resistance to the *Bt*-toxin. This threatens the long-term effectiveness of natural *Bt* sprays, which are used as a natural pest conrol method.

Finally, promoting genetic engineering as a solution to world hunger diverts much needed research dollars into expensive GMO development and away from more appropriate technologies. Hans Herren, director of the International Centre for Insect Physiology and Ecology in Nairobi, says, "What Africa most needs is investment in 'soft' biotechnologies such as alternative natural pesticides."[22]

Miguel A. Altieri   "Agricultural biotechnology innovations (i.e., *Bt* crops and herbicide resistant crops) are profit-driven rather than need-driven. The real thrust of the genetic engineering industry is not to make agriculture more productive but to generate profits. In the case of herbicide tolerance the goal is to win greater herbicide market-share for a proprietary product, and to boost seed sales at the cost of damaging the usefulness of a key pest management product (*Bt*) that is relied on as an alternative to insecticides . . . Genetically modified seeds are under corporate control and patent protection, consequently they are very expensive. Since many developing countries still lack the institutional infrastructure and low-interest credit necessary to deliver these new seeds to poor farmers, biotechnology will only exacerbate marginalization."[23]

Increasing crop productivity does not, in itself, eradicate hunger

Lack of food is not the fundamental reason why so many millions of people go to bed hunger every night. According to the 1998 book, *World Hunger: Twelve Myths*, "The world today produces enough grain alone to provide every human being on the planet with 3,500 calories a day. That's enough to make most people fat! And this estimate does not even count many other commonly eaten foods—vegetables, beans, nuts, root crops, fruits, grass-fed meats, and fish. In fact, if all foods are considered together, enough is available to provide at least 4.3 pounds per person per day. That includes 2.5 pounds of grain, beans, and nuts; about a pound of fruits and vegetables; and nearly another pound of meat, milk, and eggs." The book cites a study showing "that 78% of all malnourished children under five in the developing world live in countries with food surpluses."[24]

The organization Stop Hunger Now says, "Abundance, not scarcity, best describes the world's food supply," and a UN report confirms that we won't be running short anytime soon.[25] The primary cause of hunger is poverty. Producing more food will not solve the problem if those who need it the most cannot afford it.

Miguel A. Altieri	"In 1999 enough grain was produced globally to feed a population of eight billion people (six billion inhabit the planet in 2000), had it been evenly distributed or not fed to animals. Seven out of ten pounds of grain are fed to animals in the USA. . . . By channeling one-third of the grain produced world-wide to needy people, hunger would cease instantly."[26]
Devinder Sharma	"In its effort to bolster the commercial interests of the biotechnology industry, the international community can't see the forest for the trees. In its enthusiasm to promote an expensive technology at the expense of the poor, it overlooks the potential of biotechnology to further deepen the great divide between the haves and have-nots. No technological fix can help bridge this monumental gap. Hunger results not only from the inability of the poor to access food, it is also the result of global policies that further marginalize the poverty-stricken, cumulatively adding on to the problem of hunger . . . "In 2000, India had a record food surplus of 44 million tons. By 2002, the surplus had grown to 65 million tons, not due to excess production, but because more and more people are unable to buy the grain that lies stockpiled."[27]

Experts and organizations worldwide have condemned biotech companies for claiming that GM crops will solve world hunger. A report by ActionAid concluded that rather than alleviating world hunger, GM crop technology "is likely to exacerbate food insecurity, leading to more hungry people not less."[28] Similarly, "Oxfam and Christian Aid have both warned that GM crops could intensify poverty in the developing world."[29] The danger that this technology poses for developing nations has, nonetheless, not stopped biotech companies and their supporters from continuing to promote the myth that GMOs are the solution.

Golden rice is the wrong way to supplement vitamin A

Proponents claim that GM crops will boost nutrition. Currently there are no commercialized GM foods in which the modified trait is even designed to improve nutrition. One experimental variety, however, has garnered considerable media attention and become the industry's poster child. It is golden rice, engineered to make beta-carotene—a precursor to vitamin A. A US TV commercial for biotechnology claimed that golden rice can "help prevent blindness and infection in millions of children" suffering from vitamin-A deficiency. *Time* magazine featured the rice on its cover, stating, "This rice could save a million kids a year." Syngenta even claimed that one month of a delay in marketing Golden Rice would cause 50,000 children to go blind.[30]

A closer look reveals some interesting omissions in the industry's numbers. According to a Greenpeace report, golden rice provides so little vitamin A, "a two-year-old child would need to eat 7 pounds per day."[31] Likewise, an adult would need to eat nearly 20 pounds to get the daily recommended dose.[32]

"This whole project is actually based on what can only be characterized as intentional deception," writes Benedikt Haerlin, former international coordinator of Greenpeace's genetic engineering campaign. "We recalculated their figures again and again. We just could not believe serious scientists and companies would do this."[33]

There are other considerations. No published study has confirmed that the human body could actually convert the beta-carotene in golden rice. Other nutrients such as fat and protein, often lacking in the diets of malnourished children, are needed in order to absorb vitamin A. David Schubert points out that "a GM plant making vitamin A precursor, such as 'golden rice,' might also produce retinoic acid derivatives." He says these might result in "direct toxicity or abnormal embryonic development."[34] In addition, one gene inserted into the rice comes from daffodils. It is possible that it will also transfer known allergens from the flower.[35]

Biotech proponents also admit that to persuade people to eat yellow rice may require an educational campaign. But if they are going to spend the time to educate, they can teach people to eat a red rice from India or brown rices, which contain more vitamin A than golden rice but without the risks. Or, as Michael Pollan asks is his *New York Times Magazine* article, "The Great Yellow Hype," why not instead teach "people how to grow green vegetables [that are rich in vitamin A and other nutrients] on the margins of their rice fields, and maybe even give them the seeds to do so? Or what about handing out vitamin-A supplements to children so severely malnourished their bodies can't metabolize beta-carotene?"[36] In fact, organizations are successfully doing these. Several groups have promoted the use of gardens in developing nations and the Vitamin Angel Alliance gives at risk children high potency vitamin A tablets, strong enough so that only two are required per year to prevent blindness. At a cost of only $.05 per tablet, only $25,000 is needed to prevent 500,000 children from going blind per year.[37] Contrast this with golden rice, which has cost more than $100 million dollars so far and is not yet ready.

Even the former president of the Rockefeller Foundation, which funded development of golden rice, said "the public-relations uses of golden rice have gone too far" and are misleading the public and media. He adds, "We do not consider golden rice the solution to the vitamin A deficiency problem."[38]

Grains of Delusion	"The main agenda for golden rice is not malnutrition but garnering greater support and acceptance for genetic engineering amongst the public, the scientific community, and funding agencies. Given this reality, the promise of golden rice should be taken with a pinch of salt."[39]
Michael Pollan	"The unspoken challenge here is that if we don't get over our queasiness about eating genetically modified food, kids in the Third World will go blind.... Yet the more one learns about biotechnology's Great Yellow Hope, the more uncertain seems its promise—and the industry's command of the moral high ground. Indeed, it remains to be seen whether golden rice will ever offer as much to malnourished children as it does to beleaguered biotech companies. Its real achievement may be to win an argument rather than solve a public-health problem. Which means we may be witnessing the advent of the world's first purely rhetorical technology."[40]

Vandana Shiva	"The 'selling' of vitamin A rice as a miracle cure for blindness is based on blindness to alternatives for eliminating vitamin A deficiency, and blindness to the unknown risks of producing vitamin A through genetic engineering.... The lower cost, accessible and safer alternative to genetically engineered rice is to increase biodiversity in agriculture. Further, since those who suffer from vitamin A deficiency suffer from malnutrition generally, increasing the food security and nutritional security of the poor—through increasing the diversity of crops and the diversity of diets of poor people who suffer the highest rates of deficiency—is the reliable means for overcoming nutritional deficiencies."[41]
Devinder Sharma	"A majority of the acutely malnourished people that the proponents of "golden rice" claim they want to help cannot afford to buy rice from the market. If these poor people cannot buy ordinary rice, how will they pay for "golden" rice? The question has been conveniently overlooked. If these hungry millions could meet their daily rice requirement, there would be no malnutrition in the first place. The problem cannot be solved by providing nutritional supplements through GE rice. The answer lies in policy changes that force governments to ensure sufficient food for all."[42]

"We need to change the focus of the debate away from the limited studies that have been done to date onto the size of the irreversible legacy that we are probably going to leave for future generations."

—Professor Vyvyan Howard, expert in fetal and infant toxico-pathology

CONCLUSION

Genetic Roulette:
Gambling with our Health and Environment

On Christmas Day 1859, the Victorian Acclimatization Society released 24 rabbits into the Australian countryside so that settlers could hunt them for sport and feel more "at home."[1] The rabbits multiplied to well over 200 million, spreading out over 4 million square kilometers. That Christmas present now costs Australian agriculture about $600 million per year.[2]

With the benefit of hindsight, the mistake was obvious. But the principle continues to be ignored. Man-made interventions that self-propagate in the environment must be handled with the utmost caution and respect.

Releasing GM food crops requires even greater care. They not only might exist for centuries, they expose millions of people to unpredictable dangers.

Instead of proceeding with caution, the biotech industry decided to gamble. Armed with an incomplete and often wrong understanding of genetics, they manipulated the most fundamental components of living systems and then rushed their creations into the market. Like true gamblers, they sought a quick pay off—at least before their patents expired.

We don't need the benefit of 150 years to see their mistakes. According to the European Commission, it is "striking that the experts confirm how little was known on so many of the relevant issues only 10–15 years ago, and how much the scientific understanding of many of these issues has developed since then." Long after GM crops were approved, experts identified "previously unsuspected areas of risks and impacts," or "flaws in the way risk assessments may have been conducted in the past."[3]

When GM technology was developed, we were at the infant stages of understanding the DNA. Describing its structure and function was straightforward. The explanation was linear, well-defined, and wrong. Expecting that DNA operates in a simplistic, easily understood manner was convenient, but was it reasonable? Consider the enormous complexity of the human body. Our theories of DNA have yet to account for this still uncharted richness. Discoveries each year force scientists to discard one "fundamental truth" after the other. In July 2006, for example, the *New York Times* reported that "Researchers believe they have found a second code in DNA in addition to the genetic code."[4] How many future codes will we find? Will we eventually discover quantum mechanical or field effects? Do we yet have the tools to learn how this amazing molecule orchestrates life?

With our understanding shifting so rapidly, it is arrogant to insist that we have sufficient knowledge to make artificial, unalterable changes that risk the health of the population and environment. It may likewise be foolish to assume that we possess enough knowledge and tools to evaluate the safety of gene altered foods. The New Zealand Institute for Gene Ecology writes, "We have the view that truly good biotechnologies will be vindicated by not just the best available science, but science adequate to the task of making a sound decision on safety. Our *a priori* view is this: it is not a given that the science of the day is adequate for the task. It is possible for an applicant to do state-of-the-art analyses and not meet a standard of risk identification or resolution that may be necessary."[5]

Microbiologist and medical doctor Richard Lacey goes further. He says "it is virtually impossible to even conceive of a testing procedure to assess the health effects of genetically engineered foods when introduced into the food chain, nor is there any valid nutritional or public interest reason for their introduction."[6]

Scientists worldwide acknowledge that GM crops were introduced long before the science was ready. Many call for a prolonged moratorium. They tell the industry to come back with their products in 50–100 years, after they have done their homework.

Biotech companies insist that the benefits of the technology justify the risk. But who benefits and who's at risk? While some farmers may have some benefit from herbicide-tolerant or pesticide-laden crops, the primary advantage is profits for the seed developers. The risks are borne by everyone else. GM crops have cost the United States billions of dollars in lost markets and an estimated $3–$5 billion per year in extra government subsidies to boost their prices.[7] Food companies and farmers in various regions fight a constant battle to keep their crops pure. Contamination from unapproved rice varieties cost hundreds of millions of dollars; unapproved corn cost over a billion.

The greater gamble is with our health. We don't know in advance who is susceptible to GM food dangers, how much they will consume or what their reaction will be. If only one in a thousand becomes ill, that's a million people for every billion exposed. The probability of serious health effects increases with each new GM crop introduced.

Without post-marketing surveillance, the chances of tracing reactions to GM food are low. The incidence of a disease would have to increase dramatically before it was noticed; tens of thousands or more may have to get sick before a change is investigated. Tracking the impact of GM foods is even more difficult in North America, where the foods are not labeled. Regulators at Health Canada announced in 2002 that they would monitor Canadians for health problems from eating GM foods. A spokesperson said, "I think it's just prudent and what the public expects, that we will keep a careful eye on the health of Canadians." But according to CBC TV news, Health Canada "abandoned that research less than a year later saying it was 'too difficult to put an effective surveillance system in place.'" The news anchor added, "So at this point, there is little research into the health effects of genetically modified food. So will we ever know for sure if it's safe?"[8]

Not with the biotech companies in charge. Consider the following statement in a report submitted to county officials in California, by pro-GM members of a task force. It is: "generally agreed that long-term monitoring of the human health risks of GM food through epidemiological studies is not necessary because there is no scientific evidence suggesting any long-term harm from these foods."[9] Note the circular logic: Because no long-term epidemiological studies are in place, we have no evidence showing long-term harm. And since we don't have any evidence of long-term harm, we don't need studies to look for it.

Type 2 diabetes, asthma, allergies, stomach conditions such as acid reflux, migraines, and obesity have all increased in the United States. All may be food-related. Are they GMO-related? Unknown. We are left to guess.

But we need not be idle. Like the planet's immune response, resistance to GMOs has surfaced worldwide. In fact, the combined efforts have virtually halted the introduction of new GM crop varieties and will likely force a withdrawal of existing GM foods from the market soon.

The collapse of GM

Monsanto seeks world domination   January 1999

At a biotech industry conference in January 1999, a speaker from Arthur Anderson Consulting Group told how Monsanto executives had described to them their ideal future—a world in which all commercial seeds were genetically modified and patented. Anderson created a plan for Monsanto to achieve it. Another biotech company apparently had the same goal; their representative showed the audience a graph that projected a 95% replacement of all natural seeds by GM varieties in just five years. Within weeks, their ideal future crashed.

Europe says no to GMOs   February 1999

In February, the UK parliament invited GMO researcher Arpad Pusztai to testify, forcing his former employer to lift their gag order (see section 1.1). When Pusztai started speaking about his controversial discoveries, the press went wild. By the week's end, they had spewed out 159 "column feet" of text, which, according to one columnist "divided society into two warring blocs."[10] An editorial stated, "Within a single week the specter of a food scare has become a full scale war."[11]

Overwhelming consumer resistance to GM foods soon compelled the food industry to respond. In April 1999, Unilever publicly committed to remove GM ingredients from its European brands. Within a week, nearly all major food companies followed suit. The rejection by manufacturers and retailers continues to this day; it has kept GM foods out of the European Union in spite of official approvals of GM varieties by the EU Commission.

Americans remain under-informed

The same corporations that removed GMOs from their European lines, however, continue to sell them in the United States, where consumers remain uninformed of the issue. According to a December 2006 poll by the Pew Initiative on Food and Biotechnology, only 26% of Americans believe they have ever eaten a GM food in their lives.[12] Thus, GMOs flourish in the United States because of consumer ignorance. This leaves the industry extremely vulnerable. If some campaign or event were to push this issue above the national radar screen causing sufficient consumer concern,

US manufacturers would respond like their European counterparts. The tipping point does not require that a majority of US shoppers reject GM foods. If even a small percentage started switching brands based on GMO content, major companies would respond.

Studies show that the more people learn about GM foods the less they trust them.[13] Thus, efforts to educate US shoppers about GMOs will likely drive them towards the tipping point. This has already started with rbGH.

US shoppers reject rbGH   2006–07

The *Boston Globe* reported in September 2006 that "The region's biggest dairies are rushing to rid their bottled milk of artificial growth hormones." They wrote "If more dairies jump on board, it could be a tipping point in the long-running debate about the safety of using synthetic hormones to spur milk production."[14]

Two weeks later, the manager of a milk producers' co-op told the *New York Times*, "It seems to be an explosion in the industry. . . . All of a sudden we have national processors like Dean Foods taking entire plants hormone-free." The *Times* reported that, "dairy companies are bowing to the natural-foods trend by shunning milk from cows treated with genetically engineered growth hormone."[15]

By December 2006, Starbucks announced that they had started "a conversion of all core dairy products" to be rbGH-free in their 5,500 company-operated locations in the United States.[16] Safeway also converted their Portland and Seattle milk processing plants, and many other dairies are not far behind.

A January 2007 *Reuters* article observed, "The debate has taken a marked turn over the last several months as a growing number of dairy producers and food industry players have begun demanding rbST-free milk, citing heightened consumer demand and new niche marketing opportunities." National Milk Producers Federation spokesman Chris Galen said, "I don't think it is a trend that shows any signs of abating."[17]

The transformation was triggered by organizations such as the Oregon Physicians for Social Responsibility, Organic Consumers Association, Center for Food Safety, National Family Farm Coalition, and Food and Water Watch. By educating consumers about the health risks of the drug, it turned the hormone into a marketing liability. Similar education efforts in the United States will likely do the same to GM food crops.

Shift away from GM food in the United States   2007

A coalition of food manufacturers, distributors, and retailers in the natural products industry, along with the Institute for Responsible Technology, launched an initiative in the spring of 2007 to remove GM ingredients from the entire natural food sector. Called the Campaign for Healthier Eating in America, this comprehensive initiative will educate consumers about the health risks of GM foods and promote non-GMO brands through shopping guides. A uniform definition for declaring a product "non-GMO" has already been established through an industry-wide collaboration, and now manufacturers will receive assistance in achieving it. After they have had a chance to make the transition, the institute will encourage thousands of health food stores to put labels on the shelves next to any remaining hold-out brands that still "may contain GMOs."

The Pew survey reported that 29% of Americans are already strongly opposed to GM foods and believe they are unsafe.[18] That represents about 87 million people. But even among the 28 million Americans who buy organic food on a regular basis,[19] many do not conscientiously avoid GM ingredients in their non-organic purchases; they usually do not know how. By educating health-conscious shoppers about the dangers of GM food *and* providing clear choices *in the store*, brands without GM ingredients will have the advantage. This campaign will promote healthier eating in America and may even achieve the tipping point that inspires the whole food industry to get on board. To learn more, go to www.ResponsibleTechnology.org.

GM-free schools

Another trend contributing to the tipping point is the growing concern among parents and schools about the effects of GM foods on children. The epidemic of obesity and diabetes, as well as ADHD and depression, has intensified the focus on kids' diet and school meals. While many are banning junk food and reducing sugar and fat, some schools are also targeting GM foods. The Seattle school board, for example, instructed their 97 schools to remove GM ingredients from the meal programs. To learn about the Institute for Responsible Technology's national GM-Free School Campaign, go to www.ResponsibleTechnology.org.

Religious opposition

Many religious groups have issued strong statements of concern about GMOs. A working group at the World Council of Churches, for example, called upon churches and Christians "to build partnerships with civil society, people's movements, small scale farmer groups, and Indigenous Peoples in opposing the science, philosophy, and practice of genetic engineering in agriculture."[20] But religions largely remain the sleeping giants in the debate, since they have not yet wielded their enormous consumer clout. Any one of several could immediately force GMOs off the market simply by encouraging their members to avoid them.

Religious concerns not only include the effects on health and the environment, but many believe that crossing genes between species will create unintended consequences and is meddling with God's design. For them, a better translation of "GMO" would be "God, Move Over."

Legislation brewing

More than three-dozen US congressmen co-sponsored a "The Genetically Engineered Food Right to Know Act" in the 2003–2004 session. The bill called for the mandatory labeling of any foods that contain GM ingredients. Although there was insufficient support at the time, there was a sea change in Congress in 2006 and efforts are underway to re-introduce the bill. In addition, lawmakers are expected to introduce bills that would institute safety testing, assign liability to biotech companies for financial losses associated with their seeds and require that all GM pharmaceutical crops be grown indoors and only in non-food crops. GMO-related legislation has also been enacted at the state, county and city levels. For more information on legislative efforts in the United States, go to www.the-campaign.org.

Food companies and farmers can protect themselves

Whether the tipping point is achieved through a new scientific finding, a national education campaign, a religious leader, legislation, or even a well-received segment on Oprah Winfrey, there is an excellent chance that US food manufacturers will abandon GM foods in the near future. Several have already taken steps to protect themselves by avoiding GM ingredients. Still, farmers and food manufacturers may need to do more than just avoid GMOs in their own operations to protect themselves.

When StarLink corn contaminated the food supply, the entire US corn industry suffered, not just those who planted GM varieties. The lost exports, recalls and lowered prices cost over $1 billion. (And StarLink represented only a tiny fraction of the GM corn in the United States.)

In August 2006, the USDA announced that an unapproved GM rice variety had somehow escaped from field trials conducted at least five years earlier and contaminated current US rice stocks. Japan stopped buying long grain US rice, products were taken off shelves in Europe, rice prices plummeted, and at least 25 lawsuits were filed by rice companies against rice developer Bayer CropScience. This debacle took the rice industry completely by surprise. Since GM rice had not been commercialized, they figured they were safe.

Now the industry must decide whether to preempt future contamination by telling the government and five multinational GM crop companies, "No more GM rice trials!" But this decision is not just for rice growers. What about those who deal in lettuce, barley, sunflowers, and plums? Most vegetables, fruits, and grains have GM counterparts in some stage of development. More than one hundred species have already been grown outdoors in field trials.

And lest they think that the rice contamination was a unique incident, *Nature* magazine lists some of the other incidents of crop contamination traced to supposedly quarantined field trials.[21] In 1997, Limagrain Seed and Monsanto recalled 60,000 bags of canola that were contaminated with an unapproved variety. In 2001, Monsanto's unapproved corn "escaped its field trial site and released pollen to a commercial crop." And corn engineered to produce a pharmaceutical, also grown in 2001, contaminated both soybean and corn fields the following year. It led to the destruction of 155 acres of corn and 500,000 bushels of soy. In 2004, windblown pollen and seeds were carried from an outdoor trial of GM bentgrass, contaminating natural grass miles away. Syngenta admitted in 2005 that an unapproved corn that was field trialed in previous years had contaminated US corn supplies. Following their announcement, at least 14 shipments of corn to Japan were rejected due to discovery of the illegal variety. And in 2005, Greenpeace reported that unapproved rice grown in China had been illegally sold in the market for the previous two years. That same rice was also found in products sold in Europe in 2006.

The liability laws vary from country to country, but in some cases industry-friendly policies let the seed producers off the hook. Thus, if for no other reason, until the biotech industry is held fully liable for damage caused by its GM crops, the food industry should insist that developers "keep it in the lab."

Deciding against GMOs

Decision makers should have sufficient information from this book to confidently ban GMOs from their jurisdiction, whether that be a country, a food brand, school meals, or food for their family. Some policy makers may want to hear from the biotech side before taking action. We have created a Web site, www.GeneticRoulette.com, specifically to promote a serious scientific debate on the details presented. There, contributors can challenge, respond, add and correct information about any of the health risks presented in the two-page spreads in part 1. These 65 risks serve as a checklist. The burden is on the industry to demonstrate that each adverse finding and each theoretical risk is responded to with good science, appropriate investigation, and evidence verifying safety. Until then, wise nations and wise families should opt-out of this high-stakes gamble by refusing GM foods.

Industry may avoid scientific debates

In the past, the biotech industry has studiously avoided debating the health risks of their foods. That is because their claims of safety do not hold up well under scrutiny. There is no trove of alternate studies, new findings, or scientific breakthroughs that get GM foods off the hook. Most of the risks outlined in this book have been countered only with assumptions—usually untested or obsolete.

The public relations firm Burson Marsteller told EuropaBio, "Public issues of environmental and human health risk are communications killing fields for bioindustries in Europe."[22] They told them to avoid all public debates. In lieu of a rational discussions we get spin. When a linguist analyzed the rhetoric offered in defense of GM crops, he discovered that GM proponents use unscientific, emotional, and irrational arguments to attack critics as unscientific, emotional, and irrational.[23]

We present below some of the strategies that the industry has used in response to scientific challenges and to books critical of their technology. This may help prepare decision makers to deal with possible responses to the information presented in Genetic Roulette. Based on a decade of experience, here are some of the common reactions we have seen:

Preemptive strike. The book *Seeds of Deception* documents how threats from biotech companies stopped the publication of a book, a magazine issue, a multi-part news series on Fox TV and critical coverage by many major US newspapers.

Silence. Once a book critical of GM crops is published, the first response is usually to not draw any attention to its allegations. It is ignored.

Sweeping dismissal. When biotech spokespersons are questioned about the book's contents, the strategy is to avoid responding to specific details. Instead, they use a sweeping dismissal to try and discredit the whole thing. Terms such as a "bunch of rubbish," "unscientific," "anecdotal," and "largely discredited" may be bandied about.

Haven't read it. Some may also claim to not have read the book in order to avoid being questioned on details.

Invoking of scientific organizations. When confronted on specific issues, advocates sometimes invoke the names of one or more scientific or governmental organizations, claiming that they have thoroughly evaluated GM foods and found them safe. The implication is that others with more knowledge have already looked at this and found no problem, so you don't have to.

Cherry picking arguments. A common technique in articles or letters to editors is for advocates to address only the most speculative and least supported arguments raised, and then imply that all the claims are similarly without foundation.

Same as other foods. Some will insist that modern methods of plant breeding *other* than genetic engineering 1) are used on a wide scale; 2) have a history of safe use; and 3) create comparable mutations in the DNA. Everything about this argument is pure speculation and is not supported by scientific literature. There is *no* evidence that these modern methods are used widely, are consistently safe, or create mutations of the same kind or frequency as genetic engineering.[24] The risks of GM crops are largely unique in character and scale.

Medicines or gene therapy needed. To confound the issue, some defend GM crops by claiming that we need genetic engineering for human gene therapy or to produce medicine such as GM insulin for diabetics. This falsely implies that to be against GM crops one must necessarily be against other forms of genetic engineering.

Personal attack. When authors or scientists are personally attacked, it can signify that they have a particularly strong argument or evidence that can damage the industry position. Rhetoric used in the attack may suggest that the biotech critic has ulterior motives such as selling books or a personal philosophy or religion that is the "real" reason they are taking a stand. The strained logic implies that on the basis of misguided motivation, one should dismiss all the evidence. If this were applied to the profit-driven biotech companies, then we should likewise dismiss their claims.

Flood of "evidence." When the Chicago school system began questioning the safety of milk from cows treated with rbGH, they received a huge box of documents from Monsanto that supposedly refuted the critics. Similarly, the rbGH documents presented to FDA regulators stacked 62 feet high. This tactic of flooding decision makers with too much material is effective because people rarely take the time to thoroughly evaluate the materials. (The titles of industry studies and reports are often carefully crafted to proclaim product safety, even if the contents show otherwise.)

These tactics are catalogued here in the hope that it will preempt their use. Or at least it can help people sort through the spin and demand real answers to urgent questions.

Taking responsibility

After finding out about GMOs, politicians, regulators, reporters, food companies, farmers, chefs, school administrators, and even consumers usually figure that someone else is taking the responsibility. This is the main reason why we still face this travesty. It is easy to assume that someone else is looking out for us or that corporations would not be so stupid as to risk our health and planet. It's easy to let the scientists deal with this. It is, after all, a complicated subject; it's their field and their products, not ours.

This book is designed to show that others are *not* looking out for us. Companies *are* risking our health and planet. And it takes the obscure, complicated science and tries to make it accessible so the dangers are unmistakable. Genetic engineering of our food supply is indeed *our* field, *our* problem, and *ours* to solve.

Protecting our selves and our children is fundamental. Strategies to avoid eating GM foods are presented in the next section. Beyond that, consider taking steps to inform and protect your community, your organizations, and our world. Although GMOs present one of the greatest dangers, with informed, motivated people, it is one of the easiest global issues to solve.

Safe eating.

APPENDIX

Gathering data and staying up-to-date on the risks of GM foods

Identifying reactions to GM foods that have been released into a nation's food supply can be very difficult. Without surveillance systems, problems may not be identified, let alone investigated. We have volunteered to gather case-study and trend data, which may be valuable for those conducting research.

Collecting case studies

We are collecting information about individuals who claim to have adverse reactions to GM foods. It needs to be clear to investigators that the reaction occurs *only* to the GM ingredient *and not* to an equivalent non-GM ingredient. For example, if someone has a reaction to products made in North America that contain soy or yellow corn, it is possible that the cause is GM soy or corn. We would only be interested in collecting the details of the reaction if the person also does not react to soy or corn products that are non-GM (e.g. organic or labeled non-GMO). We do not encourage anyone to conduct dangerous experiments by exposing themselves to allergens. Rather, if an individual happens to notice such a pattern of reaction, please contact us at submit@GeneticRoulette.com. If we see any pattern in these cases studies, we will present the evidence to health authorities and researchers and will push for a full investigation.

Identifying trends

If health practitioners or population health monitors notice increases in any symptom, disease or illness after the introduction of GM ingredients, please also contact us. In the United States, rbGH was introduced in 1994. GM crops appeared in 1996.

Check for new material, challenges, and updates

The Web site www.GeneticRoulette.com will post new findings on the safety of GM foods. For example, as this book was going to press, a report was released about organ damage and other adverse effects in rats fed Monsanto's GM NewLeaf potatoes. The study had been conducted in 1998 by the Institute of Nutrition of the Russian Academy of Medical Sciences, but results were made public only recently, after Greenpeace won two successive court cases. The details will be posted at www.GeneticRoulette.com after the study and write-up have been reviewed by a group of scientists.

The Web site will also include challenges and responses to the material presented in this book. We are dedicated to a transparent and scientific debate on this important topic.

How to avoid eating genetically modified foods

There are a few ways to identify GMOs in order to avoid them.

1. Mandatory labeling

The United States and Canada do not have GM labeling requirements, but most other industrialized nations do. Some laws do not require labeling if a processed GM-derived ingredient no longer contains GM DNA or GM protein. This ignores risks of toxins and other substances produced in the GM transformation process, which may be found in the processed ingredient. The EU law closed this loophole and does require labeling if GM crops were used in production, irrespective of whether it is detectable in the final product. The European Union and others, however, still have the loophole of not requiring labeling of milk and meat from animals fed GM feed.

The Campaign for Healthier Eating in America is introducing in-store, on-shelf labeling of GM products in health food stores, planned for late 2008.

2. Voluntary "Non-GMO" labels

Many products in the United States and elsewhere are labeled by manufacturers as "Non-GMO." Although this is not defined and varies between producers, the Campaign for Healthier Eating in America is promoting a uniform standard and its verification.

3. Shopping guides

Shopping guides identifying GM vs non-GM food brands are popular in many countries. For US brands, go to www.ResponsibleTechnology.org to access online shopping guides and to find out about the availability of printed guides.

4. Organic

Organic products are not allowed to knowingly use GM ingredients (although tiny contamination does sometimes occur).

5. Avoiding "at-risk" ingredients

If a product is not identified as non-GMO using the criteria above, you may wish to avoid all ingredients derived from the GM crops used in your nation. The following list identifies those grown and consumed in the United States. Not all of these are available around the world.

List of GM crops

Currently commercialized GM crops in the US
(Number in parentheses represents the estimated percent that is genetically modified.)

>Soy (89%)
>Cotton (83%)
>Canola (75%)
>Corn (60%)
>Hawaiian papaya (more than 50%)
>Alfalfa, zucchini, and yellow squash (small amount)
>Tobacco (Quest® brand)

Other sources of GMOs
- Dairy products from cows injected with rbGH
- Food additives, enzymes, flavorings, and processing agents, including the sweetener aspartame (NutraSweet®) and rennet used to make hard cheeses
- Meat, eggs, and dairy products from animals that have eaten GM feed
- Honey and bee pollen that may have GM sources of pollen
- Contamination or pollination caused by GM seeds or pollen

Some of the ingredients that may be genetically modified
Vegetable oil, vegetable fat, and margarines (soy, corn, cottonseed, and/or canola)

GM Soy: Soy flour, soy protein, vegetable proteins, and isolates, textured vegetable protein (TVP), tofu, tamari, tempeh, protein supplements, defoaming agents used in the manufacturing of yeast and sugar, antioxidants (vitamin E), natural flavors.

GM Corn: Cornmeal, corn syrup, high-fructose corn syrup (HFCS), baking powder, white vinegar, caramel, malt, confectioner's sugar, vanilla extract (contains corn syrup), and table salt (may contain a small amount of dextrose).

The following is a list of additives that may be derived from corn or soybeans:
Ascorbic acid, ascorbate (vitamin C), citric acid, cobalamin (vitamin B12), cyclodextrin, cystein, dextrin, dextrose (added to table salt to prevent iodide sticking—very small amount), diacetyl, diglycerides (diaclyglycerol, fructose especially crystaline fructose, glucose, glutamate, glutamic acid, gluten, glycine, glycerides (mono, di, tri) glycerol, glycerol monooleate, glycerine, hemicellulose, hydrolyzed vegetable protein or starch, hydrogenated starch hydrolyates, inositol, invert sugar or inverse syrup (inversol, colorose), isomalt, lactic acid, lecithin (often specified: soy lecithin), leucine, lysine, maltodextrin, maltose (hydrogenated maltose is called maltitol), mannitol, milo starch, modified starch, monoglycerides, monosodium glutamate (MSG), oleic acid, phenylalanine, phytic acid, sorbitol, stearic acid, threonine, tocopherols (vitamin E), trehalose, xanthan gum, and zein. (In addition, cellulose and methylcellulose may be derived from cotton.)

Check www.GeneticRoulette.com for a more up-to-date list, including an indication about how frequently these products are derived from corn or soy.

Some foods that may contain GM ingredients
Infant formula, salad dressing, bread, cereal, hamburgers and hotdogs, margarine, mayonnaise, cereals, crackers, cookies, chocolate, candy, fried food, chips, veggie burgers, meat substitutes, ice cream, frozen yogurt, tofu, tamari, soy sauce, soy cheese, tomato sauce, protein powder, baking powder, alcohol, vanilla, powdered sugar, peanut butter, enriched flour, and pasta. Non-food items include cosmetics, soaps, detergents, shampoo, and bubble bath.

Food Enzymes
from Genetically Modified Organisms

Enzyme Name	GM Organism	Use (Examples)
alpha-acetolactate decarboxylase	bacteria	removes bitter substances from beer
alpha-amylase	bacteria	converts starch to simple sugars
catalase	fungi	reduces food deterioration, particularly egg-based products
chymosin	bacteria or fungi	clots milk protein to make cheese
cyclodextrin-glucosyl transferase	bacteria	starch/sugar modification
beta-glucanase	bacteria	improves beer filtration
glucose isomerase	bacteria	converts glucose fructose sugar
glucose oxidase	fungi	reduces food deterioration, particularly egg-based products
glucose oxidase	fungi	reduces food deterioration, particularly egg-based products
lipase	fungi	oil and fat modification
maltogenic amylase	bacteria	slows staling of breads
pectinesterase	fungi	improves fruit juice clarity
protease	bacteria	improves bread dough structure
pullulanase	bacteria	converts starch to simple sugars
xylanase (hemicellulase)	bacteria or fungi	enhances rising of bread dough

Reproduced with permission from GEO-PIE.

In addition, GMOs can be used to produce lactoflavin/riboflavin (vitamin B2), yeast is available for making wine, and the FDA "approved" the following enzymes: laccase, phospholipase, bacteriophage P100, asparaginase, and lactoferrin (pending).[1]

Special alert on aspartame,
a genetically engineered sweetener

The sweetener aspartame, (also known as NutraSweet, Equal, Spoonful, Canderel, Benevia, and E951) is genetically engineered.[2] The amino acids are grown using GM *E. coli* bacteria. Although numerous studies and thousands of consumer complaints have linked this controversial sweetener to serious illnesses, it is unclear if the genetic engineering contributes to the problems.

Aspartame is a molecule composed of three sub-units. The first is methyl ester, which, according to food science professor Woodrow Monte, immediately converts to methyl (wood) alcohol, a deadly poison that can bioaccumulate in the body. A single ounce can be fatal. Monte, who is the author of "Aspartame: Methanol and the Public Health" in the *Journal of Applied Nutrition*,[3] says, "Methyl alcohol then converts to two other known toxins—formaldehyde and formic acid."

The other two sub-units are amino acids (aspartic acid and phenylalanine). These may be harmless when part of protein, but according to physician H. J. Roberts, author of the medical text, *Aspartame Disease: An Ignored Epidemic*, in aspartame the amino acids are isolated and in a dangerous configuration (*L. stereoisomer*). In addition, they interact with free methyl alcohol. These factors make the amino acids particularly harmful. Roberts says the isolated phenylalanine lowers the seizure threshold and triggers psychiatric and behavioral problems, as well as other symptoms and diseases. Neuroscientist John Olney, who founded the field of neuroscience called excitotoxicity, says that aspartic acid is an excitotoxin that stimulates neurons into hyperactivity until they exhaust and die.

Psychiatrist Ralph G. Walton, medical director of Safe Harbor Behavioral Health, had to abruptly stop his own human clinical trial on aspartame when some of the subjects had serious reactions. One participant, the hospital's administrator, suffered a detached retina and went blind in one eye. Another had bleeding of the eye and others reported being poisoned.[4] Walton says that "Aspartame is a multipotential toxin and carcinogen," which also lowers seizure thresholds, produces "carbohydrate craving," and in vulnerable individuals, can cause "panic, depressive, and cognitive symptoms."[5]

There are up to 10 breakdown products of aspartame.[6] The largest (diketopiperazine) appears to be the cause for brain tumors in animal feeding studies. Olney says when it is processed (nitrosated) by the gut it produces a compound closely resembling a powerful chemical (N-nitrosourea)[7] that causes brain tumores. Author and neurosurgeon Russell Blaylock, suggests that a jump in brain tumors in the US population in the 1980s is linked to the introduction of aspartame.[8] Blaylock refers to an Italian rat study[9] in which "they fed animals aspartame throughout their lives and let them die a natural death. They found a dramatic and statistically significant increase in the related cancers of lymphoma and leukemia, along with several histological types of lymphomas." He said, "What the Italian study found is that if you take these same animals and expose them to formaldehyde in the same doses, they developed the same leukemias and lymphomas."[10] The FDA compiled a list of 92 symptoms from the more than 10,000 consumer complaints they received about aspartame. These included four kinds of seizures, blindness, memory loss, fatigue, change in heart rate, difficulty breathing, joint, bone, and chest pain, speech impairment, tremors, change in body weight, lumps, blood and lymphatic problems, developmental retardation and problems with pregnancy, anemia, conjunctivitis, male sexual dysfunction, and death. Roberts' medical text also identifies neurodegenerative disease, cancer, diabetes, obesity, and sudden cardiac death, among others.

To learn more about efforts around the world to recall aspartame—as well as the health issues, rigged research, and political maneuvering that got it approved—consult the following resources:

Organizations:

- Mission Possible International, Betty Martini, Bettym19@mindspring.com
- World Natural Health Organization, www.wnho.net
- DORway to Discovery, www.dorway.com
- Aspartame Information Group, www.mpwhi.com
- Aspartame Toxicity Center, www.holisticmed.com/aspartame

Books and DVDs:

- *Aspartame Disease: An Ignored Epidemic* by H. J. Roberts, M.D.,
- *Excitotoxins: The Taste That Kills*, by Russell Blaylock, M.D.
- *Sweet Misery: A Poisoned World*, DVD available at www.seedsofdeception.com

INSTITUTE FOR RESPONSIBLE TECHNOLOGY

The Institute for Responsible Technology was founded by Jeffrey Smith. Its priority program is to end the genetic engineering of our food supply and the outdoor release of GM crops. The Institute works all over the world to educate decision makers, media, and the public, and organize campaigns such as those described in the previous pages. In addition, we are starting to fund much needed independent safety research on GM foods.

Stay informed
…with our free monthly e-newsletter, *Spilling the Beans*, written by founding director Jeffrey Smith.

Volunteer
…to help with a GM-Free school campaign or other programs.

Become a member
…for $25 per year and receive discounts on products and a free gift.

Donate
… and help to protect ourselves, our children, and our environment from the risks of this infant technology.

And when you are finished with this book, please share it with others.

www.ResponsibleTechnology.org
info@ResponsibleTechnology.org
+1.641.209.1765

Institute for Responsible Technology
P.O. Box 469
Fairfield, IA 52556 USA

Credentials of those cited often in the text

For brevity, the credentials of scientists and authorities cited in this book are often abbreviated or omitted. The following is a list of those who are referred to often:

Arpad Pusztai, PhD, experimental biologist, formerly of the Rowett Institute, consultant to GENOK (Norwegian Institute of Gene Ecology) Tromso, Fellow of the the Royal Society of Edinburgh, the top expert in his field of lectin proteins, and one of the leading experts on GMO safety assessments. He has published over 300 primary scientific papers and 16 books.

Susan Bardocz, PhD, DSc, biochemist and nutritionist, professor at University of Debrecen (Hungary), consultant to GENOK, Tromso, and a leading expert on GMO safety assessments and author of 119 primary scientific papers in refereed international journals, 118 book chapters, and authored and edited 14 books.

Michael Antoniou, PhD, molecular geneticist researching human gene therapy at King's College London, member of the scientific review committee of the GM Nation debate, author of many articles on the use of GM in medicine and especially agriculture for the lay public.

Judy Carman, PhD, nutritional biochemist and epidemiologist, director of the Institute of Health and Environmental Research and expert on GMO safety assessments, who has been commissioned by the government of Western Australia to conduct independent assessments on GM foods.

David Schubert, PhD, molecular biologist and protein chemist and professor at the Salk Institute for Biological Studies, author of several seminal articles on GM food safety.

Joseph Cummins, PhD, professor emeritus of genetics, University of Western Ontario, author of more than 200 scientific and popular articles, many on GM food safety about which he has written since 1988.

Doug Gurian-Sherman, PhD, senior scientist at the Union of Concerned Scientists, formerly worked at the EPA on GM crops and was a science adviser to the FDA.

Mae-Wan Ho, PhD, biophysicist and geneticist, director of the Institute of Science in Society, author of 14 books and more than 400 articles, many of which highlight newly identified shortcomings of GM food safety theories and assessments.

Giles Eric Seralini, PhD, toxicologist and professor at the University of Caen, France, president of the Scientific Council of the Committee for Independant Research and Information on Genetic Engineering, and member of two French commissions for GMO evaluation, and an expert panel for the European authorities.

Michael Hansen, PhD, is a researcher and spokesperson for the Consumer Policy Institute, a division of the Consumers Union of the United States (the organization that publishes *Consumer Reports* magazine), who works on biotechnology issues and is considered an authority on safety and assessment issues.

William Freese is with the Center for Food Safety and formerly a research analyst with Friends of the Earth, and author of key papers identifying shortcomings in the US safety assessment procedures for GM crops.

Jonathan R. Latham, PhD, is a molecular biologist and plant virologist and director of Programmes and Outreach of the Bioscience Resource Project. He is currently investigating the use of plant virus genes to make GM plants.

Ricarda A. Steinbrecher, PhD, molecular geneticist and co-director of EcoNexus, writes and lectures about genetic engineering in food and farming, its risks and potential consequences on health, food security, and the environment.

ENDNOTES

INTRODUCTION

1. Kirk Azevedo, personal communication, 2006.
2. U. S. FDA, "Statement of Policy: Foods Derived from New Plant Varieties," *Federal Register* 57, no. 104 (May 29, 1992): 22991.
3. Linda Kahl, Memo to James Maryanski about *Federal Register* Document "Statement of Policy: Foods from Genetically Modified Plants," Alliance for Bio-Integrity (January 8, 1992) www.biointegrity.org.
4. Steven M. Druker, "How the US Food and Drug Administration approved genetically engineered foods despite the deaths one had caused and the warnings of its own scientists about their unique risks," Alliance for Bio-Integrity, http://www.biointegrity.org/ext-summary.html
5. Ian F. Pryme and Rolf Lembcke, "In Vivo Studies on Possible Health Consequences of Genetically Modified Food and Feed—with Particular Regard to Ingredients Consisting of Genetically Modified Plan Materials," *Nutrition and Health* 17 (2003): 1–8.
6. Christopher Preston, Peer Reviewed Publications on the Safety of GM Foods: Results of a Search of the PubMed Database for Publications on feeding Studies for GM Crops, AgBioWorld (December 2004) http://www.agbioworld.org/biotech-info/articles/biotech-art/peer-reviewed-pubs.html (Note: Preston claimed in his paper that 42 studies existed, but his list showed only 41).
7. Arpad Pusztai responds to safety research claims by Christopher Preston. Arpad Pusztai, "Pusztai Demolishes Preston and Monsanto's Safety Study Claims," GMWatch (December 15, 2004) http://www.gmwatch.org/archive2.asp?arcid=4729
8. Compiled by Wayne Parrot, "General Safety and Safety Assessment of Specific Genetically Modified Crops from Scientific Journal Articles," AgBioWorld (October, 2005) http://www.agbioworld.org/biotech-info/articles/biotech-art/gen_safety.html
9. Judy Carman, "Report on a List of Abstracts On GM Crop Safety," (July 2006) http://www.munlochygmvigil.org.uk/GMCropSafety.pdf
10. Environmental Working Group, "Monsanto Knew about PCB Toxicity for Decades," Chemical Industry Archives http://www.chemicalindustryarchives.org/dirtysecrets/annistonindepth/toxicity.asp
11. J.T.Garrett, Memo to H.B.Patrick, Chemical Industry Archives (November 14,1955) http://www.chemicalindustryarchives.org/search/pdfs/anniston/19551114_494.pdf
12. Confidential Report of Aroclor "Ad Hoc" Committee, Chemical Industry Archives (October 2, 1969) http://www.chemicalindustryarchives.org/search/pdfs/anniston/19691002_141.pdf
13. Kelly, memo to Papageorge, Chemical Industry Archives (March 30, 1970) http://www.chemicalindustryarchives.org/search/pdfs/anniston/19700330_207.pdf
14. Minutes of Aroclor Ad   690905_200.pdf
15. Monsanto Chemical Company (St. Louis), "Pollution Letter," Chemical Industry Archives (February 16, 1970) http://www.chemicalindustryarchives.org/search/pdfs/anniston/19700216_205.pdf
16. In 2005, Monsanto was fined $1.5 million for giving bribes and questionable payments to at least 140 Indonesian officials. Antje Lorch, "Monsanto Bribes in Indonesia, Monsanto Fined For Bribing Indonesian Officials to Avoid Environmental Studies for *Bt* Cotton," ifrik 1sep2005, http://www.mindfully.org/GE/2005/Monsanto-Bribes-Indonesia1sep05.htm
17. Azevedo, pers. comm.
18. "Global Seed Industry Concentration–2005," *ETC Group Communiqué* 90 (September/October 2005).
19. "Oligopoly, Inc. 2005," *ETC Group Communiqué* 91 (November/December 2005).
20. Charles Benbrook, "Genetically Engineered Crops and Pesticide Use in the United States: The First Nine Years," AG BioTech InfoNet (October 2004) http://www.biotech-info.net/Technical_Paper_6.pdf
21. Clive James, Executive summary of "Global status of commercialised biotech/GM crops: 2006," ISAAA Brief 35. 2006 www.isaaa.org/Resources/Publications/briefs/35/executivesummary/default.html
22. Louis J. Pribyl, "Biotechnology Draft Document, 2/27/92," Alliance for Bio-Integrity (March 6, 1992) www.biointegrity.org
23. Kahl, Memo to James Maryanski, January 8, 1992.
24. Dr. David Schubert, "Response to Bradford et al." found in Mike Zelina, et al., "The Health Effects of Genetically Engineered Crops on Sna Luis Obispo County," *A Citizen Response to the SLO Health Commission GMO Task Force Report, 2006*
25. Robert Mann, "GM-Eggplant Challenged in Supreme Court of India," Press Release (August 7, 2006) http://www.scoop.co.nz/stories/WO0608/S00085.htm
26. B. S., Ahloowalia, et al., "Global Impact of Mutation-Derived Varieties. *Euphytica* 135 (2004): 187–204.

27. Dr. David Schubert, "Response to Bradford et al." found in Mike Zelina, et al., "The Health Effects of Genetically Engineered Crops on Sna Luis Obispo County," *A Citizen Response to the SLO Health Commission GMO Task Force Report, 2006*

28. William Freese and David Schubert, "Safety Testing and Regulation of Genetically Engineered Foods," *Biotechnology and Genetic Engineering Reviews* 21 (November 2004).

29. Judy Carman, "Is GM Food Safe to Eat?," In: Hindmarsh R, Lawrence G, editors. *Recoding Nature Critical Perspectives on Genetic Engineering,* Sydney: UNSW Press; 2004. p. 82-93.

30. European Communities submission to World Trade Organization dispute panel, 28 January 2005, cited in Friends of the Earth Europe and Greenpeace, "Hidden Uncertainties What the European Commission doesn't want us to know about the risks of GMOs," April 2006

PART 1, SECTION 1: EVIDENCE OF REACTIONS

1. *GM Free Cymru,* "New Evidence of Harm from GM FoodTriggers Call for Immediate Ban," *Press Release, November 25, 2005.*

2. Joel Bleifuss, "No Small (Genetic) Potatoes," In These Times.com (January 10, 2000) http://www.inthesetimes.com/issue/24/03/bleifuss2403.html

3. Ian F. Pryme and Rolf Lembcke, "In Vivo Studies on Possible Health Consequences of Genetically Modified Food and Feed—with Particular Regard to Ingredients Consisting of Genetically Modified Plan Materials," *Nutrition and Health* 17(2003): 1–8.

4. Arpad Pusztai, "Can science give us the tools for recognizing possible health risks of GM food," Nutrition and Health, 2002, Vol 16 Pp 73-84

5. Stanley W. B. Ewen and Arpad Pusztai, "Effect of diets containing genetically modified potatoes expressing Galanthus nivalis lectin on rat small intestine," Lancet, 1999 Oct 16; 354 (9187): 1353-4.

6. A. Pusztai, S. W. B. Ewen, G. Grant, W. J. Peumans, E. J. M. van Damme, L. Rubio, and S. Bardocz, "Relationship Between Survival and Binding of Plant Lectins during Small Intestinal Passage and Their Effectiveness as Growth Factors," *Digestion* 46, suppl. 2 (1990): 308–316.

7. Pryme and Lembcke, "In Vivo Studies on Possible Health Consequences of Genetically Modified Food and Feed," 1–8.

8. Arpad Pusztai, "Facts Behind the GM Pea Controversy: Epigenetics, Transgenic Plants & Risk Assessment," *Proceedings of the Conference, December 1st 2005* (Frankfurtam Main, Germany: Literaturhaus, 2005).

9. Robert J. Scheuplein, Memo to the FDA Biotechnology Coordinator and others, "Response to Calgene Amended Petition," Alliance for Bio-Integrity (October 27, 1993) http://www.biointegrity.org

10. Department of Veterinary Medicine, FDA, correspondence June 16, 1993. As quoted in Fred A. Hines, Memo to Dr. Linda Kahl. "Flavr Savr Tomato:... Pathology Branch's Evaluation of Rats with Stomach Lesions From Three Four-Week Oral (Gavage) Toxicity Studies ... and an Expert Panel's Report," Alliance for Bio-Integrity (June 16, 1993) http://www.biointegrity.org/FDAdocs/17/view1.html

11. Scheuplein, "Response to Calgene Amended Petition," October 27, 1993.

12. Carl B. Johnson to Linda Kahl and others, "Flavr Savr™ Tomato: Significance of Pending DHEE Question," Alliance for Bio-Integrity (December 7, 1993) http://www.biointegrity.org

13. Fred Hines to Linda Kahl, "Flavr Savr Tomato ... Pathology Branch's Remarks to Calgene Inc.'s Response to FDA Letter of June 29, 1993," Alliance for Bio-Integrity, http://www.biointegrity.org

14. Dr. Fred Hines, Memo to Dr. Linda Kahl. "Flavr Savr Tomato: ... Pathology Branch's Evaluation of Rats with Stomach Lesions From Three Four-Week Oral (Gavage) Toxicity Studies ... and an Expert Panel's Report," Alliance for Bio-Integrity (June 16, 1993) http://www.biointegrity.org/FDAdocs/17/view1.html

15. Arpad Pusztai, "Can Science Give Us the Tools for Recognizing Possible Health Risks for GM Food?" *Nutrition and Health* 16 (2002): 73–84.

16. "Conclusions of the Expert Panel Regarding the Safety of the Flav-Savr Tomato," Environ report number: 17, Arlington, VA, USA, pp. 2355-2382; Four week oral (intubation) toxicity study in rats by IRDC, pp. 2895-3000.

17. Pusztai, "Can Science Give Us the Tools for Recognizing Possible Health Risks for GM food?" 73–84.

18. Arpad Pusztai, "Genetically Modified Foods: Are They a Risk to Human/Animal Health?" June 2001 Action Bioscience http://www.actionbioscience.org/biotech/pusztai.html

19. Scheuplein, "Response to Calgene Amended Petition," October 27, 1993.

20. Steven Druker organized the lawsuit that uncovered the memos of the FDA experts. He notes that FDA regulations explicitly require that any additive to the food supply that lacks a history of safe use prior to 1958 must be demonstrated to be safe according to the same level of proof that is required for a formal food additive petition, regardless of whether such a petition is being filed. Thus, the memo indicates a violation of the law. Steven M. Druker, Advisory on US Law and

Genetically Engineered Food," Alliance for Bio-Integrity, 2004 http://www.biointegrity.org/Advisory.html

21. *Code of Federal Regulations*, Title 21, Sec. 170.30(b)

22. Herve Kempf, "L'expertise confidentielle sur un inquiétant maïs transgénique" (Confidential report on a worrying GM corn)," Le Monde, April 22, 2004. Translation by Claire Robinson, http://www.lemonde.fr/web/article/0,1-0@2-3226,36-362061,0.html.

23. John M. Burns, "13-Week Dietary Subchronic Comparison Study with MON 863 Corn in Rats Preceded by a 1-Week Baseline Food Consumption Determination with PMI Certified Rodent Diet #5002," December 17, 2002 http://www.monsanto.com/monsanto/content/sci_tech/prod_safety/fullratstudy.pdf

24. Stéphane Foucart, "Controversy Surrounds a GMO," *Le Monde*, 14 December 2

25. R. Hindmarsh, G. Lawrence, eds, *Recoding Nature Critical Perspectives on Genetic Engineering*, Judy Carman, "Is GM Food Safe to Eat?" (Sydney: UNSW Press; 2004): 82–93; citing documents from FSANZ (Food Safety Australia and New Zealand).

26. R. I. Vazquez-Padron et al. "Cry1Ac Protoxin from *Bacillus thuringiensis* sp. Kurstaki HD73 Binds to Surface Proteins in the Mouse Small Intestine," *Biochemical and Biophysical Research Communications* 271 (2000): 54–58.

27. Nagui H. Fares, Adel K. El-Sayed, "Fine Structural Changes in the Ileum of Mice Fed on Endotoxin Treated Potatoes and Transgenic Potatoes," *Natural Toxins* 6, no. 6 (1998): 219–233.

28. Fares and El-Sayed, "Fine Structural Changes in the Ileum of Mice Fed on Endotoxin Treated Potatoes and Transgenic Potatoes," 219–233.

29. Joe Cummins, PhD, personal communication, 2006

30. Ashish Gupta et. al., "Impact of *Bt* Cotton on Farmers' Health (in Barwani and Dhar District of Madhya Pradesh)," *Investigation Report*, Oct–Dec 2005.

31. Ibid.

32. "Mortality in Sheep Flocks after Grazing on *Bt* Cotton Fields—Warangal District, Andhra Pradesh" *Report of the Preliminary Assessment*, April 2006, http://www.gmwatch.org/archive2.asp?arcid=6494

33. Ibid.

34. Ibid.

35. Vazquez-Padron, et al, "Cry1Ac Protoxin from *Bacillus thuringiensis* sp. Kurstaki HD73 Binds to Surface Proteins in the Mouse Small Intestines," 54–58.

36. Ibid.

37. G. V. Ramanjaneyulu (Centre for Sustainable Agriculture) and Sagari Ramdas (ANTHRA), letter to Shri Bir Singh Parsheera, Chairperson, Genetic Engineering Approval Committee, India, July 28, 2006.

38. C. S. Pawar, "Study in Khammam district, Andhra Pradesh, India, 2005–2006," *BT Versus Non-BT Cotton: A Critical Analysis of On-farm Data, Impressions and Opinions*, World Wildlife Fund (WWF) International

39. Ramanjaneyulu and Ramdas (ANTHRA), letter to Shri Bir Singh Parsheera, India, July 28, 2006.

40. "Study Result Not Final, Proof *Bt* Corn Harmful to Farmers," *BusinessWorld*, 02 Mar 2004.

41. "Genetically Modified Crops and Illness Linked," *Manila Bulletin*, 04 Mar 2004.

42. Ibid.

43. Ibid.

44. Mae-Wan Ho, "GM Ban Long Overdue, Dozens Ill & Five Deaths in the Philippines," ISIS Press Release, June 2, 2006.

45. Ibid.

46. Ibid.

47. Allen V. Estabillo, "Farmer's Group Urges Ban on Planting *Bt* Corn; Says It Could Be Cause of Illnesses," *Mindanews*, October 19, 2004.

48. N. Tomlinson of UK MAFF's Joint Food Safety and Standards Group 4, December 1998 letter to the U.S. FDA, commenting on its draft document, "Guidance for Industry: Use of Antibiotic Resistance Marker Genes in Transgenic Plants," http://www.food.gov.uk/multimedia/pdfs/acnfp1998.pdf; (see pages 64–68).

49. Jerry Rosman, personal communication, 2006

50. Barry M. Markaverich et al, "A Novel Endocrine-Disrupting Agent in Corn with Mitogenic Activity in Human Breast and Prostatic Cancer Cells," *Environmental Health Perspectives* 110, no. 2 (February 2002).

51. Ibid.

52. Barry M. Markaverich et al, "Leukotoxin Diols from Ground Corncob Bedding Disrupt Estrous Cyclicity in Rats and Stimulate MCF-7 Breast Cancer Cell Proliferation," *Environmental Health Perspectives* 113, no. 12 (December 2005).

53. Henning Strodthoff and Christoph Then, "Is GM maize responsible for deaths of cows in Hesse?," Greenpeace Report, Greenpeace e.V. 22745 Hamburg. December 2003.

54. Ibid.

55. Mae-Wan Ho and Sam Burcher, "Cows Ate GM Maize & Died," ISIS Press Release, January 13, 2004, http://www.isis.org.uk/CAGMMAD.php

56. Ibid.

57. Strodthoff and Then, "Is GM maize responsible for deaths of cows in Hesse?," December 2003.

58. "Report on the Molecular Characterisation of the Genetic Map of Event *Bt*-176," Scientific Institute of Public Health, Service of Biosafety and Biotechnology IPH/1520/SBB/03-0408, June 16, 2003.

59. Ho and Burcher, "Cows Ate GM Maize & Died," January 13, 2004.

60. M. Malatesta, C. Caporaloni, S. Gavaudan, M. B. Rocchi, S. Serafini, C. Tiberi, G. Gazzanelli, "Ultrastructural Morphometrical and Immunocytochemical Analyses of Hepatocyte Nuclei from Mice Fed on Genetically Modified Soybean," *Cell Struct Funct.* 27 (2002): 173–180.

61. Ibid.

62. M. Malatesta, C. Tiberi, B. Baldelli, S. Battistelli, E. Manuali, M. Biggiogera, "Reversibility of Hepatocyte Nuclear Modifications in Mice Fed on Genetically Modified Soybean," *Eur J Histochem,* 49 (2005): 237-242.

63. Malatesta et al. "Ultrastructural Morphometrical," 173–180.

64. Ibid.

65. A. I. Lamond and J. E. Sleeman, Nuclear Substructure and Dynamics. *Current Biology* 13 (2003): R825–828.

66. T. Misteli, "Concepts in nuclear architecture." *Bioessays* 27 (2000): 477–487.

67. Malatesta et al., "Ultrastructural Morphometrical," 173–180.

68. E. Izaurralde and D. L. Spector, "Nucleus and Gene Expression: The interplay of transcriptional and post-transcriptional mechanisms that regulate gene expression," *Current Opinion Cell Biology* 16 (2004): 219–222.

69. Misteli, "Concepts in nuclear architecture," 477–487.

70. Malatesta, et al, "Reversibility of Hepatocyte Nuclear Modifications in Mice Fed on Genetically Modified Soybean," 237–242.

71. R. Tudisco, P. Lombardi, F. Bovera, D. d'Angelo, M. I. Cutrignelli, V. Mastellone, V. Terzi, L. Avallone, F. Infascelli, "Genetically Modified Soya Bean in Rabbit Feeding: Detection of DNA Fragments and Evaluation of Metabolic Effects by Enzymatic Analysis," *Animal Science* 82 (2006): 193–199.

72. Malatesta, et al, "Ultrastructural Analysis of Pancreatic Acinar Cells from Mice Fed on Genetically modified Soybean," 409.

73. M. Bendayan, A. Bruneau, J. Morisset, "Morphometrical and Immunocytochemical Studies on Rat Pancreatic Acinar Cells Under Control and Experimental Conditions," *Biol. Cell* 54 (1995): 227–234.

74. S. Grégoire, M. Bendayan, "Immunocytochemical Studies of Pancreatic Acinar Cells from Spontaneously Diabetic BB Wistar rats." *Pancreas* 2 (1987): 205–211.

75. M. Malatesta, M. Biggiogera, E. Manuali, M. B. L. Rocchi, B. Baldelli, G. Gazzanelli, "Fine Structural Analyses of Pancreatic Acinar Cell Nuclei from Mice Fed on GM Soybean," *Eur J Histochem* 47 (2003): 385–388.

76. M. Malatesta, B. Baldelli, S. Battistelli, C. Tiberi, E. Manuali, M. Biggiogera, "Nuclear Changes Induced in Hepatocytes after GM Diet are Reversible," *7th Multinational Congress on Microscopy—European Extension* (2005): 267–268.

77. S. S. Guraya, *Biology of Spermatogenesis and Spermatozoa in Mammals* (Springer Verlag, Berlin, Heidelberg, NewYork, London, Paris, Tokyo, 1987).

78. L. Vecchio et al, "Ultrastructural Analysis of Testes from Mice Fed on Genetically Modified Soybean," *European Journal of Histochemistry* 48, no. 4 (Oct–Dec 2004):449–454.

79. Ibid.

80. Ibid.

81. S. Fakan, "Ultrastructural Cytochemical Analyses of Nuclear Functional Architecture" *Eur J Histochem* 48 (2004): 5–14.

82. L. Vecchio et al, "Ultrastructural analysis of testes."

83. Ibid.

84. S. Fakan and E. Puvion. "The Ultrastructural Visualization of Nuclear and Extranucleolar RNA Synthesis and Distribution," *Int Rev Cytol* 65 (1980): 255–99.

85. Oliveri et al., "Temporary Depression of Transcription in Mouse Pre-implantion Embryos from Mice Fed on Genetically Modified Soybean," *48th Symposium of the Society for Histochemistry, Lake Maggiore (Italy), September 7–10, 2006.*

86. Tudisco et al, "Genetically Modified Soya Bean in Rabbit Feeding: Detection of DNA Fragments and Evaluation of Metabolic Effects by Enzymatic Analysis," 193–199.

87. Ibid.

88. I.V. Ermakova, "Diet with the Soya Modified by Gene EPSPS CP4 Leads to Anxiety and Aggression in Rats," *14th European Congress of Psychiatry. Nice, France, March 4-8, 2006.*

89. "Genetically modified soy affects posterity: Results of Russian scientists' studies," *REGNUM,* October 12, 2005; http://www.regnum.ru/english/526651.html

90. Irina Ermakova, "Genetically modified soy leads to the decrease of weight and high mortality of rat pups of the first generation. Preliminary studies," *Ecosinform* 1 (2006): 4–9.

91. I.V.Ermakova, "Genetically Modified Organisms and Biological Risks," *Proceedings of International Disaster Reduction Conference (IDRC) Davos, Switzerland August 27th – September 1st, 2006*: 168–172.

92. I.V.Ermakova "GMO: Life itself intervened into the experiments," Letter, *EcosInform* N2 (2006): 3–4.

93. Mark Townsend, "Why soya is a hidden destroyer," *Daily Express*, March 12, 1999.

94. Ibid.

95. Ibid.

96. Hye-Yung Yum, Soo-Young Lee, Kyung-Eun Lee, Myung-Hyun Sohn, Kyu-Earn Kim, "Genetically Modified and Wild Soybeans: An immunologic comparison," *Allergy and Asthma Proceedings* 26, no. 3 (May–June 2005): 210-216(7).

97. Cummins, pers. comm.

98. Arpad Pusztai, PhD, personal communication, 2006.

99. See for example, Scott H. Sicherer et al., "Prevalence of peanut and tree nut allergy in the United States determined by means of a random digit dial telephone survey: A 5-year follow-up study," *Journal of allergy and clinical immunology*, March 2003, vol. 112, n 6, 1203-1207); and Ricki Helm et al., "Hypoallergenic Foods—Soybeans and Peanuts," *Information Systems for Biotechnology News Report*, October 1, 2002.

100. John Boyles, MD, personal communication, 2007.

101. Comments to ANZFA about Applications A346, A362 and A363 from the Food Legislation and Regulation Advisory Group (FLRAG) of the Public Health Association of Australia (PHAA) on behalf of the PHAA, "Food produced from glyphosate-tolerant canola line GT73," http://www.iher.org.au/

102. Ibid.

103. U.K. Advisory Committee on Releases to the Environment, "Advice on a notification for marketing of herbicide tolerant GM oilseed rape," 24 September 2003, http://www.defra.gov.uk/environment/acre/advice/pdf/acre_advice36.pdf

104. Eva Novotny, "Report for the Chardon LL Hearing, Non-Suitability of Genetically Engineered Feed for Animals," Presented by Scientists for Global Responsibility, May 2002.

105. S. Leeson, "The Effect of Glufosinate Resistant Corn on Growth of Male Broiler Chickens," Department of Animal and Poultry Sciences, University of Guelph, Report No. A56379, July 12, 1996.

106. Comments to ANZFA about Applications A372, A375, A378 and A379 from the Food Legislation and Regulation Advisory Group (FLRAG) of the Public Health Association of Australia (PHAA) on behalf of the PHAA. http://www.iher.org.au/

107. Steve Kestin and Toby Knowles, Department of Clinical Veterinary Science, University of Bristol, testimony on behalf of Friends of the Earth, before the Chardon LL Hearings of the Advisory Committee on Releases to the Environment, November 2000.

108. Novotny, "Report for the Chardon LL Hearing, Non-Suitability of Genetically Engineered Feed for Animals," May 2002.

109. V. E. Prescott, et al, "Transgenic Expression of Bean r-Amylase Inhibitor in Peas Results in Altered Structure and Immunogenicity," *Journal of Agricultural Food Chemistry* (2005): 53.

110. Gundula Meziani and Hugh Warwick, "Seeds of Doubt," Soil Association (UK), September 17, 2002.

111. Ibid.

112. Ibid.

113. Mark Newhall, "He Says Geese Don't Like Roundup Ready Beans," *Farm Show* 24, no. 5 (2000).

114. Steve Sprinkel, "When the Corn Hits the Fan," *Acres, U.S.A.*, September 18, 1999.

115. Howard Vlieger, personal communication, 2003.

116. Bill Lashmett, personal communication, 2003.

117. Vlieger, pers. comm.

118. Steve Sprinkel, "When the Corn Hits the Fan."

119. Vlieger, pers. comm.

120. Sprinkel, "When the Corn Hits the Fan."

121. Hinze Hogendoorn, "Genetically Modified Corn (Zea mays) and Soya (Glycine soja) or Their Natural Varieties - Do Mice Have a Preference?"; http://www.talk2000.nl/mice/talk-Extended.htm

122. Meziani and Warwick, "Seeds of Doubt."

123. Hinze Hogendoorn, "Genetically Modified Corn (Zea mays) and Soya (Glycine soja) or Their Natural Varieties - Do Mice Have a Preference?"; http://www.talk2000.nl/mice/talk-Extended.htm

124. Rick Weiss, "Biotech Food Raises a Crop of Questions," *Washington Post*, August 15, 1999: A1.

125. L. R. B. Mann, D. Straton and W. E. Crist, "The Thalidomide of Genetic Engineering," Revised April 2001 from the GE issue of 'Soil & Health (NZ)' Aug '99, connectotel, http://www.connectotel.com/gmfood/trypto.html

126. William E. Crist, "The Toxic L-Tryptophan Epidemic," as quoted in A. N. Mayeno and G. J. Gleich, eds, "Eosinophilia-Myalgia Syndrome and Tryptophan Production: A Cautionary Tale." *Trends Biotechnol* 12 (1994): 346–352; (also see

www.seedsofdeception.com).

127. James Maryanski, FDA Biotechnology Coordinator, speaking to investigator William E. Crist's, "The Toxic L-Tryptophan Epidemic," see www.seedsofdeception.com/Public/L-tryptophan/index.cfm

128. Edwin M. Kilbourne, et al, "Tryptophan Produced by Showa Denko and Epidemic Eosinophilia-Myalgia Syndrome," *Journal of Rheumatology Supplement* 23, no. 46 (October 1996): 81–92.

129. National Eosinophilia-Myalgia Syndrome Network, position statement, approved quote by Gerald J. Gleich, Mayo Clinic and Foundation, May 25, 2000.

PART 1, SECTION 2: GENE INSERTION DISRUPTS THE DNA

1. Cesare Gessler, from the ETH Swiss Federal Institute of Technology, quoted in "Florianne Koechlin: Opening Speech," *Epigenetics, Transgenic Plants & Risk Assessment, Proceedings of the Conference, December 1st 2005*, (Frankfurtam Main, Germany: Literaturhaus, 2005).

2. "Elements of Precaution: Recommendations for the Regulation of Food Biotechnology in Canada; An Expert Panel Report on the Future of Food Biotechnology prepared by The Royal Society of Canada at the request of Health Canada Canadian Food Inspection Agency and Environment Canada" The Royal Society of Canada, January 2001.

3. J. R. Latham, et al., "The Mutational Consequences of Plant Transformation," *The Journal of Biomedicine and Biotechnology* 2006, Article ID 25376: 1-7; see also Allison Wilson, et. al., "Transformation-induced mutations in transgenic plants: Analysis and biosafety implications," *Biotechnology and Genetic Engineering Reviews* – Vol. 23, December 2006.

4. Allison Wilson, et al., "Regulatory Regimes for Transgenic Crops," *Nature Biotechnology* 23 (2005): 785; citing the following: M. Hernandez, et al., *Transgenic Res.* 12 (2003): 179–189; P. Windels, I. Tavernier, A. Depicker, E. Van Bockstaele, and M. De Loose, *M. Eur. Food Res. Technol.* 213 (2001): 107–112; W. Freese and D. Schubert, *Biotechnol. Genet. Eng. Rev.* 21 (2004): 299–324; and A. Spok, et al., "Risk Assessment of GMO Products in the European Union," (Bundesministerium fur Gesundheit und Frauen, Vienna, 2004) http://www.bmgf.gv.at

5. A. Forsbach, D. Shubert, B. Lechtenberg, M. Gils, R. Schmidt. "A Comprehensive Characterisation of Single-Copy T-DNA Insertions in the *Arabidopsis thaliana* Genome," *Plant Mol Biol* 52 (2003): 161–176.

6. F. E. Tax, D. M. Vernon, "T-DNA-Associated Duplication/Translocations in *Arabidopsis*: Implications for mutant analysis and functional genomics," *Plant Physiol* 126 (2001): 1527–1538.

7. H. Kaya, S. Sato, S. Tabata, Y. Kobayashi, M. Iwabuchi, T. Araki, "*Hosoba toge toge*, a syndrome caused by a large chromosomal deletion associated with a T-DNA insertion in *Arabidopsis*," Plant Cell Physiol 41, no. 9 (2000): 1055–1066.

8. Wilson, et. al., "Transformation-induced mutations in transgenic plants: Analysis and biosafety implications."

9. S. K. Svitashev, W. P. Pawlowski, I. Makarevitch, D. W. Plank, D. A. Somers, "Complex Transgene Locus Structures Implicate Multiple Mechanisms for Plant Transgene Rearrangement," *Plant Journal* 32 (2002): 433–445.

10. Allison Wilson, PhD, Jonathan Latham, PhD, and Ricarda Steinbrecher, PhD, "Genome Scrambling—Myth or Reality? *Transformation-Induced Mutations in Transgenic Crop Plants Technical Report—October 2004*, http://www.econexus.info; see also J. R. Latham, et al., "The Mutational Consequences of Plant Transformation," *The Journal of Biomedicine and Biotechnology* 2006, Article ID 25376: 1–7.

11. I. Makarevitch, S. K. Svitashev and D. A. Somers, "Complete sequence analysis of transgene loci from plants transformed via microprojectile bombardment," *Plant Mol Biol* 52 (2003): 421–432.

12. Latham, et al., "The Mutational Consequences of Plant Transformation," 1–7; see also John Innes Centre, "Study G02002—Methods for the analysis of GM wheat and barley seed for unexpected consequences of the transgene insertion," September 2001 to January 2005.

13. U.S. FDA, "Premarket notice concerning bioengineered foods: Proposed rule," Federal Register 66:4706-38. http://www.cfsan.fda.gov/~lrd/fr010118.html

14. John Innes Centre, "Study G02002," September 2001 to January 2005.

15. Robert Mann, "GM-eggplant Challenged in Supreme Court of India," Press Release, August 7, 2006; http://www.scoop.co.nz/stories/WO0608/S00085.htm

16. S. M. Jain, "Tissue culture-derived variation in crop improvement," *Euphytica* 118 (2001): 153–166.

17. Latham, et al., "The Mutational Consequences of Plant Transformation," 1-7; see also Wilson, "Genome Scrambling—Myth or Reality?"

18. P. H. Bao, S. Granata, S. Castiglione, G. Wang, C. Giordani, E. Cuzzoni, G. Damiani, C. Bandi, S. K. Datta, K. Datta, I. Potrykus, A. Callegarin and F. Sala, "Evidence for genomic changes in transgenic rice (*Oryza sativa* L.) recovered from protoplasts" *Transgen Res* 5 (1996): 97–103.

19. M. Labra, C. Savini, M. Bracale, N. Pelucchi, L. Colombo, M. Bardini and F. Sala, "Genomic changes in transgenic rice (Oryza sativa L.) plants produced by infecting calli with *Agrobacterium tumefaciens*," *Plant Cell Rep* 20 (2001): 325–330.

20. Scottish Crop Research Institute, "Study GO2001: Transcriptome, proteome and metabolome analysis to detect

unintended effects in genetically modified potato," September 2001 to January 2005; and John Innes Centre, "Study G02002—Methods for the analysis of GM wheat and barley seed for unexpected consequences of the transgene insertion, September 2001 to January 2005.

21. Ibid.

22. NRC/IOM: Committee on Identifying and Assessing Unintended Effects of Genetically Engineered Foods on Human Health, *Safety of Genetically Engineered Foods: Approaches to assessing unintended health effects* (Washington, DC: The National Academies Press, 2004).

23. D. A. Kessler, M. R. Taylor, J. H. Maryanski, E. L. Flamm, L. S. Kahl, "The safety of foods developed by biotechnology," *Science* 256 (1992): 1747–1832.

24. Wilson, et al, "Genome Scrambling—Myth or Reality?"

25. David Schubert, "A Different Perspective on GM Food," *Nature Biotechnology* 20, no. 10 (October 2002): 969.

26. Srivastava, et al, "Pharmacogenomics of the cystic fibrosis transmembrane conductance regulator (CFTR) and the cystic fibrosis drug CPX using genome microarray analysis," *Mol Med.* 5, no. 11(Nov 1999):753–67.

27. Ibid.

28. "Elements of Precaution," The Royal Society of Canada, January 2001.

29. Srivastava, et al, "Pharmacogenomics of the cystic fibrosis transmembrane conductance regulator (CFTR) and the cystic fibrosis drug CPX using genome microarray analysis," 753–67.

30. David Schubert, "A Different Perspective on GM Food," *Nature Biotechnology* 20, no. 10 (October 2002): 969.

31. Ibid.

32. Ibid.

33. E. Ann Clark, "Parliamentarians and Technology: Meeting the Challenges for the New Millenium, Workshop on Ensuring Food Safety," uoguelph.ca, (May 9, 2000), http://www.uoguelph.ca/plant/research/homepages/eclark/Hc.htm

34. D. B. Kohn et al., "Occurrence of leukaemia following gene therapy of X-linked SCID," *Nature Reviews Cancer* 3 no. 7 (July 2003): 477–88.

35. Clark, "Parliamentarians and Technology."

36. Joe Cummins, Mae-Wan Ho, Angela Ryan, "Hazardous CaMV promoter?" *Nature Biotechnology* 18 (April 1, 2000): 363–363; http://www.nature.com/nbt/journal/v18/n4/full/nbt0400_363a.html

37. A. Pusztai and S. Bardocz, "GMO in animal nutrition: potential benefits and risks," Chapter 17, *Biology of Nutrition in Growing Animals*, R. Mosenthin, J. Zentek and T. Zebrowska (Eds.) Elsevier, October 2005

38. M. W. Ho and J. Cummins, "Hazards of transgenic plants containing the cauliflower mosaic viral promoter: Authors' reply to critiques of "*The Cauliflower Mosaic Viral Promoter - a Recipe for Disaster?*," *Microbial Ecology in Health and Disease* 12, no. 1, (26 September 2000): 6–11(6)

39. Clark, "Parliamentarians and Technology."

40. A. Kohli, S. Griffiths, N. Palacios, R. M. Twyman, P. Vain, D. A. Laurie, and P. Christou, "Molecular characterization of transforming plasmid rearrangements in transgenic rice reveals a recombination hotspot in the CaMV 35S promoter and confirms the predominance of microhomology mediated recombination," *Plant J* 17 (1999): 591–601.

41. S. P. Kumpatla and T. C. Hall, "Organizational complexity of a rice transgenic locus susceptible to methylation-based silencing. *IUBMB Life* 48 (1999): 459–467.

42. C. Collonier, G. Berthier, F. Boyer, M. N. Duplan, S. Fernandez, N. Kebdani, A. Kobilinsky, M. Romanuk, Y. Bertheau, "Characterization of commercial GMO inserts: a source of useful material to study genome fluidity," poster courtesy of Pr. Gilles-Eric Seralini, Président du Conseil Scientifique du CRII-GEN, www.crii-gen.org

43. Mae-Wan Ho, "Transgenic Lines Proven Unstable," Institute for Science in Society, http://www.i-sis.org.uk/TLPU.php; For further discussion, see Ho et al, "CaMV 35S promoter fragmentation hotspot confirmed, and it is active in animals," *Microbial Ecology in Health and Disease* 2000:13, http://www.i-sis.org.uk/mehd3.php

44. Terje Traavik and Jack Heinemann, *Genetic Engineering and Omitted Health Research: Still No Answers to Ageing Questions*, TWN Biotechnology & Biosafety Series 7, 2007

45. David Schubert, PhD, personal communication, 2006.

46. Ho, "Transgenic Lines Proven Unstable," and Rönning et al., "Event specific real-time quantitative PCR for genetically modified *Bt* 11 maize (Zea Mays)," *Eur Food Res Technol* 216 (2003): 347–354.

47. Traavik and Heinemann, *Genetic Engineering and Omitted Health Research: Still No Answers to Ageing Questions*.

48. Ibid.

49. William Freese and David Schubert "Safety Testing and Regulation of Genetically Engineered Foods," *Biotechnology and Genetic Engineering Reviews* 21 (November 2004).

50. Jack Heinemann et al, "Submission on Application A549 Food Derived from High Lysine Corn LY038: to permit the use in food of high lysine corn," Submitted to Food Standards Australia/New Zealand (FSANZ) by New Zealand Institute of Gene Ecology, January 22, 2005.

51. FANTOM Consortium and RIKEN Genome Exploration Research Group and Genome Science Group (Genome Network Project Core Group), *Science* 309 (2005): 1559–1563; and RIKEN Genome Exploration Research Group and Genome Science Group (Genome Network Project Core Group) and the FANTOM Consortium, *Science* 309 (2005): 1564–1566.

52. Helen Pearson, "What is a Gene?" *Nature* 441 (May 25, 2006).

53. B.P Lewis, C. B. Burge, and D. P. Bartel, "Conserved seed pairing, often flanked by adenosines, indicates that thousands of human genes are microRNA targets," *Cell 120* (2005): 15–20.

54. C. Cogoni and G. Macino, "Post-transcriptional gene silencing across kingdoms," *Curr. Opin. Genet. Develop.* 10 (2005): 638–643; and G. J. Hannon, "RNA interference," *Nature* 418 no. 6894 (2002): 244–251.

55. M. Cretenet, J. Goven, J. A. Heinemann, B. Moore, and C. Rodriguez-Beltran, Submission on the DAR for Application A549 Food Derived from High-Lysine Corn LY038: to permit the use in food of high-lysine corn (2006) http://www.inbi.canterbury.ac.nz; with citations for S. Altuvia and E. G. H. Wagner, "Switching on and off with RNA," *Proc. Natl. Acad. Sci. USA* 97 no. 18 (2000): 9824–9826; and G. Faugeron, "Diversity of homology-dependent gene silencing strategies in fungi," *Curr. Opin. Microbiol.* 3(2000): 144–8; and N. A. Tchurikov, L. G. Chistyakova, et al. "Gene-specific Silencing by Expression of Parallel Complementary RNA in Escherichia coli," *J. Biol. Chem.* 275, no 34 (2000): 26523–26529; and Hannon, "RNA interference," 244–251.

56. T. Gura, "A silence that speaks volumes." *Nature* 404, no.678 (2000): 804–808.

57. Cretenet, et al., Submission on the DAR for Application A549 Food Derived from High-Lysine Corn LY038.

58. Cogoni and Macino, "Post-transcriptional gene silencing across kingdoms," 244–251, and L. Timmons, D. L. Court, et al, "Ingestion of bacterially expressed dsRNAs can produce specific and potent genetic interference in Caenorhabditis elegans," *Gene* 263 (2001):103–112.

59. L. Timmons, et al., "Ingestion of bacterially expressed dsRNAs," 103–112.

60. Minoo Rassoulzadegan et al, "RNA-mediated non-mendelian inheritance of an epigenetic change in the mouse," *Nature* 441 (May 25, 2006): 469–474.

61. Susan J. Lolle et al., "Genome-wide non-mendelian inheritance of extra-genomic information in Arabidopsis," *Nature* 434 (March 24, 2005): 505–509.

62. S. Hirotsune, N. Yoshida, et al., "An expressed pseudogene regulates the messenger-RNA stability of its homologous coding gene," *Nature* 423 (2003): 91–96.

63. Z. Zhao, Y. Cao, et al., "Double-Stranded RNA Injection Produces Nonspecific Defects in Zebrafish." *Develop. Biol.* 229 (2001): 215–223.

64. Heinemann et al, Submission on Application A549 Food Derived from High Lysine Corn LY038.

65. Ibid.

66. Ibid.

67. M. Stevenson, "Therapeutic potential of RNA interference," *N. Engl. J. Med.* 351 (2004): 1772–1777.

68. E. A. Brisibe, N. Okada, H. Mizukami, H. Okuyama, and Y. R. Fujii, "RNA interference: potentials for the prevention of HIV infections and the challenges ahead," *Trends Biotechnol.* 21(2003): 306–311.

69. D. L. Lewis, J. E.Hagstrom, A. G. Loomis, J. A. Wolff, H. and Herweijer, "Efficient delivery of siRNA for inhibition of gene expression in postnatal mice," *Nat. Genet.* 32 (2002): 107–108.

70. E. Check, "Hopes rise for RNA therapy as mouse study hits target," *Nature* 432 (2004):136; and P. D. Zamore and N.Aronin, "siRNAs knock down hepatitis," *Nat. Med.* 9(2003): 266–267.

71. Cretenet, et al, Submission on the DAR for Application A549 Food Derived from High-Lysine Corn LY038.

72. S. Xiang, J. Fruehauf, and C. J. Li, "Short hairpin RNA–expressing bacteria elicit RNA interference in mammals." *Nat. Biotechnol.* 24no. 6(June 2006):697–702.

73. Cretenet, et al, Submission on the DAR for Application A549 Food Derived from High-Lysine Corn LY038.

74. Andreas Rang, et al, "Detection of RNA variants transcribed from the transgene in Roundup Ready soybean," *Eur Food Res Technol* 220 (2005): 438–443.

75. P. Windels, I. Taverniers, et al. "Characterisation of the Roundup Ready soybean insert," *Eur. Food Res. Technol.* 213 (2001): 107–112.

76. Rang et al, "Detection of RNA variants transcribed," 438–443.

77. P. Windels, I. Taverniers, et al. "Characterisation of the Roundup Ready soybean insert."

78. Jack Heinemann et al, Submission on Application A549 Food Derived from High Lysine Corn LY038

79. Andreas Rang et al, "Detection of RNA variants transcribed."

80. Monsanto Company, comments of Windels, et al., Publication Regarding Roundup Ready® Soybeans, August 16, 2001.

81. Monsanto Company, "Additional Characterization and Safety Assessment of the DNA Sequence Flanking the 3' End of the Functional Insert of Roundup Ready® Soybean Event 40-3-2," MSL-17632, February 2002; http://www.food.gov.uk/multimedia/pdfs/RRSsafetysummary.pdf

82. G. Meister, and T. Tuschl, "Mechanisms of gene silencing by double-stranded RNA," *Nature* 431 (2004): 343–349; and C. Mello, C. C. and D. Conte, Jr., "Revealing the world of RNA interference," *Nature* 432 (2004): 338–342.

83. "Elements of Precaution," The Royal Society of Canada, January 2001.

84. Richard D. Firn. "The genetic manipulation of Natural Product composition—risk assessment when a system is predictably unpredictable," *Epigenetics, Transgenic Plants & Risk Assessment, Proceedings of the Conference, December 1st 2005*, (Frankfurtam Main, Germany: Literaturhaus, 2005).

85. Ibid.

86. U. Roessner, et al., "Metabolic Profiling Allows Comprehensive Phenotyping of Genetically or Environmentally Modified Plant Systems," *Plant Cell* 13 (2001): 11–29.

87. Susan Benson, Mark Arax, and Rachel Burstein, "Growing Concern: As biotech crops come to market, neither scientists—who take industry money—nor federal regulators are adequately protecting consumers and farmers," *Mother Jones*, January/February 1997; http://www.motherjones.com/mother_jones/JF97/biotech_jump2.html

88. Royal Holloway, University of London, "Study G02005: The application of metabolic profiling to the safety assessment of GM foods," October 2001 to October 2004.

89. Mark Rasmussen, "Pest Resistant Plants: A New Frontier for Animal Nutrition," Iowa State University, hand out for *Animal Science* 519 (Digestive Physiology and Metabolism in Ruminants), 2006.

90. "Elements of Precaution," The Royal Society of Canada, January 2001.

91. B. Meldrum, "Amino acids as dietary excitotoxins: a contribution to understanding neurodegenerative disorders," *Brain Res* 18 (1993): 293–314.

92. Rasmussen, "Pest Resistant Plants: A New Frontier for Animal Nutrition."

93. N. J. Bate, J. Orr, W. Ni, A. Meromi, T. Nadler-Hassar, P. W. Doerner, R. A. Dixon, C. J. Lamb, Y. Elkind, "Quantitative relationship between phenylalanine ammonia-lyase levels and phenylpropanoid accumulation in transgenic tobacco identifies a rate-determining step in natural product synthesis," *Proc. Natl. Acad. Sci. USA* 91 (1994): 7608–12.

94. "Elements of Precaution," The Royal Society of Canada, January 2001.

95. S. L. Franck-Oberaspach, and B. Keller, "Consequences of classical and biotechnological resistance breeding for food toxicology and allergenicity. *Plant Breeding* 116 (1997): 1–17.

96. Richard D. Firn, "The genetic manipulation of Natural Product composition."

97. Mark Rasmussen, "Pest Resistant Plants: A New Frontier for Animal Nutrition."

98. Schubert, "A Different Perspective on GM Food," 969.

99. U.S. Department of Agriculture, "Phytonutrients Take Center Stage," Agricultural Research Service Web site, http://www.ars.usda.gov/is/AR/archive/dec99/stage1299.htm

100. Freese and Schubert, "Safety Testing and Regulation of Genetically Engineered Foods."

101. Marc A. Lappé, et al, "Alterations in Clinically Important Phytoestrogens in Genetically Modified, Herbicide-Tolerant Soybeans," *Journal of Medicinal Food* 1, no. 4.

102. Life Sciences Network, "Food can be 'More Powerful than Drugs,'" December 13, 2002; reporting on Barbara Demmig-Adams and William W. Adams, III "Antioxidants in Photosynthesis and Human Nutrition," *Science* 13 (December 2002): 2149-2153.

103. European Communities submission to World Trade Organization dispute panel, 28 January 2005 , cited in Friends of the Earth Europe and Greenpeace, "Hidden Uncertainties What the European Commission doesn't want us to know about the risks of GMOs," April 2006

104. Doug Gurian-Sherman, "Holes in the Biotech Safety Net, FDA Policy Does Not Assure the Safety of Genetically Engineered Foods," Center for Science in the Public Interest, http://www.cspinet.org/new/pdf/fda_report__final.pdf

105. W. K. Novak, and A. G. Haslberger, "Substantial equivalence of antinutrients and inherent plant toxicants in genetically modified foods," *Food Chem. Toxicol.* 38(2000):473-483.

106. Ibid.

107. Ibid.

108. National Research Council. "Genetically Modified Pest-Protected Plants: Science and Regulation" (Washington, DC: National Academy Press, 2000).

109. U. Roessner, et al., "Metabolic Profiling Allows Comprehensive Phenotyping of Genetically or Environmentally Modified Plant Systems," *Plant Cell* 13(2001): 11–29.

110. David Schubert, "Regulatory regimes for transgenic crops," letter in *Nature Biotechnology* 23(2005): 785–787, citing E. Grotewold, "Plant metabolic diversity: A regulatory perspective," *Trends Plant Sci.* 10: 57–6.

111. D. Saxena, and G. Stotzky, "*Bt* Corn Has a Higher Lignin Content than Non-*Bt* Corn." *American Journal of Botany* 88, no.9 (2001), 1704–1706.

112. For an excellent discussion of these type of changes, see William Freese and David Schubert, "Safety Testing and Regulation of Genetically Engineered Foods," *Biotechnology and Genetic Engineering Reviews* 21 (November 2004); and

David Schubert, "Regulatory regimes for transgenic crops," letter in *Nature Biotechnology* 23 (2005): 785–787.

113. R. Betarbet, T. B. Sherer, G. MacKenzie, et al., "Chronic systemic pesticide exposure reproduces features of Parkinson's disease," *Nature Neuroscience* 3(2000): 1301–1306.

114. Schubert, "Regulatory regimes for transgenic crops," 785–787.

115. A. S. Reddy and T. L. Thomas, "Modification of plant lipid composition: Expression of a cyanobacterial D6-desaturase gene in transgenic plants," *Nature BioTechnology* 14 (1996): 639–642.

116. T. Inose and K. Murata, "Enhanced accumulation of toxic compound in yeast cells having high glycolytic activity: A case study on the safety of genetically engineered yeast," *International Journal of Food Science and Technology* 30 (1995): 141–146.

117. U.K. Biotechnology and Biological Sciences Research Council, "Making Crops Make More Starch," *BBSRC Business*, January 1998: 6–8.

118. W. Hashimoto, K. Momma, T. Katsube, Y. Ohkawa, T. Ishige, M. Kito, S. Utsumi, K. Murata, "Safety Assessment of Genetically Engineered Potatoes With Designed Soybean Glycinin: Compositional Analyses of the Potato Tubers and Digestibility of the Newly Expressed Protein in Transgenic Potatoes," *Journal of the Science of Food and Agriculture* 79 (1999): 1607–1612.

119. S. C. H. J. Turk, S. C. M. Smeekens, "Genetic modification of plant carbohydrate metabolism," as quoted in V. L. Chopra, V. S. Malik, S. R. Bhat, eds, *Applied Plant Biotechnology* (Enfield: Science Publishers, 1999), 71–100.

120. Th. A. Dueck, A. van der Werf, L. A. P. Lotz, W. Jordi, "Methodological Approach to a Risk Analysis for Polygene-Genetically Modified Plants (GMPs): a Mechanistic Study, *AB Nota* 50 (Wageningen: Research Institute for Agrobiology and Soil Fertility (AB-DLO), 1998).

121. E. Delhaize, D. M. Hebb, K. D. Richards, J. M. Lin, P. R. Ryan, R. C. Gardner, "Cloning and expression of a wheat (Triticum aestivum) phosphatidylserine synthase cDNA: Overexpression in plants alters the composition of phospholipids," *Journal of Biological Chemistry* 274 (1999): 7082–7088.

122. F. Murray, D. Llewellyn, H. McFadden, D. Last, E. S. Dennis, W. J. Peacock, "Expression of the Talaromyces flavus glucose oxidase gene in cotton and tobacco reduces fungal infection, but is also phytotoxic," *Mol. Breed* 5 (1999): 219–232.

123. K. Momma, W. Hashimoto, S. Ozawa, S. Kawai, T. Katsube, F. Takaiwa, M. Kito, S. Utsumi, K. Murata, "Quality and safety evaluation of genetically engineered rice with soybean glycinin: analyses of the grain composition and digestibility of glycinin in transgenic rice," *Bioscience Biotechnology and Biochemistry* 63 (1999): 314–318.

124. X. Ye, S. Al Babili, A. Kloeti, J. Zhang, P. Lucca, P. Beyer, I, Potrykus, "Engineering the provitamin A (beta-carotene) biosynthetic pathway into (carotenoid-free) rice endosperm," *Science* 287 (2000): 303–305.

125. Arpad Pusztai, "Facts behind the GM pea controversy," *Epigenetics, Transgenic Plants & Risk Assessment, Proceedings of the Conference, December 1st 2005* (Frankfurtam Main, Germany: Literaturhaus, 2005)

126. USDA Application # 95-352-01, cited in Latham et al, "The Mutational Consequences of Plant Transformation, Journal of Biomedicine and Biotechnology 2006:1-7, article ID 25376, http://www.hindawi.com/journals/JBB/index.html

127. Stephen R. Padgette et al, Table 2 in "The Composition of Glyphosate-Tolerant Soybean Seeds Is Equivalent to That of Conventional Soybeans," *The Journal of Nutrition* 126, no. 4 (April 1996).

128. Stephen R. Padgette et al, "The Composition of Glyphosate-Tolerant Soybean Seeds Is Equivalent to That of Conventional Soybeans," *The Journal of Nutrition* 126, no. 4, (April 1996); including data in the journal archives from the same study.

129. Pusztai and Bardocz, "GMO in animal nutrition: potential benefits and risks."

130. Padgette et al, "The Composition of Glyphosate-Tolerant Soybean Seeds Is Equivalent to That of Conventional Soybeans."

131. Lisa K. Karr-Lilienthal, et. al., "Chemical Composition and Protein Quality Comparisons of Soybeans and Soybean Meals from Five Leading Soybean-Producing Countries," J. Agric. Food Chem. 2004, 52, 6193-6199

132. Food Legislation and Regulation Advisory Group (FLRAG) of the Public Health Association of Australia (PHAA) on behalf of the PHAA, Comments to ANZFA about Applications A346, A362 and A363; http://www.iher.org.au/

133. Ibid.

134. Ibid.

135. Food Legislation and Regulation Advisory Group (FLRAG) of the Public Health Association of Australia (PHAA) on behalf of the PHAA, Comments to ANZFA about Applications A372, A375, A378 and A379; http://www.iher.org.au/

136. Cretenet, et al, Submission on the DAR for Application A549 Food Derived from High-Lysine Corm LY038.

137. C. K. Shewmaker, J. A. Sheely, M. Daley, S. Colburn, D. Y. Ke, "Seed-specific overexpression of phytoene synthase: increase in carotenoids and other metabolic effects," *Plant Journal* 22, (1999): 401–412.

138. Food Legislation and Regulation Advisory Group (FLRAG) of the Public Health Association of Australia (PHAA) on behalf of the PHAA, "Food produced from glyphosate-tolerant canola line GT73," Comments to ANZFA about Applications A346, A362 and A363; http://www.iher.org.au/

139. FLRAG, comments to ANZFA about Applications A346, A362 and A363.

140. Derek Matthews, et al, "Toxic Secondary Metabolite Production in Genetically Modified Potatoes in Response to Stress," *J. Agric. Food Chem.*, ASAP Article 53 (20), 7766 -7776, 2005. Web Release Date: September 2, 2005

141. Patrick D. Colyer, et al, "Plant Pathology and Nematology: Root-Knot Nematode Reproduction and Root Galling Severity on Related Conventional and Transgenic Cotton Cultivars," *The Journal of Cotton Science* 4 (2000): 232–236; www.jcotsci.org

142. A. R. Myerson, "Seeds of discontent: cotton growers say strain cuts yields," *New York Times* Nov. 19, 1997; K. L. Edmisten, and A.C. York, "Concerns with Roundup Ready Cotton," North Carolina Cooperative Extensive Service, 1999. [Extracts] http://www.biotech-info.net/Cotton_agronomic_problems.html

143. C. M. Benbrook, "Troubled Times Amid Commercial Success for Roundup Ready Soybeans: Glyphosate Efficacy is Slipping and Unstable Transgene Expression Erodes Plant Defenses and Yields" (Sandpoint, Idaho: Northwest Science and Environmental Policy Center, 2001), http://www.biotech-info.net/troubledtimes.html; J. Fernandez-Cornejo and W. D. McBride, "Adoption of Bioengineered Crops," USDA ERS Agricultural Economic Report No. AER810 (2002), http://www.ers.usda.gov/publications/aer810/

144. R. W. Elmore, F. W. Roeth, L.A. Nelson, C. A. Shapiro, R. N. Klein, S. Z. Knezevic, and A. Martin, "Glyphosate-Resistant Soybean Cultivar Yields Compared with Sister Lines," *Agron. J.* 93 (2001): 408–412; see also R. W. Elmore, F.W. Roeth, R.N. Klein, S.Z. Knezevic, A. Martin, L.A. Nelson, and C.A. Shapiro, "Glyphosate-resistant soybean cultivar response to glyphosate," *Agron. J.* 93 (2001): 404–407.

145. A. Aumaitre, et al., "New feeds from genetically modified plants: substantial equivalence, nutritional equivalence, digestibility, and safety for animals and the food chain," *Livest. Prod. Sci.* 74 (2002): 223–238.

146. Pusztai and Bardocz, "GMO in animal nutrition: potential benefits and risks."

147. John Innes Centre, "Study G02002," September 2001 to January 2005.

148. Ibid.

149. Royal Holloway, University of London, "Study G02005," October 2001 to October 2004.

150. Lehesranta Satu, et al., "Comparison of tuber proteomes of potato varieties, landraces, and genetically modified lines," *Plant Physiol.* 138 no. 3(July 2005): 1690–1699.

151. Firn, "The genetic manipulation of Natural Product composition—risk assessment when a system is predictably unpredictable."

152. European Communities submission to World Trade Organization dispute panel, 28 January 2005 , cited in Friends of the Earth Europe and Greenpeace, "Hidden Uncertainties What the European Commission doesn't want us to know about the risks of GMOs," April 2006

153. Firn, "The genetic manipulation of Natural Product composition—risk assessment when a system is predictably unpredictable."

154. Rothamsted Research Centre, "Study G02003: Comparison of the metabolome and proteome of GM and non-GM wheat: Defining substantial equivalence," September 2001 to January 2005; see also Institute of Food Research, Norwich Research Park, "Study GO2004: Development and comparison of molecular profiling methods for improved safety evaluation using GM brassicas," September 2001 to January 2005.

PART 1, SECTION 3: THE PROTEIN MAY CREATE PROBLEMS

1. Michael Pollan, "Playing God in the Garden," *New York Times Magazine*, Oct. 25, 1998.

2. Rick Weiss, "Biotech Food Raises a Crop of Questions," *Washington Post*, August 15, 1999: A1.

3. Ibid.

4. Julie A. Nordlee et al, "Identification of a Brazil-Nut Allergen in Transgenic Soybeans," *N Engl J Med* 334 (1996):688–92.

5. Louis J. Pribyl, "Biotechnology Draft Document, 2/27/92," March 6, 1992, Alliance for Bio-Integrity, http://www.biointegrity.org

6. Food and Drug Administration, "Statement of Policy: Foods Derived from New Plant Varieties," Docket No. 92N-0139, 1992.

7. US EPA "Biopesticides Registration Action Document (BRAD)—*Bacillus thuringiensis* Plant-Incorporated Protectants: Product Characterization & Human Health Assessment," EPA BRAD (2001b) (October 15, 2001); http://www.epa.gov/pesticides/biopesticides/pips/bt_brad2/2-id_health.pdf

8. William Freese and David Schubert, "Safety Testing and Regulation of Genetically Engineered Foods," *Biotechnology and Genetic Engineering Reviews* 21 (November 2004); and David Schubert, "Regulatory regimes for transgenic crops," letter in *Nature Biotechnology* 23 (2005): 785–787.

9. FAO-WHO, "Evaluation of Allergenicity of Genetically Modified Foods. Report of a Joint FAO/WHO Expert Consultation on Allergenicity of Foods Derived from Biotechnology," Jan. 22–25, 2001; http://www.fao.org/es/ESN/

food/pdf/allergygm.pdf

10. D. D. Metcalfe et al, "Assessment of the Allergenic Potential of Foods Derived from Genetically Engineered Crop Plants," *Critical Reviews in Food Science and Nutrition* 36(S) (1996): S165–186.

11. Gendel, "The use of amino acid sequence alignments to assess potential allergenicity of proteins used in genetically modified foods," *Advances in Food and Nutrition Research* 42 (1998), 45–62.

12. US EPA, "Biopesticides Registration Action Document (BRAD)—*Bacillus thuringiensis* Plant-Incorporated Protectants."

13. G. A. Kleter and A. A. C. M. Peijnenburg, "Screening of transgenic proteins expressed in transgenic food crops for the presence of short amino acid sequences indentical to potential, IgE-binding linear epitopes of allergens," *BMC Structural Biology* 2 (2002): 8–19.

14. R. I. Vazquez Padron, L. Moreno Fierros, L. Neri Bazan, G. A. De la Riva, R. Lopez Revilla, "Intragastric and intraperitoneal administration of Cry1Ac protoxin from *Bacillus thuringiensis* induces systemic and mucosal antibody responses in mice," *Life Sci.* 64 (1999): 1897–1912; and R. I. Vazquez Padron, J. Gonzalez Cabrera, C. Garcia Tovar, L. Neri Bazan, R. Lopez Revilla, M. Hernandez, L. Morena Fierros, G.A. De la Riva, "Cry1Ac protoxin from *Bacillus thuringiensis* sp. *kurstaki* HD73 binds to surface proteins in the mouse small intestine," *Biochem. Biophys. Res. Commun.* 271 (2000): 54–58.

15. T. J. Fu, "Digestion Stability as a Criterion for Protein Allergenicity Assessment," *Ann. NY. Acad. Sci.* 964 (2002): 99–110; and references within this article.

16. M. Cretenet, J. Goven, J. A. Heinemann, B. Moore, and C. Rodriguez-Beltran, Submission on the DAR for Application A549 Food Derived from High-Lysine Corn LY038: to permit the use in food of high-lysine corn, 2006, www.inbi. canterbury.ac.nz

17. Cretenet, et al., Submission on the DAR for Application A549 Food Derived from High-Lysine Corn LY038.

18. SAP Report No. 2000-06, "December 1, 2000 REPORT FIFRA Scientific Advisory Panel Meeting, A Set of Scientific Issues Being Considered by the Environmental Protection Agency Regarding: Assessment of Scientific Information Concerning StarLink™ Corn," November 28, 2000.

19. H. P. J. M. Noteborn, "Assessment of the Stability to Digestion and Bioavailability of the LYS Mutant Cry9C Protein from Bacillus thuringiensis serovar tolworthi," Unpublished study submitted to the EPA by AgrEvo, EPA MRID No. 447343-05 (1998); and H. P. J. M. Noteborn et al, "Safety Assessment of the *Bacillus thuringiensis* Insecticidal Crystal Protein CRYIA(b) Expressed in Transgenic Tomatoes," in *Genetically modified foods: safety issues*, American Chemical Society Symposium Series 605, eds. K.H. Engel et al., (Washington, DC, 1995): 134–47.

20. Ibid.

21. Mae-Wan Ho and Joe Cummins, "GM Food & Feed Not Fit for Man or Beast," Press Release, Institute of Science in Society, (based on a paper presented at an ISP Briefing to Parliament, House of Commons, 29 April 2004); citing as the source, E. H. Chowdhury, H. Kuribara, A. Hino, P. Sultana, O. Mikami, N. Shimada, K. S. Guruge, M. Saito, Y. Nakajima. "Detection of corn intrinsic and recombinant DNA fragments and CrylAb protein in the gastrointestinal contents of pigs fed genetically modified corn *Bt* 11," *J. Anim. Sci.* 81 (2003): 2546–51.

22. Noteborn, "Assessment of the Stability to Digestion and Bioavailability of the LYS Mutant Cry9C Protein from Bacillus thuringiensis serovar tolworthi."

23. US EPA, "Biopesticides Registration Action Document (BRAD)—*Bacillus thuringiensis* Plant-Incorporated Protectants."

24. Ho and Cummins, "GM Food & Feed Not Fit for Man or Beast," 29 April 2004.

25. Washington State Department of Health, "Report of health surveillance activities: Asian gypsy moth control program," (Olympia, WA: Washington State Dept. of Health, 1993).

26. M. Green, et al., "Public health implications of the microbial pesticide *Bacillus thuringiensis*: An epidemiological study, Oregon, 1985-86," *Amer. J. Public Health* 80, no. 7(1990): 848–852.

27. M.A. Noble, P.D. Riben, and G. J. Cook, "Microbiological and epidemiological surveillance program to monitor the health effects of Foray 48B BTK spray" (Vancouver, B.C.: Ministry of Forests, Province of British Columbi, Sep. 30, 1992).

28. I.L. Bernstein et al, "Immune responses in farm workers after exposure to *Bacillus thuringiensis* pesticides," *Environmental Health Perspectives* 107, no. 7(1999): 575–582.

29. J. R. Samples, and H. Buettner, "Ocular infection caused by a biological insecticide," *J. Infectious Dis.* 148, no. 3 (1983): 614; as reported in Carrie Swadener, "*Bacillus thuringiensis (B.t.)*", *Journal of Pesticide Reform* 14, no. 3 (Fall 1994)

30. Green, et al., "Public health implications of the microbial pesticide *Bacillus thuringiensis*: An epidemiological study, Oregon, 1985-86," 848–852.

31. A. Edamura, MD, "Affidavit of the Federal Court of Canada, Trial Division. Dale Edwards and Citizens Against Aerial Spraying vs. Her Majesty the Queen, Represented by the Minister of Agriculture," (May 6, 1993); as reported in Swadener, "*Bacillus thuringiensis (B.t.)*."

32. Bernstein et al, "Immune responses in farm workers after exposure to *Bacillus thuringiensis* pesticides," 575–582.

33. Swadener, "*Bacillus thuringiensis (B.t.)."*

34. *Health effects of B.t.: Report of surveillance in Oregon, 1985-87. Precautions to minimize your exposure* (Salem, OR: Oregon Departmentof Human Resources, Health Division, April 18, 1991).

35. *Material Safety Data Sheet for Foray 48B Flowable Concentrate* (Danbury, CT: Novo Nordisk, February, 1991).

36. R. E. Bryant, J. A. Mazza, and L. R. Foster, "Effect of cyclophosphamide-induced neutropenia on susceptibility of mice to lethal infection with *Bacillus thuringiensis*," (Unpublished abstract) (Oregon Health Sciences University, 1993).

37. J. P. Siegel, J. A. Shadduck, and J. Szabo, "Safety of the entomopathogen *Bacillus thuringiensis* var. *israelensis* for mammals," *J. Econ. Ent.* 80 (1987):717–723.

38. Vazquez et al, "Intragastric and intraperitoneal administration of Cry1Ac protoxin from *Bacillus thuringiensis* induces systemic and mucosal antibody responses in mice," 1897–1912; Vazquez et al, "Characterization of the mucosal and systemic immune response induced by Cry1Ac protein from *Bacillus thuringiensis* HD 73 in mice," *Brazilian Journal of Medical and Biological Research* 33 (2000): 147–155.

39. Vazquez et al, "*Bacillus thuringiensis* Cry1Ac protoxin is a potent systemic and mucosal adjuvant," *Scandanavian Journal of Immunology* 49 (1999): 578–584. See also Vazquez-Padron et al., 147 (2000b).

40. L.Moreno-Fierros, N.Garcia, R.Lopez-Revilla, R.I.Vazquez-Padron, "Intranasal, rectal and intraperitoneal immunization with protoxin Cry1Ac from *Bacillus thuringiensis* induces compartmentalized serum, intestinal, vaginal, and pulmonary immune responses in Balb/c mice," *Microbes and Infection* 2 (2000): 885–90.

41. EPA Scientific Advisory Panel, "*Bt* Plant-Pesticides Risk and Benefits Assessments," March 12, 2001: 76. Available at: http://www.epa.gov/scipoly/sap/2000/october/octoberfinal.pdf

42. Vazquez et al, "Cry1Ac protoxin from *Bacillus thuringiensis sp. kurstaki* HD73 binds to surface proteins in the mouse small intestine," 54–58.

43. Noteborn et al, "Safety Assessment of the *Bacillus thuringiensis* Insecticidal Crystal Protein CRYIA(b) Expressed in Transgenic Tomatoes," 134–47.

44. Terje Traavik and Jack Heinemann, *Genetic Engineering and Omitted Health Research: Still No Answers to Ageing Questions*, TWN Biotechnology & Biosafety Series 7, 2007. Cited in their quote was: G. Stotzky, "Release, persistence, and biological activity in soil of insecticidal proteins from *Bacillus thuringiensis*," found in Deborah K. Letourneau and Beth E. Burrows, *Genetically Engineered Organisms. Assessing Environmental and Human Health Effects* (cBoca Raton, FL: CRC Press LLC, 2002), 187–222.

45. "BT: An Alternative to Chemical Pesticides," Environmental Protection Division, Ministry of Environment, Government of British Columbia, Canada, http://www.env.gov.bc.ca/epd/epdpa/ipmp/fact_sheets/BTfacts.htm

46. C. M. Ignoffo, and C. Garcial, "UV-photoinactivation of cells and spores of *Bacillus thuringiensis* and effects of peroxidase on inactivation," *Environmental Entomology* 7 (1978): 270–272.

47. "BT: An Alternative to Chemical Pesticides."

48. US EPA, "Biopesticides Registration Action Document (BRAD)—*Bacillus thuringiensis* Plant-Incorporated Protectants."

49. M. Mendelsohn et al, "Are *Bt* Crops Safe?" *Nature Biotechnology* 21, no. 9 (2003): 1003–1009 (see p. 1009, Table 6).

50. A. Hilbeck, M. S.Meier, and A. Raps, "Non-Target Organisms and *Bt* Plants: Report to Greenpeace International," *EcoStrat GmbH*, April 2000, http://www.greenpeaceusa.org/media/press_releases/gmo-report-complete.pdf

51. A. Dutton, H. Klein, J. Romeis, and F. Bigler, "Uptake of *Bt*-toxin by herbivores feeding on transgenic maize and consequences for the predator *Chrysoperia carnea*," *Ecological Entomology* 27 (2002): 441–7; and J. Romeis, A. Dutton, and F. Bigler, "*Bacillus thuringiensis* toxin (Cry1Ab) has no direct effect on larvae of the green lacewing *Chrysoperla carnea* (Stephens) (Neuroptera: Chrysopidae)," *Journal of Insect Physiology* 50, no.2–3 (2004): 175–183.

52. "Assessment of Additional Scientific Information Concerning StarLink Corn," EPA's Scientific Advisory Panel, SAP Report No. 2001-09, from meeting held July 17-18, 2001. Available at: http://www.epa.gov/scipoly/sap/2001/july/julyfinal.pdf.

53. William Ryberg, "Growers of biotech corn say they weren't warned: StarLink tags appear to indicate it's suitable for human food products," *Des Moines Register*, October 25, 2000.

54. EPA Preliminary Evaluation of Information Contained in the October 25, 2000 Submission from Aventis CropScience, Appendix 1; as cited in Bill Freese, "The StarLink Affair, Submission by Friends of the Earth to the FIFRA Scientific Advisory Panel considering Assessment of Additional Scientific Information Concerning StarLink Corn," July 17–19, 2001.

55. William Freese, "The StarLink Affair, Submission by Friends of the Earth to the FIFRA Scientific Advisory Panel considering Assessment of Additional Scientific Information Concerning StarLink Corn," July 17–19, 2001.

56. Ibid.

57. "Life-Threatening Food?" CBSNews.com, May 17, 2001, quoting Marc Rothenberg, allergy expert and adviser to the

government in the StarLink investigation.

58.   William Freese, "The StarLink Affair."

59.   Weiss, "Biotech Food Raises a Crop of Questions."

60.   "Assessment of Additional Scientific Information Concerning StarLink Corn," FIFRA Scientific Advisory Panel Report No. 2001-09, July 2001.

61.   Marc Kaufman, "EPA Rejects Biotech Corn as Human Food; Federal Tests Do Not Eliminate Possibility That It Could Cause Allergic Reactions, Agency Told," *Washington Post*, July 28, 2001: A02.

62.   J. Byard, "Cry9C protein: The digestibility of the Cry9C protein by simulated gastric and intestinal fluids," submitted to the EPA by Aventis CropScience. EPA MRID No. 451144-01 (2000): 17, as reported in William Freese, "Genetically Engineered Crop Health Impacts Evaluation: A Critique of U.S. Regulation of Genetically Engineered Crops and Corporate Testing Practices, with a Case Study of *Bt* Corn," Friends of the Earth U.S., http://www.foe.org/camps/comm/safefood/gefood/index.html

63.   Freese and Schubert, "Safety Testing and Regulation of Genetically Engineered Foods."

64.   T. Prior, S. Kunwar, and I. Pastan, "Studies on the activity of barnase toxins in vitro and in vivo," *Biocong Chem* 7 (1996): 23–9.

65.   Food Legislation and Regulation Advisory Group (FLRAG) of the Public Health Association of Australia (PHAA) on behalf of the PHAA, Comments to ANZFA about Applications A372, A375, A378 and A379, http://www.iher.org.au/

66.   Ilinskaya and Vamvakas "Nephrotic effect of bacterial ribonucleases in the isolated and perfused rat kidney," *Toxicology* 120 (1997): 55–63.

67.   Freese and Schubert, "Safety Testing and Regulation of Genetically Engineered Foods."

68.   Michiels et al, "Method to obtain male sterile plants," U.S. Patent 6,344,602 awarded to Aventis CropScience, February 5, 2002.

69.   Freese, "Genetically Engineered Crop Health Impacts Evaluation—GAPS Analysis."

70.   FLRAG, comments to ANZFA about Applications A372, A375, A378 and A379.

71.   Joseph Cummins, "Expanding terminator," Sustainable Agriculture Network Discussion Group (August 30, 2000), http://lists.ifas.ufl.edu/cgi-bin/wa.exe?A2=ind0008&L=sanet-mg&D=0&O=A&P=69745

72.   Joe Cummins, "Barnase Ribonuclease is toxic to Humans and other Mammals," Submission to Indian Supreme Court, October 18, 2006; citing P. Kirkharn, et al., "Towards the design of an antibody that recognizes a given protein epitope, *J. Mol. Biol.* 285 (1999): 909–15.

73.   Jack Heinemann et al, "Submission on Application A549 Food Derived from High Lysine Corn LY038: to permit the use in food of high lysine corn," Submitted to Food Standards Australia/New Zealand (FSANZ) by New Zealand Institute of Gene Ecology, January 22, 2005.

74.   M. Chamruspollert, G. M. Pesti, et al, "Dietary interrelationships among arginine, methionine, and lysine in young broiler chicks," *Br. J. Nutr.* 88 (2002): 655–660 (see p. 660).

75.   Jack Heinemann et al, "Submission on Application A549 Food Derived from High Lysine Corn LY038: to permit the use in food of high lysine corn," Submitted to Food Standards Australia/New Zealand (FSANZ) by New Zealand Institute of Gene Ecology, January 22, 2005.

76.   I. Giroux, E. M. Kurowska, et al, "Role of dietary lysine, methionine, and arginine in the regulation of hypercholesterolemia in rabbits," *J. Nutr. Biochem.* 10, no 3(1999): 166–171.

77.   M. Cretenet et al., "Submission on the DAR for Application A549 Food Derived from High-Lysine Corn LY038"

78.   P. Rozan, Y. H. Kuo, and F. Lambein, "Nonprotein amino acids in edible lentil and garden pea," *Amino Acids* 20 (2001): 319–324.

79.   T. Fujita, M. Fujita, T. Kodama, T. Hada, and K. Higashimo, "Determination of D- and L-pipecolic acid in food samples including processed foods," *Ann. Nutr. Met.*, 47 (2003): 165–169.

80.   Cretenet, et al, "Submission on the DAR for Application A549 Food Derived from High-Lysine Corn LY038."

81.   Ibid.

82.   J. W. J. Heijst, H. W. M. Niessen, K. Hoekman, and C. G. Schalkwijk, "Advanced Glycation End Products in Human Cancer Tissues: Detection of N-(Carboxymethyl)lysine and Argpyrimidine," *Ann. NY Acad. Sci.* 1043(2005): 725–733.

83.   T. Goldberg, W. Cai, M. Peppa, V. Dardaine, B. S. Baliga, J. Uribarri, and H. Vlassara, "Advanced glycoxidation end products in commonly consumed foods," *J. Am. Diet. Assoc.* 104(2004): 1287–1291.

84.   R. B. Elliott, "Diabetes—A man made disease," *Med. Hypoth*eses, 67 (March 9, 2006): 388-91.

85.   M. Peppa, H. Brem, P. Ehrlich, J. G. Zhang, W. Cai, Z. Li, A. Croitoru, S. Thung, and H. Vlassara, "Adverse Effects of Dietary Glycotoxins on Wound Healing in Genetically Diabetic Mice," *Diabetes* 52(2003): 2805–2813.

86.   Elliott, "Diabetes—A man made disease," 388-91.

87.   T. Henle, "Protein-bound advanced glycation endproducts (AGEs) as bioactive amino acid derivatives in foods," *Am. Acid* 29(2005): 313–322.

88. M. Freixes, A. Rodriguez, E. Dalfo, and I. Ferrer, "Oxidation, glycoxidation, lipoxidation, nitration, and responses to oxidative stress in the cerebral cortex in Creutzfeldt-Jakob disease," *Neurobiol. Aging*, Nov 23 2005; [E-pub ahead of print]

89. S. E. Fayle, and J. A. Gerrard, *The Maillard Reaction* (London: Royal Society of Chemistry, 2002).

90. J. A. Gerrard, "The Maillard reaction in food: progress made, challenges ahead-Conference report from the Eighth International Symposium on the Maillard Reaction," *Trends Food Sci. Tech.* 17 (2006): 324–330; and T. Henle, "Protein-bound advanced glycation endproducts (AGEs) as bioactive amino acid derivatives in foods," *Am. Acid* 29 (2005): 313–322.

91. S. Panigrahi, L. A. Bestwick, R. H. Davis, and C. D. Wood, "The nutritive value of stackburned yellow maize for livestock: tests in vitro and in broiler chicks," *Br. J. Nut.* 76 (1996), 97–108.

92. Cretenet, et al, "Submission on the DAR for Application A549 Food Derived from High-Lysine Corn LY038."

93. Ibid.

94. Ibid.

95. CAC (p. 18 paragraph 47); as cited in M. Cretenet, et al, "Submission on the DAR for Application A549 Food Derived from High-Lysine Corn LY038"

96. Cretenet, et al, "Submission on the DAR for Application A549 Food Derived from High-Lysine Corn LY038."

97. Ibid.

98. Jack Heinemann, letter to Hon. Kim Chance MLC, Centre for Integrated Research in Biosafety, July 31, 2006.

99. C. Mennella, M. Visciano, A. Napolitano, M. D. Del Castillo, and V. Fogliano, V, "Glycation of lysine-containing dipeptides," *J. Pep. Sci.* 12 (2006): 291–296.

100. Cretenet, et al, "Submission on the DAR for Application A549 Food Derived from High-Lysine Corn LY038."

101. Goldberg, et al, "Advanced glycoxidation end products in commonly consumed foods," 1287–1291.

102. Cretenet, et al, "Submission on the DAR for Application A549 Food Derived from High-Lysine Corn LY038."

103. Goldberg, et al, "Advanced glycoxidation end products in commonly consumed foods."

104. J. Heinemann, "Guess who's coming to dinner, A new kind of GM food may be about to join you at the dinner table, *The Press*, May 5, 2006.

105. Econexus, the Five Year Freeze, Friends of the Earth, GeneWatch UK, Greenpeace, the Soil Association, and Dr Michael Antoniou, Comments on GM Science Review, October 14th 2003.

106. M. E. Taliansky, and F. Garcia-Arenal, "Role of cucumovirus capsid protein in long-distance movement within the infected plant," *J Virol* 69, no. 2, 9162–2; R. W. Briddon, M. S. Pinner, J. Stanley, and P. G. Markham, "Geminivirus coat protein gene replacement alters insect specificity," *Virology* 177 no. 1 (1990): 85–94.

107. B. Cooper, et al., "A defective movement protein of TMV in transgenic plants confers resistance to multiple viruses whereas the functional analog increases susceptibility," *Virology* 206, no. 1 (1995): 307–13; V. Ziegler-Graff, P. J. Guilford, and D. C. Baulcombe, "Tobacco rattle virus RNA-1 29K gene product potentiates viral movement and also affects symptom induction in tobacco," *Virology* 182 no. 1(1991): 145–55.

108. R. W. Siegel, S. Adkins, and C. C. Kao, "Sequence-specific recognition of a subgenomic RNA promoter by a viral RNA polymerase," *Proc Natl Acad Sci USA* 94 no. 21(1997): 11238–43; P. Y. Teycheney, et al., "Synthesis of (-)-strand RNA from the 3' untranslated region of plant viral genomes expressed in transgenic plants upon infection with related viruses," *J Gen Virol* 81, no. 4(2000): 1121–6.

109. G. Pruss, et al, "Plant viral synergism: the potyviral genome encodes a broad-range pathogenicity enhancer that transactivates replication of heterologous viruses," *Plant Cell* 9, no. 6(1997), 859–68; S. Sonoda, et al. "The helper component-proteinase of sweet potato feathery mottle virus facilitates systemic spread of potato virus X in Ipomoea nil," *Phytopathology* 90 (2000): 944–950.

110. A. A. Agranovsky, et al, "Beet yellows closterovirus HSP70-like protein mediates the cell-to-cell movement of a potexvirus transport-deficient mutant and a hordeivirus-based chimeric virus," *J Gen Virol* 79, pt 4 (1998): 889–95; G. Sunter, J. L. Sunter, and D. M. Bisaro, "Plants expressing tomato golden mosaic virus AL2 or beet curly top virus L2 transgenes show enhanced susceptibility to infection by DNA and RNA viruses," *Virology* 285, no. 1 (2001): 59–70.

111. Hao et al, "The plant cell," 15 (2003): 1034–1048; Kong et al, *EMBO journal* 19 (2000): 3485–3495; Rubino et al *Journal of General Virology* 81 (2000) 279–286; and Dalmay et al, *EMBO Journal* 20 (2001): 2069–2077.

112. Jonathan Latham, PhD, personal communication, 2006

113. Joe Cummins, "Transgenic virus resistant plums," June 11, 2006.

PART 1, SECTION 4: THE FOREIGN PROTEIN MAY BE DIFFERENT THAN INTENDED

1. Doug Gurian-Sherman, "Holes in the Biotech Safety Net," FDA Policy Does Not Assure the Safety of Genetically Engineered Foods, Center for Science in the Public Interest, http://www.cspinet.org/new/pdf/fda_report_final.pdf

2. J. M. WAL, "Strategies for Assessment and Identification of Allergenicity in (Novel) Foods." *International Dairy Journal* 8, (1998) 413-423.

3. David Schubert, "A different perspective on GM food," *Nature Biotechnology* 20 (2002): 969.

4. Gurian-Sherman, "Holes in the Biotech Safety Net, FDA Policy Does Not Assure the Safety of Genetically Engineered Foods."

5. David Schubert, "A different perspective on GM food."

6. FIFRA Scientific Advisory Panel, "Mammalian Toxicity Assessment Guidelines for Protein Plant Pesticides," SAP Report No. 2000-03B: 23, http://www.epa.gov/scipoly/sap/2000/june/finbtmamtox.pdf

7. Barry Commoner, "Unraveling the DNA Myth: The spurious foundation of genetic engineering," *Harper's*, February 2002, http://www.mindfully.org/GE/GE4/ DNA-Myth-CommonerFeb02.htm

8. M. Cretenet, et al, "Submission on the DAR for Application A549 Food Derived from High-Lysine Corn LY038" citing, for example, M. Bucciantini, et al., "Inherent toxicity of aggregates implies a common mechanism for protein misfolding diseases," *Nature* 416 (2002): 507–511.

9. Ibid.

10. Demonstrated in a series of recent articles, e.g. Bucciantini et al. "Prefibrillar amyloid protein aggregates share common features of cytotoxicity," *J. Biol Chem* 279 (2004): 31374–31382; Kayed et al., "Common structure of soluble amyloid oligomers implies common mechanisms of pathogenesis," *Science* 300 (2003): 486-489.

11. Terje Traavik and Jack Heinemann, *Genetic Engineering and Omitted Health Research: Still No Answers to Ageing Questions*, TWN Biotechnology & Biosafety Series 7, 2007.

12. Cretenet, "Submission on the DAR for Application A549 Food Derived from High-Lysine Corn LY038."

13. Gurian-Sherman, "Holes in the Biotech Safety Net, FDA Policy Does Not Assure the Safety of Genetically Engineered Foods."

14. Latham et al, "The Mutational Consequences of Plant Transformation, *Journal of Biomedicine and Biotechnology* 2006:1-7, article ID 25376, http://www.hindawi.com/journals/JBB/index.html

15. "Draft risk analysis report application A378, Food derived from glyphosate-tolerant sugarbeet line 77 (GTSB77)," ANZFA, March 7, 2001, www.agbios.com/docroot/decdocs/anzfa_gtsb77.pdf

16. Food Legislation and Regulation Advisory Group (FLRAG) of the Public Health Association of Australia (PHAA) on behalf of the PHAA, Comments to ANZFA about Applications A372, A375, A378 and A379, http://www.iher.org.au/

17. E. Levine et al., "Molecular Characterization of Insect Protected Corn Line MON 810." Unpublished study submitted to the EPA by Monsanto, EPA MRID No. 436655-01C (1995).

18. Allison Wilson, PhD, Jonathan Latham, PhD, and Ricarda Steinbrecher, PhD, "Genome Scrambling—Myth or Reality? Transformation-Induced Mutations in Transgenic Crop Plants Technical Report—October 2004," www.econexus.info.

19. Gilles-Eric Seralini, "Genome Fluidity and Health Risks for GMOs," *Epigenetics, Transgenic Plants & Risk Assessment, Proceedings of the Conference, December 1st 2005* (Frankfurtam Main, Germany: Literaturhaus, 2005).

20. Latham et al, "The Mutational Consequences of Plant Transformation."

21. "Food Derived from Insect-Protected Mon 863 Corn, A Safety Assessment," *Technical Report Series* No. 34, Food Standards Australia New Zealand, June 2004.

22. Mae-Wan Ho and Sam Burcher, "Cows Ate GM Maize & Died," ISIS Press Release, 13/01/04, http://www.i-sis.org.uk/CAGMMAD.php

23. J. M.Wal, "Strategies for assessment and identification of allergenicity in (novel) foods." *International Dairy Journal* 8 (1998): 413–423.

24. National Research Council, "Environmental Effects of Transgenic Plants: The Scope and Adequacy of Regulation." (Washington, DC: National Academy Press, 2002).

25. Doug Gurian-Sherman, "Holes in the Biotech Safety Net, FDA Policy Does Not Assure the Safety of Genetically Engineered Foods, Center for Science in the Public Interest," http://www.cspinet.org/new/pdf/fda_report_final.pdf

26. EPA's Scientific Advisory Panel, "Mammalian Toxicity Assessment Guidelines for Protein Plant Pesticides," SAP Report No. 2000-03B (Sept. 28, 2000): 10, 14, http://www.epa.gov/scipoly/sap/2000/june/finbtmamtox.pdf.

27. EPA's review of Mycogen/Pioneer's *Bt* (Cry1F) corn. (Only 5 of the 605 amino acids were sequenced.) "Biopesticides Registration Action Document—*Bacillus thuringiensis* Cry1F Corn," US EPA, August 2001, http://www.epa.gov/pesticides/biopesticides/ingredients/tech_docs/brad_006481.pdf.

28. William Freese, "Genetically Engineered Crop Health Impacts Evaluation: A Critique of U.S. Regulation of Genetically Engineered Crops and Corporate Testing Practices, with a Case Study of *Bt* Corn," Friends of the Earth U.S., http://www.

foe.org/camps/comm/safefood/gefood/index.html

29. William Freese, "A Critique of the EPA's Decision to Reregister *Bt* Crops and an Examination of the Potential Allergenicity of *Bt* Proteins," adapted from comments of Friends of the Earth to the EPA, Dec. 9, 2001, www.foe.org/safefood/comments.pdf.

30. Mae-Wan Ho, Letter to José Maurício Bustani, on behalf of the Independent Science Panel, 15 August 2005.

31. C. Collonier, G. Berthier, F. Boyer, M. N. Duplan, S. Fernandez, N. Kebdani, A. Kobilinsky, M. Romanuk, Y. Bertheau, "Characterization of commercial GMO inserts: a source of useful material to study genome fluidity," Poster presented at ICPMB: International Congress for Plant Molecular Biology (n°VII), Barcelona, 23-28th June 2003. Poster courtesy of Dr. Gilles-Eric Seralini, Président du Conseil Scientifique du CRII-GEN, www.crii-gen.org; also "Transgenic lines proven unstable" by Mae-Wan Ho, ISIS Report, 23 October 2003, www.i-sis.org.uk

32. Seralini, "Genome Fluidity and Health Risks for GMOs."

33. Mae-Wan Ho, "Transgenic Lines Proven Unstable," Institute for Science in Society, http://www.i-sis.org.uk/TLPU.php

34. Seralini, "Genome Fluidity and Health Risks for GMOs."

35. Ibid.

36. Mae-Wan Ho, "Unstable Transgenic Lines Illegal," Institute for Science in Society, Press Release 03/12/03, http://www.isis.org.uk/UTLI.php

37. Hernandez et al., "A specific real-time quantitative PCR detection system for event MON810 in maize YieldGuard based on the 3'-transgene integration sequence," *Transgenic Research* 12 (2003):179–189; Holck et al., "5'-Nuclease PCR for quantitative event-specific detection of the genetically modified MON810 MaisGard maize," *Eur Food Res Technol* 214 (2002): 449–453; Collonnier et al. "Characterization of commercial GMO-inserts: A source of useful material to study genome fluidity?," 2003; Windels et al., "Characterisation of the Roundup Ready soybean insert," *Eur Food Res Technol* 213 (2001): 107–112; Rönning et al., "Event specific real-time quantitative PCR for genetically modified *Bt* 11 maize (Zea Mays)," *Eur Food Res Technol* 216 (2003): 347–354.

38. Traavik and Heinemann, *Genetic Engineering and Omitted Health Research: Still No Answers to Ageing Questions.*

39. Takano et al, "The structures of integration sites in transgenic rice," The Plant Journal 11, no. 3 (1997): 353–361; Collonnier et al. "Characterization of commercial GMO-inserts: A source of useful material to study genome fluidity?"; and Hernandez et al, "A specific real-time quantitative PCR detection system for event MON 810 in maize YieldGuard based on the 3'-transgene integration sequence," *Transgenic Research* 12 (2003): 179–189.

40. Traavik and Heinemann, *Genetic Engineering and Omitted Health Research: Still No Answers to Ageing Questions.*

41. Mae-Wan Ho and Joe Cummins, "GM Food & Feed Not Fit for Man or Beast," Press Release, Institute of Science in Society, (based on a paper presented at an ISP Briefing to Parliament, House of Commons, 29 April 2004); citing as the source, E. H. Chowdhury, H. Kuribara, A. Hino, P. Sultana, O. Mikami, N. Shimada, K. S. Guruge, M. Saito, Y. Nakajima. "Detection of corn intrinsic and recombinant DNA fragments and CrylAb protein in the gastrointestinal contents of pigs fed genetically modified corn *Bt* 11," *J. Anim. Sci.* 81 (2003): 2546–51.

42. Commoner, "Unraveling the DNA Myth: The spurious foundation of genetic engineering."

43. Marcello Buiatti, "Epigenetic Processes and the 'Unintended Effects' of Genetic Engineering," *Epigenetics, Transgenic Plants & Risk Assessment, Proceedings of the Conference, December 1st 2005* (Frankfurt-am-Main, Germany: Literaturhaus, 2005).

44. "Syngenta's GM Maize Scandals: A trail of unstable GM maize varieties, dead cows, cross-contamination and misinformation," ISIS Press Release, March 30, 2005.

45. William Freese, "Organic, not Genetically Engineered," Comments of Friends of the Earth before the FIFRA Scientific Advisory Panel (SAP), Open Meeting on *Bt* Crop Re-Registrations, October 20, 2000.

46. "Elements of Precaution: Recommendations for the Regulation of Food Biotechnology in Canada; An Expert Panel Report on the Future of Food Biotechnology prepared by The Royal Society of Canada at the request of Health Canada Canadian Food Inspection Agency and Environment Canada" The Royal Society of Canada, January 2001.

47. Ibid.

48. Freese, "Organic, not Genetically Engineered," October 20, 2000.

49. Terje Traavik, Conference presentation to delegates of the Cartagena Protocol for Biosafety, Kuala Lumpur, sponsored by the Third World Network, February 22, 2004. http://www.seedsofdeception.com/utility/showArticle/?objectID=36

50. P. Meyer, F. Linn, I. Heidmann, H. Meyer, I. Niedenhof, and H. Saedler, "Endongenous and environmental factors influence 35S promoter methylation of a maize A1 gene construct in transgenic petunia and its colour phenotype," *Molecular Genes and Genetics* 231, no. 3 (1992): 345–352.

51. George Gallepp , "Scientists Find Compound that Makes *Bt* Pesticide More Effective," College of Agriculture and Life Sciences, University of Wisconsin, May 21, 2001, http://www.cals.wisc.edu/media/news/05_01/zwitter_*Bt*.html

52. W. K. Novak, and A. G. Haslberger, "Substantial equivalence of antinutrients and inherent plant toxicants in genetically modified foods," *Food Chem. Toxicol.* 38 (2000): 473–483.

53. Joe Cummins and Mae-Wan Ho For Independent Science Panel, Reply to Questionnaire Codex Guideline for the Conduct

of Food Safety Assessment of Foods Derived from Recombinant-DNA Plants, ISIS Press Release, December 19, 2005.

54. "Elements of Precaution," The Royal Society of Canada, January 2001.

55. Florianne Koechlin, "Opening Speech," Epigenetics, Transgenic Plants & Risk Assessment, Proceedings of the Conference, December 1st 2005 (Frankfurtam Main, Germany: Literaturhaus).

56. Cummins and Ho, Reply to Questionnaire Codex Guideline for the Conduct of Food Safety, December 19, 2005.

57. Laurence D. Hurst, Csaba Pál and Martin J. Lercher, The Evolutionary Dynamics of Eukaryotic Gene Order, Nature Reviews Genetics 5(2004): 299–310.

58. Helen Pearson, "What is a Gene?" *Nature* 441 (May 25, 2006).

59. Bill Lambrecht, *Dinner at the New Gene Café: How Genetic Engineering Is Changing What We Eat, How We Live, and the Global Politics of Food* (New York: St. Martin's Press, 2001).

60. Eran Segal, et al., "A genomic code for nucleosome positioning," *Nature* (2006). Aug 17, 2006; 442(7104):772-8.

61. Nicholas Wade, "Scientists Say They've Found a Code Beyond Genetics in DNA," *The New York Times*, July 25, 2006, http://www.nytimes.com/2006/07/25/science/25dna.html

PART 1, SECTION 5: TRANSFER OF GENES

1. Autumn Fiester, "Why the omega-3 piggy should not go to market," *Nature Biotechnology* – 24 (2006): 1472–1473.

2. Ricarda A. Steinbrecher, "The CaMV 35S Promoter Government and Corporate Scientific Incompetence: Failure to assess the safety of GM crops," *Econexus Report*, December 2002.

3. Terje Traavik and Jack Heinemann, *Genetic Engineering and Omitted Health Research: Still No Answers to Ageing Questions*, TWN Biotechnology & Biosafety Series 7, 2007.

4. L. Maturin, and R. Curtiss, "Degradation of DNA by nucleases in intestinal tract of rats," Science 196 (1977): 216–218.

5. A. B. McAllan, "The fate of nucleic acids in ruminants," *Progress in Nutrional Science* 41 (1982): 309–317.

6. Ricarda A. Steinbrecher and Jonathan R. Latham, "Horizontal gene transfer from GM crops to unrelated organisms," GM Science Review Meeting of the Royal Society of Edinburgh on "GM Gene Flow: Scale and Consequences for Agriculture and the Environment," January 27, 2003.

7. Traavik and Heinemann, *Genetic Engineering and Omitted Health Research*; citing Schubbert, et al, "Ingested foreign (phage M13) DNA survives transiently in the gastrointestinal tract and enters the bloodstream of mice," *Mol Gen Genet.* 242, no. 5 (1994): 495–504; Schubbert et al, "Foreign (M13) DNA ingested by mice reaches peripheral leukocytes, spleen, and liver via the intestinal wall mucosa and can be covalently linked to mouse DNA," *Proc Natl Acad Sci USA* 94, no. 3 (1997): 961–6; Schubbert et al, "On the fate of orally ingested foreign DNA in mice: chromosomal association and placental transmission to the fetus, *Mol Gen Genet.* 259, no. 6 (1998): 569–76; Hohlweg and Doerfler, "On the fate of plants or other foreign genes upon the uptake in food or after intramuscular injection in mice," *Mol Genet Genomics* 265 (2001): 225–233; Palka-Santani, et al., "The gastrointestinal tract as the portal of entry for foreign macromolecules: fate of DNA and proteins," *Mol Gen Genomics* 270 (2003): 201–215; Einspanier, et al, "The fate of forage plant DNA in farm animals; a collaborative case-study investigating cattle and chicken fed recombinant plant material," *Eur Food Res Technol* 212 (2001): 129–134; Klotz, et al, "Degradation and possible carry over of feed DNA monitored in pigs and poultry," Eur Food Res Technol 214 (2002): 271–275; Forsman, et al, "Uptake of amplifiable fragments of retrotransposon DNA from the human alimentary tract," *Mol Gen Genomics* 270 (2003): 362–368; Chen, et al, "Transfection of mEpo gene to intestinal epithelium in vivo mediated by oral delivery of chitosan-DNA nanoparticles," *World Journal of Gastroenterology* 10, no 1(2004): 112–116; Phipps, et al, "Detection of transgenic and endogenous plant DNA in rumen fluid, duodenal digesta, milk, blood, and feces of lactating dairy cows," *J Dairy Sci.* 86, no. 12(2003): 4070-8.

8. Schubbert, et al, "On the fate of orally ingested foreign DNA in mice," 569–576; and R. Schubbert, et al, "Ingested foreign (phage M13) DNA survives transiently in the gastrointestinal tract and enters the bloodstream of mice," 495-504.

9. Chowdhury, et al, "Detection of genetically modified maize DNA fragments in the intestinal contents of pigs fed StarLink CBH351," *Vet Hum Toxicol.* 45 , no. 2 (March 2003): 95–6.

10. P. A. Chambers, et al, "The fate of antibiotic resistance marker genes in transgenic plant feed material fed to chickens," *J. Antimic. Chemother.* 49 (2000): 161–164.

11. Paula S. Duggan, et al, "Fate of genetically modified maize DNA in the oral cavity and rumen of sheep," *Br J Nutr.* 89, no 2 (Feb.2003): 159–66.

12. Einspanier, et al, "The fate of forage plant DNA in farm animals: A collaborative case-study investigating cattle and chicken fed recombinant plant material," *European Food Research and Technology*, 212 (2001): 129–34.

13. Forsman, et al, "Uptake of amplifiable fragments of retrotransposon DNA from the human alimentary tract," *Mol Genet Genomics* 270, no 3 (Dec. 2003): 362–8.

14. Martin-Orue, et al, "Degradation of transgenic DNA from genetically modified soya and maize in human intestinal simulations," *British Journal of Nutrition* 87 (2002): 533–42.

15. Steinbrecher and Latham, "Horizontal gene transfer from GM crops to unrelated organisms."

16. Traavik and Heinemann, *Genetic Engineering and Omitted Health Research.*

17. Steinbrecher and Latham, "Horizontal gene transfer from GM crops to unrelated organisms."

18. M. G. Kidwell "Lateral transfer in natural populations of eukaryotes," *Annual Reviews in Genetics* 27 (1993): 235–256; J. Wostemeyer, A. Wostemeyer, K. Voigt "Horizontal gene transfer in the rhizosphere: A curiosity or a driving force in evolution?" *Advances in Botanical Research Incorporating Advances in Plant Pathology* 24 (1997): 399–429; and F. Bertolla and P. Simonet "Review. Horizontal gene transfers in the environment: natural transformation as a putative process for gene transfers between transgenic plants and microorganisms," *Research in Microbiology* 150, no 6 (1999): 375–384 (includes (2) and (14)).

19. A. A. Salyers, N. B. Shoemaker, "Resistance gene transfer in anaerobes: New insights, new problems," Clinical Infectious Diseases 23, Suppl. 1 (1996): S36–S43; and M. P. Nikolich, G. Hong, N. B. Shoemaker, A. A. Salyers, "Evidence for natural horizontal transfer of tetq between bacteria that normally colonize humans and bacteria that normally colonize livestock," *Applied and Environmental Microbiology* 60, no 9 (1994): 3255–3260.

20. J. A. Colanduoni and J. J.Villafranca, "Inhibition of Escherichia coli glutaminesynthetase by phosphinothricin," *Bioorganic Chemistry* 14, no 2 (1986): 163–169; I. Ahmad I and D. Malloch, "Interaction of soil microflora with the bioherbicide phosphinothricin," *Agriculture, Ecosystems, and Environment* 54 (1995): 165–174; I. Ahmad, J. Bissett, and D. Malloch, "Effect of phosphinothricin on nitrogen metabolism of Trichoderma species and its implications for their control of phytopathogenic fungi," *Pesticide Biochemistry and Physiology* 53 (1995a): 49–59; and I. Ahmad, J. Bissett, and D. Malloch, "Influence of the bioherbicide phosphinothricin on interactions between phytopathogens and their antagonists," *Canadian Journal of Botany* 73 (1995b): 1750–1760.

21. Steinbrecher and Latham, "Horizontal gene transfer from GM crops to unrelated organisms."

22. K. M. Nielsen, "Review. Barriers to horizontal gene transfer by natural transformation in soil bacteria," APMIS 106, no 84(1998): 77–84.

23. Steinbrecher and Latham, "Horizontal gene transfer from GM crops to unrelated organisms."

24. Ibid.

25. Ibid.

26. Schubert, "Response to Bradford, et al."

27. F. Assad, and E. R. Signer, "Cauliflower mosaic virus P35S promoter activity in *E. coli.*" *Mol. Gen. Genet.* 223 (1990): 517–520; and D. Jacob, et al., "Plant-specific promoter sequences carry elements that are recognised by the eubacterial transcription machinery," *Transgenic Research* 11, no. 3 (June 2002): 291–303(13). (Other studies show functioning of CaMV 35S in yeast. See H. Hirt, M. Kogl, T. Murbacher, E. Heberlebors, *Curr Genet* 17 (1990): 473–479; J. Ruth, H. Hirt, R. J. Schweyen, *Mol Gen Genet* 235 (1992): 365–372; H. Gmunder, J. Kohli, *Mol Gen Genet* 220 (1989): 95–101; and N. Pobjecky, G. H. Rosenberg, G. nter-Gottlieb, N. F. Kaufer, *Mol Gen Genet* 220 (1990): 314–316).

28. U.K. Department of the Environment, Food and Rural Affairs and the Advisory Committee on Releases into the Environment (ACRE) February 2002: "In the unlikely event that the T25 maize pat gene is transferred to a soil bacterium then it would not be expressed. This is because it is linked to the cauliflower mosaic virus promoter that expresses genes in plants—not bacteria." As cited in Steinbrecher and Latham, "Horizontal gene transfer from GM crops to unrelated organisms."

29. Colanduoni and Villafranca, "Inhibition of *Escherichia coli* glutamine-synthetase by phosphinothricin," 163–169; and Pline, et al, "Antibacterial activity of the herbicide glufosinate on Pseudomonas syringae pathovar glycinea," *Pesticide Biochemistry and Physiology* 71, no. 1 (2001): 48–55.

30. Antony Barnett, "GM genes 'jump' species barrier," Observer May 28, 2000; also reported on German TV (ZDF), May 21, 2000. The findings at the time had not been published.

31. Schubert, "Response to Bradford, et al."

32. Netherwood et al, "Assessing the survival of transgenic plant DNA in the human gastrointestinal tract," *Nature Biotechnology* 22 (2004): 2.

33. Harry Gilbert, personal communication.

34. H. Flint, D. Mercer, K. Scott, C. Melville, and L. Glover, L, "Survival of Ingested DNA in the Gut and the Potential for Genetic Transformation of Resident Bacteria," Food Standards Agency Project Reference FSG01007 (United Kingdom, Food Standards Agency, 2001), http://www.foodstandards.gov.uk/multimedia/pdfs/rowett1.pdf

35. Mae-Wan Ho, "Recent evidence confirms risks of horizontal gene transfer," ISIS contribution to ACNFP/Food Standards Agency Open Meeting, 13 November 2002, Institute of Science in Society, London.

36. Food Standards Agency (UK). nd. "Technical report on the Food Standards Agency Project G010008 evaluating the risks associated with using GMOs in human foods," University of Newcastle, Food Standards Agency, United Kingdom, http://www.foodstandards.gov.uk/multimedia/pdfs/gmnewcastlereport.PDF

37. Murray Lumpkin to Bruce Burlington, "The tomatoes that will eat Akron," Internal memo between FDA scientists, made

public due to a lawsuit, Alliance for Bio-Integrity, December 17, 1992, www.biointegrity.org

38. Albert Sheldon to James Maryanski, Biotechnology Coordinator, "Use of Kanamycin Resistance Markers in Tomatoes," March 30, 1993, www.biointegrity.org

39. The American Medical Association, the UK Royal Society, the World Health Organization, the United Nations Food and Agriculture Organization, Pasteur Institute, European Food Safety Authority, Codex Alimentarius, Indian Council of Medical Research and others, have expressed concern that the use of ARM genes might quicken the development of antibiotic resistant diseases. The British Medical Association even cited ARM genes as one of their reasons for proposing a ban of GM crops. See for example, "Submission of the British Medical Association to the Health And Community Care Committee On The Impact Of GM Crop Trials," The Scottish Parliament HC/02/30/A November 20, 2002 http://www.mindfully.org/GE/GE4/BMA-GM-Crop-Trials20nov02.htm

40. Ricki Lewis, "The Rise of Antibiotic-Resistant Infections," FDA Consumer magazine, September 1995, http://www.fda.gov/fdac/features/795_antibio.html

41. Lumpkin to Burlington, "The tomatoes that will eat Akron."

42. "Guidance For Industry: Use of Antibiotic Resistance Marker Genes in Transgenic Plants," Draft released for comment on: September 4, 1998, http://vm.cfsan.fda.gov/%7Edms/opa-armg.html

43. F. Gebhard, and K. Smalla, K. "Monitoring field releases of genetically modified sugar beets for persistence of transgenic plant DNA and horizontal gene transfer," FEMS Microbiology Ecology 28 (1999): 261–272.

44. Steinbrecher and Latham, "Horizontal gene transfer from GM crops to unrelated organisms."

45. "Opinion of the Scientific Panel on Genetically Modified Organisms on the use of antibiotic resistance genes as marker genes in genetically modified plants," The EFSA Journal 48 (2004): 1–18, http://www.efsa.eu.int 10

46. K. L. Goodyear, et al. "Comment on: An assessment of the risks associated with the use of antibiotic resistance genes in genetically modified plants: report of the Working Party of the British Society for Antimicrobial Chemotherapy," J. Antimicrob. Chemother. 54 (2004): 959.

47. 1995 Annual Report of the UK Advisory Committee on Novel Foods and Processes (ACNFP) on Ciba Geigy maize line CG00526-176, also known as Maximizer.

48. "Spain to ban Syngenta corn, EU's biggest biotech crop," Checkbiotech.org, (Bloomberg), 30 Apr 2004, http://www.checkbiotech.org/root/index.cfm?

49. Traavik and Heinemann, Genetic Engineering and Omitted Health Research.

50. Joe Cummins, "Kanamycin Still Used and Cross-Reacts with New Antibiotics," http://www.i-sis.org.uk/kanomycin.php

51. H. Ishikawa, A. Ikuko, T. Minami, Y. Shinmoura, H. Ojo, and T. Otani, "Prevention of infectious complications subsequent to endoscopic treatment of the colon and rectum," J Infect Chemother 5 (1999): 86–90.

52. E. Hehl, R. Beck, K. Luthard, R. Guthoff, and B. Drewelow, "Improved penetration of amonoglycosides and fluoroquininolones into the aqueous humour of patients by means of acuvue contact lenses," Eur J Pharmacol 55 (1999): 317–323.

53. J. Yelon, J. Green, and J. Evans, "Efficacy of an interperitoneal antibiotic to reduce incidence of infection in the trauma patient a prospective randomized study," J AmCollSurg 182 (1996): 5091–4.

54. T. Ito, E. Akino, and K. Hiramatsu , "Evaluation of antibiotics for enterohemorrhagic Escherichia coli 0157 enteritis effect of various antibiotics on extracellular release of verotoxin," Kansenshogaku Zasshi 71 (1997): 130–5.

55. J. Onaolapo J, "Cross-resistance between some aminoglycoside antibiotics," Afr J Med Sci. 23 (1994): 215–9.

56. N. Mikkelsen, M. Brannvali, A.Virtanen, and L. Kirsebom, "Inhibition of P RNA cleavage by aminoglycosides," Proc. Natnl Acad Sci USA 96 (1999): 6155–60; and T. Yamamoto, G. Nair and Y. Takeda, "Emergence of tetracycline resistance due to a multiple drug resistance plasmid in Vibrio cholerae 0139," FEMS Immunol Med Microbiol 11 (1995): 131–6.

57. Joe Cummins, personal correspondence.

58. Pusztai and Bardocz, "GMO in animal nutrition."

59. Ricarda A. Steinbrecher, "The CaMV 35S Promoter, Government and Corporate Scientific Incompetence: Failure to assess the safety of GM crops," ECONEXUS Briefing, December 2002.

60. Joseph Cummins, "Eating Cauliflower Mosaic Virus infected vegetables does not prove that that Cauliflower Mosaic Virus Promoter in genetically modified crops is safe," ISIS Press Release, February 18, 2001, http://www.i-sis.org.uk/eatingcamv-pr.php

61. See for example, O. P. Rekvig, et al, "Antibodies to eukaryotic, including autologous, native DNA are produced during BK virus infection, but not after immunization with non-infectious BK DNA," Scand. J. Immunol. 36 (1992): 487–95.

62. S. Covey, et al, "Host regulation of the cauliflower mosaic virus multiplication cycle," Proc. Nat. Acad. Sci. USA 87 (1990): 1633–7, as cited in J. Cummins, et al, "Hazards of CaMV Promoter," Nature Biotechnology (April 2000).

63. Assaad and Signer, "Cauliflower mosaic-virus p35S promoter activity in Escherichia-coli," 517–520.

64. N. Pobjecky, G. H. Rosenberg, G. Dintergottlieb, N. F. Kaufer, "Expression of the beta-glucuronidase gene under the control of the CaMV-35S promoter in Schizosaccharomyces-pombe," Molecular & General Genetics 220, no. 2 (1990): 314–316.

65. H. Guilley, R. K. Dudley, G. Jonard, E. Balazs, and K. E. Richards, "Transcription of Cauliflower Mosaic Virus DNA: Detection of promoter sequences, and characterization of transcripts," *Cell* 30 (1982):763–773.

66. A. Lewin, D. Jacob, B. Freytag, B. Appel B, "Gene expression in bacteria directed by plant-specific regulatory sequences," *Transgenic Research* 7 (1998): 403–411.

67. M. Tepfer et al, "Transient expression in mammalian cells of transgenes transcribed from the Cauliflower mosaic virus 35S promoter," *Environ Biosafety Res.* 3 no. 2 (Apr-Jun 2004): 91–7.

68. C. Burke, X-B Yu, L. Marchitelli, E. A. Davis, and S. Ackerman, "Transcription Factor IIA of wheat and human function similarly with plant and animal viral promoters," *Nucleic Acid Research* 18, no. 12(1990): 3611–3620; and R. Cooke and P. Penon, "In vitro transcription from cauliflower mosaic virus promoters by a cell-free extract from tobacco cells," *Plant Molecular Biology* 14 (1990): 391–405; and J. Vlasak, et al, "Comparison of hCMV immediate early and CaMV 35S promoters in both plant and human cells," *J Biotechnol* 103, no. 3 (Aug. 2003): 197–202.

69. R. Marit, et al, "The 35S CaMV plant virus promoter is active in human enterocyte-like cells," *Eur Food Res Technol* 222 (2006): 185–193.

70. Ibid.

71. Terje Traavik presented findings by the Norwegian Institute for Gene Ecology to delegates of the UN Cartagena Protocol for Biosafety, in advance of their February 2004 meeting in Kuala Lumpur, Malaysia. See Jeffrey M. Smith, "GM Food Promoter Transfers to Rat Cells," Press release and backgrounder, Feb 24, 2004, http://www.seedsofdeception.com/Public/AboutGeneticallyModifiedFoods/GMFoodPromoterTransferstoRatCells/index.cfm

72. Paula S. Duggan, et al, "Fate of genetically modified maize DNA in the oral cavity and rumen of sheep," *British Journal of Nutrition* 89 (2003): 159–166; see other section on transgene survival in the digestive tract.

73. Steinbrecher and Latham, "Horizontal gene transfer from GM crops to unrelated organisms."

74. "Meningitis fear over GM food," BBC News, April 26, 1999.

75. Paula S. Duggan et al, "Fate of genetically modified maize DNA in the oral cavity and rumen of sheep," 159–66.

76. H. Flint, K. Scott, G01011 Dissemination of GM DNA and antibiotic resistance genes via rumen microorganisims (United Kingdom: Rowett Research Institute, Food Standards Agency, 2002).

77. D. K. Mercer, K. P. Scott, W. A. Bruce-Johnson, L. A. Glover, and H. J. Flint, "Fate of free DNA and transformation of oral bacterium Streptococcus gordonii DL1 plasmid DNA in human saliva," *Applied and Environmental Microbiology* 65 (1999): 6–10.

78. Ibid.

79. "Scientists Warn of GM Crops Link to Meningitis," *Daily Mail* (UK), April 26, 1999.

PART 1, SECTION 6: ENVIRONMENTAL AND BIOACCUMULATED TOXINS

1. Ricarda A. Steinbrecher, "Risks associated with ingestion of Chardon LL maize, The reversal of N-acetyl-L- glufosinate to the active herbicide L-glufosinate in the gut of animals," Chardon LL Hearing, London, May 2002.

2. Colanduoni and Villafranca,"Inhibition of *Escherichia coli* glutamine-synthetase by phosphinothricin," *Bioorganic Chemistry* 14, no. 2(1986): 163–169l; and W. A. Pline, G.H. Lacy, V. Stromberg, K. K. Hatzios, "Antibacterial activity of the herbicide glufosinate on Pseudomonas syringae pathovar glycinea," *Pesticide Biochemistry and Physiology* 71, no 1(2001): 48–55.

3. C. A. Liu, H. Zhong, J. Vargas, D. Penner, M. Sticklen," Prevention of fungal diseases in transgenic, bialaphos- and glufosinate-resistant creeping bentgrass (*Agrostis palustrls*), *Weed Science* 46, no.1(1998): 139–146; and T. Tada, H. Kanzaki, E. Norita, H. Uchimiya, I. Nakamura, "Decreased symptoms of rice blast disease on leaves of bar-expressing transgenic rice plants following treatment with bialaphos," *Molecular Plant-Microbe Interactions* 9, no. 8(1998): 762–764.

4. Y-J Ahn, Y-J Kim and J-K Yoo, "Toxicity of the herbicide glufosinate-ammonium to predatory insects and mites of Tetranychus urticae (*Acari: Tetranychidae*) under laboratory conditions," *Journal of Economic Entomology* 94, no. 1 (2001): s157–161.

5. T. Watanabe and T. Sano, "Neurological effects of glufosinate poisoning with a brief review," *Human & Experimental Toxicology* 17, no. 1 (1998): 35–39.

6. I-N Bremmer, and K-H Leist, *Disodium-N-acetyl-L-glufosinate; AE F099730 - Hazard evaluation of Lglufosinate produced intestinally from N-acetyl-L-glufosinate* (Frankfurt: Hoechst Schering AgrEvo GmbH, Safety Evaluation, 1997), unpublished; (see FAO publication on www.fao.org/ag/agp/agpp/pesticid/jmpr/Download/98/glufosi3.pdf)

7. H-M Kellner, K. Stumpf, and R. Braun, "Hoe 099730-14C Pharmacokinetics in rats following single oral and intravenous administration of3 mg/kg body," (Germany: Hoechst RCL, 1993), unpublished.

8. M. N. Huang, and S. M. Smith, "Metabolism of [14C]-N-acetyl glufosinate in a lactating goat," AgrEvo USA Co., Pikeville, PTRL East Inc., USA, 1993. Project 502BK. Study U012A/A524. Report A54155, unpublished, http://www.fao.org/WAICENT/FAOINFO/AGRICULT/AGP/AGPP/Pesticid/JMPR/Download/98_eva/glufosi.pdf

9. In one study, for example, protein produced from a gene found in *E. coli* turned NAG into glufosinate. G. Kriete, et al,

"Male sterility in transgenic tobacco plants induced by tapetum-specific deacetylation of the externally applied non-toxic compound N-acetyl-L-phosphinothricin," *Plant Journal* 9, no 6 (1996): 809–818.

10. Bremmer and Leist, "Disodium-N-acetyl-L-glufosinate (AE F099730, substance technical) - Toxicity and metabolism studies summary and evaluation."

11. Huang and Smith, "Metabolism of [14C]-N-acetyl glufosinate in a lactating goat."

12. Steinbrecher, "Risks associated with ingestion of Chardon LL maize." (Note: This work is an excellent summary of the risks associated with NAG conversion within the gut.)

13. T. Fujii, "Transgenerational effects of maternal exposure to chemicals on the functional development of the brain in the offspring," *Cancer Causes and Control* 8, no. 3 (1997): 524–528.

14. H. Takahashi, et al., "A Case of Transient Diabetes Isipidus Associated with Poisoning by a Herbicide Containing Glufosinate," *Clinical Toxicology* 38, no. 2 (2000): 153–156.

15. "Bayer's GE Crop Herbicide, Glufosinate, Causes Brain Damage," *The Japan Times*, 7 December 2004.

16. Bayer's GE Crop Herbicide, Glufosinate, Causes Brain Damage, *The Japan Times*, 7 December 2004

17. T. Watanabe, and T. Iwase, "Development and dymorphogenic effects of glufosinate ammonium on mouse embryos in culture." *Teratogenesis carcinogenesis and mutagenesis*, 16, no. 6 (1996): 287–299.

18. T. Watanabe, "Apoptosis induced by glufosinate ammonium in the neuroepithelium of developing mouse embryos in culture," Neuroscientific Letters 222, no. 1(1997): 17–20, as cited in Glufosinate ammonium fact sheet, *Pesticides News*, no.42 (December 1998): 20–21.

19. T. Fujii, "Transgenerational effects of maternal exposure to chemicals on the functional development of the brain in the offspring," 524-528.

20. T. Fujii, T. Ohata, M. Horinaka, "Alternations in the response to kainic acid in rats exposed to glufosinate-ammonium, a herbicide, during infantile period," *Proc. Of the Japan Acad. Series B-Physical and Biological Sciences* 72, no. 1 (1996): 7–10.

21. "Bayer's GE Crop Herbicide, Glufosinate, Causes Brain Damage."

22. Steinbrecher, "Risks associated with ingestion of Chardon LL maize."

23. FLRAG, comments to ANZFA about Applications A372, A375, A378 and A379.

24. Charles Benbrook, "Genetically Engineered Crops and Pesticide Use in the United States: The First Nine Years," BioTech InfoNet, Technical Paper Number 7, October 2004.

25. Benbrook, "Genetically Engineered Crops and Pesticide Use in the United States: The First Nine Years," October 2004; The paper states: "This large increase reflects the slipping efficacy of the Roundup Ready system, the emergence of tolerant and resistance weeds, and the falling price of soybean herbicides, and the progressively lower-rate herbicides used on conventional acres."

26. M. A. Lappe, E.B. Bailey, C. Childress, and K D. R. Setchell, "Alterations in clinically important phytoestrogens in genetically modified, herbicide-tolerant soybeans," *J. Med. Foods* 1 (1999): 241–245

27. Anders Legarth Schmidt, "Poisonous Spray [Roundup] on a Course Towards Drinking Water," *Politiken*, May 10, 2003.

28. M. R. Fernandez, et al., "Crop Production Factors Associated with Fusarium Head Blight in Spring Wheat in Eastern Saskatchewan," *Crop Science*, 45 (2005):1908–1916

29. Andy Coghlan, "Roundup Weedkiller May Encourage Blight," *New Scientist*, August 14, 2003.

30. Adrian Ewins,"Scientists eye glyphosate-fusarium link,"Saskatoon Newsroom,July 10,2003,http://www.organicconsumers. org/ge/071403_ge_wheat.cfm

31. R.J.Kremer,P.A.Donald,and A.J.Keaster"Herbicide Impact on Fusarium spp. and Soybean Cyst Nematode in Glyphosate-Tolerant Soybean," *American Society of Agronomy*, 2000, http://www.biotech-info.net/fungi_buildup_abstract.html

32. European Communities submission to World Trade Organization dispute panel, 28 January 2005.

33. EPA Rule, "Pesticide Tolerances and Food and Feed Additive Regulations for Glyphosate: Final Rule," *Federal Register* 57 (1992): 42700.

34. Judy Carman, "The Problem with the Safety of Round-Up Ready Soybeans," from Diverse Women for Diversity, 8th August 1999, http://members.iinet.net.au/~rabbit/notjcsoy.htm

35. S. O. Duke, et al, "Isoflavone, glyphosate and aminomethylphosphonic acid levels in seeds of glyphosate-treated, glyphosateresistant soybean," *J. Agric. Food Chem.* 51 (2003): 340–344.

36. Heinrich Sandermann, "Plant biotechnology: ecological case studies on herbicide resistance," *Trends in Plant Science* 11, no. 7 (July 2006): 324–328.

37. Lennart Hardell and Mikael Eriksson, "A case-control study of non-Hodgkin lymphoma and exposure to pesticides," *Cancer* 85, no. 6 (Mar. 15, 1999).

38. Caroline Cox, "Herbicide Fact Sheet: Glyphosate," *Journal of Pesticide Reform* 24, no. 4 (Winter 2004).

39. Maria do Desterro Leiros da Costa, et al., "Neuroimaging abnormalities in parkinsonism: study of five cases," *Arq Neuropsiquatr.* 61, no 2B (June 2003): 381–6.

40. L.P. Walsh, "Roundup inhibits steroidogenesis by disrupting steroidogenic acute regulatory (StAR) protein expression,"

Environmental Health Perspectives 108 (2000), 769–776.

41. Sophie Richard, Safa Moslemi, Herbert Sipahutar, Nora Benachour, and Gilles-Eric Seralini, "Differential Effects of Glyphosate and Roundup on Human Placental Cells and Aromatase," *Environmental Health Perspectives* 113, no. 6 (June 2005), http://ehp.niehs.nih.gov/members/2005/7728/7728.html

42. Jorgelina Daruich, et al., "Effect of the Herbicide Glyphosate on Enzymatic Activity in Pregnant Rats and Their Fetuses," *Environmental Research* 85, no. 3 (March 2001): 226–231.

43. Caroline Cox and Michael Surgan, "Unidentified Inert Ingredients in Pesticides: Implications," *Environmental Health Perspectives* Aug 18 2006, http://www.mindfully.org/Pesticide/2006/Inert-Ingredients-Pesticides18aug06.htm

44. Sophie Richard, et al, "Differential Effects of Glyphosate and Roundup on Human Placental Cells and Aromatase."

45. Julie Marc, et al., "Pesticide Roundup Provokes Cell Division Dysfunction at the Level of CDK1/Cyclin B Activation," *Chemical Research in Toxicology*, 15, no. 3 (Mar 2002): 326–31.

46. F. Peixoto, "Comparative effects of the Roundup and glyphosate on mitochondrial oxidative phosphorylation," *Chemosphere* 61 (2005): 1115–1122.

47. Sophie Richard, et al, "Differential Effects of Glyphosate and Roundup on Human Placental Cells and Aromatase"

48. Ibid.

49. Wade V. Welshons, et al, "Large Effects from Small Exposures. I. Mechanisms for Endocrine-Disrupting Chemicals with Estrogenic Activity, Table 2," *Environmental Health Perspectives* 111, no. 8 (June 2003)

50. "Glufosinate Ammonium; Pesticide Tolerance, Environmental Protection Agency, 40 CFR Part 180, ACTION: Final rule," *Federal Register* 68, no. 188 (September 29, 2003), http://www.epa.gov/fedrgstr/EPA-PEST/2003/September/Day-29/p24565.htm

51. Sophie Richard, et al, "Differential Effects of Glyphosate and Roundup on Human Placental Cells and Aromatase."

52. Ibid.

53. Schmidt, "Denmark Bans Glyphosates, The Active Ingredient In Roundup," *Politiken*, May 10, 2003.

54. Gilles-Eric Seralini, "Genome Fluidity and Health Risks for GMOs."

55. Division of Food Chemistry and Technology and Division of Contaminants Chemistry, "Points to Consider for Safety Evaluation of Genetically Modified Foods: Supplemental Information," November 1, 1991, www.biointegrity.org

56. Ibid.

57. Rui Yukui, et al, "Heavy metals content in transgenic soybean oil from Beijing Market," AgroFOOD Industry Hi-Tech 17, no 2 (March/April 2006).

58. Ibid.

59. Gerald B. Guest to James Maryanski, "Regulation of Transgenic Plants—FDA Draft Federal Register Notice on Food Biotechnology," Alliance for BioIntegrity, February 5, 1992, www.biointegrity.org

60. "Plant Toxins and Antinutrients, Genetically Engineered Organisms," Public Issues Education Project, http://www.geo-pie.cornell.edu/issues/toxins.html

61. European Communities submission to World Trade Organization dispute panel, 28 January 2005.

62. A. Agodi, et al., "Detection of genetically modified DNA sequences in milk from the Italian Market," *Int J Hyg Environ-Health* 209 (2006):81–88.

63. D. W. Brewster, J. Warren, W. E. Hopkins II, "Metabolism of glyphosate in Sprague-Dawley rats: tissue distribution, identification, and quantitation of glyphosate-derived materials following a single oral dose," *Fundam Appl Toxicol* 17 (1991): 43–51; and G. M. Williams, R. Kroes, I. C. Munro, "Safety evaluation and risk assessment of the herbicide Roundup and its active ingredient, glyphosate, for human," *Regul Toxicol Pharmacol* 31 (2000): 117–165.

64. Sophie Richard, et al, "Differential Effects of Glyphosate and Roundup on Human Placental Cells and Aromatase."

65. Yei-Shung Wang, et al., "Accumulation of 2,4-D and glyphosate in fish and water hyacinth," *Water, Air, & Soil Pollution* 74, nos. 3–4 (April, 1994).

66. M.I. Yousef, M. H. Salem, H.Z. Ibrahim, S. Helmi, M. A. Seehy, K. Bertheussen, "Toxic effects of carbofuran and glyphosate on semen characteristics in rabbits," *J Environ Sci Health B* 30: 513–534.

67. Gilles-Eric Seralini, "Genome Fluidity and Health Risks for GMOs"

68. European Communities submission to World Trade Organization dispute panel, 28 January 2005.

69. R. Dasgupta, B. H. Garcia, II, and R. M. Goodman, "Systemic spread of an RNA insect virus in plants expressing plant viral movement protein genes," *Proc Natl Acad Sci USA* 98, no 9 (2001), 4910–5.

70. G.A. De Zoeten, "Risk assessment: Do we let history repeat itself?" *Phytopathology* 81 (1991): 585–86; R. Hull, "Risks in using transgenic plants?" *Science* 264 (1994): 1649–50, author reply 1651–2; M. Gibbs "Risks in using transgenic plants?" Science 264 (1994): 1650–1651; R. F. Allison, A. Greene, and W. L. Schneider, "Significance of RNA recombination in capsid protein-mediated virus-resistant transgenic plants," in M. Tepfer, and E. Balazs, eds., *Virus-resistant transgenic plants: potential ecological impact* (Versailles/Heidelberg: INRA and Springer-Verlag); and M. Gibbs, J. Armstrong, E. Weiller, and A. Gibbs, Virus evolution; the past, a window on the future?" in Tepfer and Balazs, eds., *Virus-resistant*

transgenic plants: potential ecological impact, 1-19.

71. Jonathan R Latham, PhD and Ricarda A Steinbrecher, PhD, "Horizontal gene transfer of viral inserts from GM plants to Viruses," GM Science Review Meeting of the Royal Society of Edinburgh on "GM Gene Flow: Scale and Consequences for Agriculture and the Environment" 27 January 2003—amended February 2004

72. Mark Varrelmann, et al, "Transgenic or Plant Expression Vector-Mediated Recombination of *Plum Pox Virus, Journal of Virology* 74, no. 16 (Aug. 2000): 747462–7469

73. M. Borja, T. Rubio, H. B. Scholthof, et al, „Restoration of wild-type virus by double recombination of tombusvirus mutants with a host transgene," *MPMI* 12 (1999): 153–162.

74. Latham, and Steinbrecher, "Horizontal gene transfer of viral inserts from GM plants to Viruses."

75. M. Gibbs, "Risks in using transgenic plants?" Science 264 (1994):1650–1651.

76. I. Weiland and M. Edwards. "A single nucleotide substitution in the alpha a gene confers oat pathogenicity to barley stripe mosaic virus strain ND18," MPMl 9 (1996): 62–67.

77. From Econexus, the Five Year Freeze, Friends of the Earth, GeneWatch UK, Greenpeace, the Soil Association, and Dr Michael Antoniou, *Comments on GM Science Review*, October 14th 2003.

78. In Gibbs, et al, 1999 PNAS 99 8022-27, there is a report of a hypbrid vertebrate/plant virus that infects plants. In De Medeiros, et al., 2005 PNAS 2005 vol 102 1175-80, Also available is de medeiros et al 2005 PNAS 2005 vol 102 1175-80, a gene from an insect was expressed in human cell lines, and allowed the cells to become infected by a plant virus (tomato spotted wilt virus).

79. Latham, and Steinbrecher, "Horizontal gene transfer of viral inserts from GM plants to Viruses."

PART 1, SECTION 7: OTHER TYPES OF GM FOODS CARRY RISKS

1. Fredrich-Wilhelm Graefe zu Baringdorf, letter to FDA Commissioner David Kessler, December 7, 1994; as cited in Robert Cohen, *Milk, the Deadly Poison* (Englewood Cliffs, New Jersey, Argus Publishing: 1998).

2. Estimates of increased milk supply vary. In Samuel Epstein's, "Potential Public Health Hazards Of Biosynthetic Milk Hormones," *International Journal of Health Services* 20 (1990):73–84, the range was -1% to 10%; The Animal Health Institute claims a 10-25% increase. See AHI Bovine Somatotropin (BST). Report No. 1-5/88-i SM, 1998.

3. APHIS Info Sheet, December 2002, http://www.aphis.usda.gov/vs/ceah/cahm/ Dairy_Cattle/Dairy02/bst-orig.pdf

4. Robert P. Heaney, et al, "Dietary changes favorably affect bone remodeling in older adults." *Journal of the American Dietetic Association* 99, no. 10 (October 1999): 1228–1233.

5. "Milk, Pregnancy, Cancer May Be Tied," *Reuters*, September 10, 2002.

6. Estimates of increased IGF-1 levels vary considerably. In Mepham et al, "Safety of milk from cows treated with bovine somatotropin," *The Lancet* 2 (1994):197, IGF-1 levels were up to 10 times higher. The methods used may also underestimate IGF-1 levels considerably. See Samuel S. Epstein, "Unlabeled Milk From Cows Treated With Biosynthetic Growth Hormones: A Case of Regulatory Abdication," *International Journal of Health Services* 26(1996): 173–185; and Samuel S. Epstein, *What's In Your Milk?* (Victoria, British Columbia, Canada:Trafford Publishing, 2006), 197–204.

7. Samuel S. Epstein, What's In Your Milk?, 197–204; including citations to Mepham, "Public health information of bovine somatotropin use in dairying: discussion paper," *Journal Royal Soc. Med.* 85(1992): 736–739.

8. For a review of literature linking elevated levels of IGF-1 with increased risks of breast, colon and prostate cancers, see Samuel S. Epstein, *What's In Your Milk?, 197–204.*

9. June M. Chan, et al, "Plasma Insulin-Like Growth Factor-1 [IGF-1] and Prostate Cancer Risk: A Prospective Study," *Science.* 279 (January 23, 1998): 563–566.

10. S. E. Hankinson, et al, "Circulating concentrations of insulin-like growth factor 1 and risk of breast cancer," *Lancet* 351, no. 9113 (1998): 1393–1396.

11. R. Torrisi et al, "Time course of fenretinide-induced modulation of circulating insulin-like growth factor (IGF)-i, IGF-II and IGFBP-3 in a bladder cancer chemoprevention trial," *International Journal of Cancer* 87, no. 4 (August 2000): 601–605.

12. Cited in Samuel S. Epstein, *What's In Your Milk?*, 197–204.

13. Geier et al, "Insulin-like growth factor-1 inhibits cell death induced by anticancer drugs in the MCF-7 cells: involvement of growth factors in drug resistance," *Cancer Invest.*13 (1995):480–486.

14. Philipps et al, "Growth of artificially fed infant rats: effect of supplementation with insulin-like growth factor I," *Am. J. Physiol.* 272 (1997): R1532-R1539

15. Lasmezas et al, "Recombinant Human Growth Hormone and Insulin-Like Growth Factor I Induce PRP Gene Expression in PC12 Cell," *Biochem, Biophys. Res. Comm.* 196 (1993):1163–1169.

16. See Samuel Epstein, "Potential Public Health Hazards Of Biosynthetic Milk Hormones," *International Journal of Health Services* 20 (1990):73–84; and Brian Tokar, "Monsanto: A Checkered History," The Ecologist 28, no. 5 (Sept/Oct 1998)

17. Erik Millstone, Eric Brunner and Ian White, "Plagiarism or protecting public health?" *Nature* 371 (October 20, 1994): 647–8.

18. Kronfeld, "Bovine somatotropin," *J. Am. Med. Assn.* 265 (1991):1389.

19. Capuco, et al, "Somatotropin increases thyroxine-5`-monodeiodinase activity in lactating mammary tissue of cow," *J. Endocrinol.* 121(1989):205–211.

20. Mepham, "Public health implications of bovine somatotropin use in dairying: discussion paper," *J. Royal Soc. Med.* 85 (1992):736–739.

21. Baer et al, "Composition and flavor of milk produced by cows injected with recombinant bovine somatotropin," *J. Dairy Sci.* 72 (1989):1424–1434.

22. Mepham, "Public health implications of bovine somatotropin use in dairying: discussion paper," 736–739.

23. Jeffrey Smith, "Spilled Milk," Chapter 3 in *Seeds of Deception* (Yes! Books, 2003).

24. Shiv Chopra, et al, "rBST (Nutrilac) 'Gaps Analysis' Report," rBST Internal Review Team, Health Protection Branch, Health Canada, Ottawa, Canada, April 21, 1998.

25. Smith, "Spilled Milk."

26. Nicholas Bakalar, "Rise in Rate of Twin Births May Be Tied to Dairy Case," *New York Times*, May 30, 2006.

27. Gary Steinman, "Mechanisms of Twinning VII. Effect of Diet and Heredity on the Human Twinning Rate," *Journal of Reproductive Medicine,* May 2006.

28. S.E. Echternkamp et al, "Ovarian Follicular Development in Cattle Selected for Twin Ovulations and Births," *Journal of Animal Science* 82 no. 2 (2004): 459–471; and S. E. Echternkamp et al, "Concentrations of insulin-like growth factor-I in blood and ovarian follicular fluid of cattle selected for twins," *Biology of Reproduction*, 43(1990): 8–14.

29. S. Lien et al, "A primary screen of the bovine genome for quantitative trait loci affecting twinning rate," *Mamm Genome* ll (2000):877–882.

30. Steinman, "Mechanisms of Twinning."

31. Robert P. Heaney et al, "Dietary changes favorably affect bone remodeling in older adults," *Journal of the American Dietetic Association* 99, no. 10 (October 1999):1228–1233.

32. N. E. Allen, et al, "The associations of diet with serum insulin-like growth factor I and its main binding proteins in 292 women meat-eaters, vegetarians, and vegans," *Cancer Epidemiol Biomarkers Prev* ll(2000):1441–1448.

33. N. E. Allen, et al, "Hormones and diet: Low insulin-like growth factor-I but normal bioavailable androgens in vegan men," *Br J Cancer* 83(2000):95–97.

34. W. H. James, "Dizygotic twinning, birth weight and latitude," *Ann Hum Biol* 12(1985):441–447.

35. M. G. Bulmer, "Twinning rate in Europe during the war," *Br Med J* 1 (1959):29–30; and M. G. Bulmer, "The twinning rate in Europe and Africa," *Ann Hum Genet* 24 (1960):121–125; and F. Parazzini, et al, "Temporal trends in twinning rates in Italy around World War II, *Hum Reprod* 13(1998):3279–3280; and I. Nakamura, et al, "Decrease in twinning rate in a hospital in Tokyo during World War II," *Acta Genet Med Gemellol (Roma)* 39 (1990):335–338.

36. Steinman, "Mechanisms of Twinning," 405–10.

37. R.A. Cushman, et al, "Effect of long-term treatment with recombinant bovine somatotropin and estradiol on hormone concentrations and ovulatory response of superovulated cattle," *Theriogenology* 55 (2001): 1533–1547; J.G. Gong, "Influence of metabolic hormones and nutrition on ovarian follicle development in cattle: Practical implications," *Domest. Anim. Endocrinol.* 23 (2002):229–241.

38. Steinman, "Mechanisms of Twinning."

39. "Study by LIJ Obstetrician Finds that a Woman's Chances of Having Twins Can Be Modified by Diet," Press release, North Shore Long Island Jewish Health System, June 07, 2006, http://www.northshorelij.com/body.cfm?id=15&action=detail&ref=808

40. Geoffrey Lean and Jonathan Owen, "The GM 99: Genetically modified ice cream could be coming to Britain," *The Independent on Sunday,* July 9, 2006.

41. "Final Assessment Report Application A544, Ice Structuring Protein as a processing Aid for Ice Crean and Edible Ices," FSANZ, 7-05, 5 October 2005.

42. Joe Cummins, et al., "GM Protein in Ice Cream," ISIS Press Release, July 4, 2006.

43. S. Wildt and T.U. Gerngross, "The humanization of N-glycosylation pathways in yeast," *Nat Rev Microbiol* 3, no.2 (2005): 119–28; and H. Li et al., "Optimization of humanized IgGs in glycoengineered Pichia pastoris, *Nat Biotechnol.* 24, no 2 (2006): 210–5.

44. U. S. Food and Drug Administration Center for Food Safety and Applied Nutrition Office of Food Additive Safety, "Agency Response Letter," GRAS Notice No. GRN 000117, April 17, 2003; an avid ice cream eater in the US, (male, age 13-20) would ingest as much as 0.33 milligrams of ISP per kilogram body weight per day. At 160 pounds, that's 23 milligrams.

45. Joe Cummins, "Environmentalists Ben and Jerry may feed children genetically modified Ice Cream," July 9, 2006 Sustainable Agriculture Network Discussion Group.

PART 1, SECTION 8: RISKS ARE GREATER FOR CHILDREN AND NEWBORNS

1. Florianne Koechlin, "Opening Speech," Epigenetics, Transgenic Plants & Risk Assessment, Proceedings of the Conference, December 1st 2005 (Frankfurtam Main, Germany: Literaturhaus).

2. William Freese and David Schubert, "Safety Testing and Regulation of Genetically Engineered Foods," *Biotechnology and Genetic Engineering Reviews* 21 (November 2004).

3. Ibid.

4. Catherine Gallou-Kabani and Claudine Junien, "Nutritional Epigenomics of Metabolic Syndrome, New Perspective Against the Epidemic," *Diabetes* 54(2005): 1899–1906.

5. Ibid.; see also J. E. Cropley, et al., "Germ-line epigenetic modification of the murine Avy allele by nutritional supplementation," *Proc Natl Acad Sci USA* 103, no. 46 (Nov 14, 2006):17308–17312.

6. "Common Nutrients Fed To Pregnant Mice Altered Their Offspring's Coat Color And Disease Susceptibility," Press release, August 1, 2003, http://www.dukemednews.org/news/article.php?id=6804

7. See for example, Andrew P. Feinberg et al., "The epigenetic progenitor origin of human cancer," *Nature Reviews Genetics*, Vol 7, January 2006, 21; and Christine B. Yoo and Peter A. Jones, "Epigenetic therapy of cancer: past, present and future," *Nature Reviews Drug Discovery*, Vol 5, January 2006, 37.

8. Allison Wilson, PhD, Jonathan Latham, PhD, and Ricarda Steinbrecher, PhD, "Genome Scrambling—Myth or Reality? *Transformation-Induced Mutations in Transgenic Crop Plants Technical Report—October 2004,* http://www.econexus.info

9. W. Doerfler, R. Schubert, "Uptake of foreign DNA from the environment: the gastrointestinal tract and the placenta as portals of entry," *Journal of Molecular Genes and Genetics* 242 (1994): 495–504.

10. Ohn J. Fialka, "EPA Scientists Pressured to Allow Continued Use of Dangerous Pesticides," *Wall Street Journal*, May 25, 2006: A4, http://online.wsj.com/article/SB114852646165862757.html

11. "EPA Scientists Potest Pending Pesticide Approvals—Unacceptable Risk to Children and Political Pressure on Scientists Decried," Press release, Public Employees for Environmental Responsibility, May 25, 2006, http://www.peer.org/news/news_id.php?row_id=691

12. Ibid.

13. *The Guardian*, Mar 13, 1998.

14. Royal Society (UK) "Genetically modified plants for food use and human health—an update," Policy document 4/02, February 2002, http://www.royalsoc.ac.uk

15. Robert Uhlig, "Fears for babies from GM milk," *Daily Telegraph*, February 5, 2002.

16. "A Snapshot of Federal Research on Food Allergy: Implications for Genetically Modified Food," a report commissioned by the Pew Initiative on Food and Biotechnology, June 2002; Luca Bucchini, Ph.D. and Lynn R. Goldman, M.D., MPH, citing H. A. Sampson, L. Mendelson, and J. P. Rosen, "Fatal and near-fatal anaphylactic reactions to food in children and adolescents," *New England Journal of Medicine* 327, no 6(1992):380–4.

17. United States Environmental Protection Agency. "Mammalian toxicity assessment guidelines for protein plant pesticides," U.S. EPA FIFRA Scientific Advisory Panel Report 2000-03B, September 28, 2000.

18. "Elements of Precaution: Recommendations for the Regulation of Food Biotechnology in Canada; An Expert Panel Report on the Future of Food Biotechnology prepared by The Royal Society of Canada at the request of Health Canada Canadian Food Inspection Agency and Environment Canada" The Royal Society of Canada, January 2001: 59.

19. Royal Society (UK) "Genetically modified plants for food use and human health—an update," Policy document 4/02, February 2002, http://www.royalsoc.ac.uk

20. Ibid.

21. Mepham, "Public health implications of bovine somatotropin use in dairying: discussion paper," *J. Royal Soc. Med.* 85 (1992):736–739.

22. Samuel Epstein, "Hormonal Milk Poses Greater Risks Than Just Twinning," Press Release, A Scribe Newswire, June 27, 2006.

23. Samuel Epstein, "Potential Public Health Hazards of Biosynthetic Milk Hormones," Report to FDA Commissioner Young, July 19, 1989.

24. Additional subgroups included, "pregnant and lactating women, the elderly and those with chronic diseases or compromised immune systems." Joint FAO/WHO Food Standard Programme, Codex Alimentarius Commission, "Draft Guideline for the conduct of food safety assessment of foods derived from recombinant-DNA plants," Report of the Third Session of the Codex Ad Hoc Intergovernmental Task Force on Food Derived from Biotechnology, ALINORM 03/34, 2002.

25. David Schubert, personal communication to H. Penfound, Greenpeace Canada, October 25, 2002.

CONNECTING THE DOTS

1. Quoted in Ashok B. Sharma, "ICMR Wants Overhaul Of GM Foods Regulation," *The Financial Express*, July 26, 2004.
2. "A Snapshot of Federal Research on Food Allergy: Impllications for Genetically Modified Food," a report commissioned by the Pew Initiative on Food and Biotechnology, June 2002; Luca Bucchini, Ph.D. and Lynn R. Goldman, M.D., MPH, citing S. A. Bock, A. Munoz-Furlong, and H. A. Sampson, "Fatalities due to anaphylactic reactions to foods," *Journal of Allergy and Clinical Immunology* 107, no 1 (2001): 191–3.
3. J. Ordlee, et al, "Identification of a Brazil-Nut Allergen in Transgenic Soybeans," *The New England Journal of Medicine*, March 14, 1996.
4. V. E. Prescott, et al, "Transgenic Expression of Bean r-Amylase Inhibitor in Peas Results in Altered Structure and Immunogenicity," *Journal of Agricultural Food Chemistry* (2005): 53.
5. A. Pusztai, et al, "Genetically Modified Foods: Potential Human Health Effects," in: *Food Safety: Contaminants and Toxins* (ed. JPF D'Mello) (Wallingford Oxon, UK: CAB International), 347–372, also additional communication with Arpad Pusztai.
6. Mark Townsend, "Why soya is a hidden destroyer," *Daily Express*, March 12, 1999.
7. G. A. Kleter and A. A. C. M. Peijnenburg, "Screening of transgenic proteins expressed in transgenic food crops for the presence of short amino acid sequences indentical to potential, IgE-binding linear epitopes of allergens," *BMC Structural Biology* 2 (2002): 8–19.
8. Netherwood et al, "Assessing the survival of transgenic plant DNA in the human gastrointestinal tract," *Nature Biotechnology*, 22, 02 (February 2004).
9. A. Pusztai and S. Bardocz, "GMO in animal nutrition: potential benefits and risks," Chapter 17, *Biology of Nutrition in Growing Animals*, R. Mosenthin, J. Zentek and T. Zebrowska (Eds.) Elsevier, October 2005.
10. See for example, Scott H. Sicherer et al., "Prevalence of peanut and tree nut allergy in the United States determined by means of a random digit dial telephone survey: A 5-year follow-up study," *Journal of allergy and clinical immunology*, March 2003, vol. 112, n 6, 1203-1207); and Ricki Helm et al., "Hypoallergenic Foods—Soybeans and Peanuts," *Information Systems for Biotechnology News Report*, October 1, 2002.
11. Andreas Rang, et al, "Detection of RNA variants transcribed from the transgene in Roundup Ready soybean," *Eur Food Res Technol* 220 (2005): 438–443.
12. Hye-Yung Yum, Soo-Young Lee, Kyung-Eun Lee, Myung-Hyun Sohn, Kyu-Earn Kim, "Genetically Modified and Wild Soybeans: An immunologic comparison," *Allergy and Asthma Proceedings* 26, no. 3 (May–June 2005): 210-216(7).
13. Ibid.
14. Caroline Cox, "Herbicide Fact Sheet: Glyphosate," *Journal of Pesticide Reform* 24, no. 4 (Winter 2004).
15. Manuela Malatesta, et al, "Ultrastructural Analysis of Pancreatic Acinar Cells from Mice Fed on Genetically modified Soybean," *Journal of Anatomy* 201, no. 5 (November 2002): 409.
16. William Freese, "Genetically Engineered Crop Health Impacts Evaluation: A Critique of U.S. Regulation of Genetically Engineered Crops and Corporate Testing Practices, with a Case Study of *Bt* Corn," Friends of the Earth U.S., http://www.foe.org/camps/comm/safefood/gefood/index.html
17. M. Green, et al., "Public health implications of the microbial pesticide *Bacillus thuringiensis*: An epidemiological study, Oregon, 1985-86," *Amer. J. Public Health* 80, no. 7(1990): 848–852; and M.A. Noble, P.D. Riben, and G. J. Cook, *Microbiological and epidemiological surveillance program to monitor the health effects of Foray 48B BTK spray* (Vancouver, B.C.: Ministry of Forests, Province of British Columbi, Sep. 30, 1992).
18. I.L. Bernstein et al, "Immune responses in farm workers after exposure to *Bacillus thuringiensis* pesticides," *Environmental Health Perspectives* 107, no. 7(1999), 575–582.
19. John M. Burns, "13-Week Dietary Subchronic Comparison Study with MON 863 Corn in Rats Preceded by a 1-Week Baseline Food Consumption Determination with PMI Certified Rodent Diet #5002," December 17, 2002 http://www.monsanto.com/monsanto/content/sci_tech/prod_safety/fullratstudy.pdf
20. "Assessment of Scientific Information Concerning StarLink™ Corn," SAP Report No. 2000-06, December 1, 2000, FIFRA Scientific Advisory Panel Meeting November 28, 2000.
21. Jeffrey M. Smith, "*Bt*-maize (corn) during pollination, may trigger disease in people living near the cornfield," Press Release, February 2004, http://www.seedsofdeception.com/Media-maizepollen.php; and Estabillo, "Farmer's group urges ban on planting *Bt* corn; says it could be cause of illnesses,"
22. "*Bt* cotton causing allergic reaction in MP; cattle dead," *Bhopal*, Nov. 23, 2005, http://news.webindia123.com/news/showdetails.asp?id=170692&cat=Health
23. "Mortality in Sheep Flocks after Grazing on *Bt* Cotton Fields—Warangal District, Andhra Pradesh" *Report of the Preliminary Assessment,* April 2006, http://www.gmwatch.org/archive2.asp?arcid=6494
24. Traavik and Heinemann, *Genetic Engineering and Omitted Health Research.*

25. Luca Bucchini, Ph.D. and Lynn R. Goldman, M.D., MPH, "A Snapshot of Federal Research on Food Allergy"

26. Charles Sheehan, "Scientists see spike in kids' food allergies," *Chicago Tribune*, 9 June 2006, http://www.montereyherald.com/mld/montereyherald/living/health/

27. Arpad Pusztai, "Can science give us the tools for recognizing possible health risks of GM food," *Nutrition and Health*, 2002, Vol 16 Pp 73-84.

28. Fares and El-Sayed, "Fine Structural Changes in the Ileum of Mice Fed on Endotoxin Treated Potatoes and Transgenic Potatoes," 219–233.

29. A. Pusztai and S. Bardocz, "GMO in animal nutrition: potential benefits and risks," Chapter 17, *Biology of Nutrition in Growing Animals*, R. Mosenthin, J. Zentek and T. Zebrowska (Eds.) Elsevier, October 2005.

30. Arpad Pusztai, "Facts Behind the GM Pea Controversy: Epigenetics, Transgenic Plants & Risk Assessment," *Proceedings of the Conference, December 1st 2005* (Frankfurtam Main, Germany: Literaturhaus, 2005).

31. Arpad Pusztai, "Can science give us the tools for recognizing possible health risks of GM food," *Nutrition and Health*, 2002, Vol 16 Pp 73-84.

32. John M. Burns, "13-Week Dietary Subchronic Comparison Study with MON 863 Corn in Rats Preceded by a 1-Week Baseline Food Consumption Determination with PMI Certified Rodent Diet #5002," December 17, 2002 http://www.monsanto.com/monsanto/content/sci_tech/prod_safety/fullratstudy.pdf

33. M. Malatesta, C. Caporaloni, S. Gavaudan, M. B. Rocchi, S. Serafini, C. Tiberi, G. Gazzanelli, "Ultrastructural Morphometrical and Immunocytochemical Analyses of Hepatocyte Nuclei from Mice Fed on Genetically Modified Soybean," *Cell Struct Funct.* 27 (2002): 173–180

34. R. Tudisco, P. Lombardi, F. Bovera, D. d'Angelo, M. I. Cutrignelli, V. Mastellone, V. Terzi, L. Avallone, F. Infascelli, "Genetically Modified Soya Bean in Rabbit Feeding: Detection of DNA Fragments and Evaluation of Metabolic Effects by Enzymatic Analysis," *Animal Science* 82 (2006): 193–199.

35. Comments to ANZFA about Applications A346, A362 and A363 from the Food Legislation and Regulation Advisory Group (FLRAG) of the Public Health Association of Australia (PHAA) on behalf of the PHAA, "Food produced from glyphosate-tolerant canola line GT73," http://www.iher.org.au/

36. "Mortality in Sheep Flocks after Grazing on *Bt* Cotton Fields—Warangal District, Andhra Pradesh" *Report of the Preliminary Assessment,* April 2006, http://www.gmwatch.org/archive2.asp

37. Traavik and Heinemann, *Genetic Engineering and Omitted Health Research.*

PART 2: THE REGULATION OF GM FOODS IS INADEQUATE

1. "Monsanto Bribery Charges in Indonesia by DoJ and USSEC," Third World Network, Malaysia, Jan 27, 2005, http://www.mindfully.org/GE/2005/Monsanto-Indonesia-Bribery27jan05.htm

2. "Greenpeace exposes Government-Monsanto nexus to cheat Indian farmers: calls on GEAC to revoke BT cotton permission," Press release, March 3, 2005, http://www.greenpeace.org/india_en/news/details?item_id=771071

3. Jeffrey M. Smith, *Seeds of Deception*, (Iowa: Yes! Books, 2003), 224.

4. See Federal Food, Drug and Cosmetic Act (FFDCA), http://www.fda.gov/opacom/laws/fdcact/fdctoc.htm

5. Kurt Eichenwald, Gina Kolata, and Melody Petersen, "Biotechnology Food: From the Lab to a Debacle," *New York Times*, January 25, 2001.

6. Dan Quayle, "Speech in the Indian Treaty Room of the Old Executive Office Building," May 26, 1992.

7. William Freese and David Schubert, "Safety Testing and Regulation of Genetically Engineered Foods," *Biotechnology and Genetic Engineering Reviews* 21 (November 2004).

8. See Smith, *Seeds of Deception*; and for copies of FDA memos, see The Alliance for Bio-Integrity, www.biointegrity.org

9. Memos 1991, 1992a, and 1992b below are 3 of 24 internal FDA documents obtained in a Freedom of Information Act request by the Alliance for Bio-Integrity. See www.bio-integrity.org

10. FDA Memo, "Points to Consider for Safety Evaluation of Genetically Modified Foods. Supplemental Information," Memo from Division of Food Chemistry and Technology and Division of Contaminants Chemistry, FDA, to James Maryanski, Biotechnology Coordinator, FDA, November 1, 1991, www.bio-integrity.org/FDAdocs/10/10.pdf

11. FDA Memo, "Revision of Toxicology Section of the *Statement of Policy: Foods Derived from Genetically Modified Plants*," Memo from Samuel I. Shibko, Director, Division of Toxicological Review and Evaluation, FDA to James Maryanski, Biotechnology Coordinator, FDA, January 31, 1992, www.bio-integrity.org/FDAdocs/03/03.pdf

12. FDA Memo, "Comments on Biotechnology Draft Document, 2/27/92." Draft memo from Dr. Louis J. Pribyl (recipient not cited), March 6, 1992, www.bio-integrity.org/FDAdocs/04/04.pdf

13. Freese and Schubert, "Safety Testing and Regulation of Genetically Engineered Foods."

14. Steven M. Druker, "How the US Food and Drug Administration approved genetically engineered foods despite the deaths one had caused and the warnings of its own scientists about their unique risks," Alliance for Bio-Integrity, http://

www.biointegrity.org/ext-summary.html

15. Linda Kahl, Memo to James Maryanski about Federal Register document "Statement of Policy: Foods from Genetically Modified Plants," January 8, 1992, www.biointegrity.org

16. Gerald B. Guest, memo to James Maryanski, "Regulation of Transgenic Plants—FDA Draft Federal Register Notice on Food Biotechnology," February 5, 1992, www.biointegrity.org

17. Louis J. Pribyl, "Biotechnology Draft Document, 2/27/92," March 6, 1992, http://www.biointegrity.org/FDAdocs/04/view1.html

18. "Statement of Policy: Foods Derived from New Plant Varieties," Federal Register 57, no. 104 (May 29, 1992): 22991.

19. William Freese, "Genetically Engineered Crop Health Impacts Evaluation: A Critique of U.S. Regulation of Genetically Engineered Crops and Corporate Testing Practices, with a Case Study of Bt Corn," Friends of the Earth U.S., http://www.foe.org/camps/comm/safefood/gefood/index.html

20. FDA Letter, Letter from Alan M. Rulis, Office of Premarket Approval, Center for Food Safety and Applied Nutrition, FDA to Dr. Kent Croon, Regulatory Affairs Manager, Monsanto Company, Sept 25, 1996. See Letter for BNF No. 34 at http://www.cfsan.fda.gov/~lrd/biocon.html

21. Doug Gurian-Sherman, "Holes in the Biotech Safety Net, FDA Policy Does Not Assure the Safety of Genetically Engineered Foods," Center for Science in the Public Interest, http://www.cspinet.org/new/pdf/fda_report__final.pdf

22. Union of Concerned Scientists, "Evidence of Political Interference, Summary of the FDA Scientist Survey," July 20, 2006 http://www.ucsusa.org/scientific_integrity/interference/fda-scientists-survey-summary.html

23. Gurian-Sherman, "Holes in the Biotech Safety Net, FDA Policy Does Not Assure the Safety of Genetically Engineered Foods."

24. "Health risks of genetically modified foods," editorial, Lancet, 29 May 1999.

25. Freese, "Genetically Engineered Crop Health Impacts Evaluation: A Critique of U.S. Regulation of Genetically Engineered Crops and Corporate Testing Practices, with a Case Study of Bt Corn."

26. Sheldon Krimsky and Nora K. Murphy, "Biotechnology at the Dinner Table: FDA's Oversight of Transgenic Food," Annals, AAPSS, 584 (November 2002).

27. "Elements of Precaution: Recommendations for the Regulation of Food Biotechnology in Canada; An Expert Panel Report on the Future of Food Biotechnology prepared by The Royal Society of Canada at the request of Health Canada Canadian Food Inspection Agency and Environment Canada" The Royal Society of Canada, January 2001.

28. "Good Enough To Eat?" New Scientist (February 9, 2002), 7.

29. Judy Carman, "Is GM Food Safe to Eat?" in R. Hindmarsh, G. Lawrence, eds., Recoding Nature Critical Perspectives on Genetic Engineering (Sydney: UNSW Press, 2004): 82–93.

30. Philip Regal, Professor of Ecology, "Evolution, and Behavior at the University of Minnesota," quoted in "Landmark Lawsuit Challenges FDA Policy on Genetically Engineered Food," http://www.biointegrity.org/Lawsuit.html

31. Suzanne Wuerthele, Sientist's Statements, gmwatch.org, May 29, 2004

32. Bill Lambrecht, Dinner at the New Gene Café (St. Martin's Press, September 2001), 139.

33. "Elements of Precaution," The Royal Society of Canada, January 2001.

34. Friends of the Earth Europe, "Throwing Caution to the Wind: A review of the European Food Safety Authority and its work on genetically modified foods and crops," November 2004.

35. Jeffrey M. Smith, "Genetically Modified Corn Study Reveals Health Damage and Cover-up," Ecologist, October 2005.

36. Ibid.

37. Friends of the Earth Europe and Greenpeace, "Hidden Uncertainties What the European Commission doesn't want us to know about the risks of GMOs," April 2006.

38. Marcello Buiatti: Epigenetic Processes and the "Unintended Effects" of Genetic Engineering, Epigenetics, Transgenic Plants& Risk Assessment, Proceedings of the Conference, December 1st 2005, Literaturhaus, Frankfurtam Main, Germany

39. Food Legislation and Regulation Advisory Group (FLRAG) of the Public Health Association of Australia (PHAA) on behalf of the PHAA, "Comments to ANZFA about Applications A372, A375, A378 and A379," http://www.iher.org.au/

40. Ashok B. Sharma, "ICMR Wants Overhaul Of GM Foods Regulation," Financial Express, New Delhi, India, July 25, 2004; see also "Regulatory Regimen for Genetically Modified Foods the Way Ahead," Indian Council of Medical Research, New Delhi, April 2004, http://icmr.nic.in/reg_regimen.pdf

41. Allison Wilson, et al., "Regulatory regimes for transgenic crops," Nature Biotechnology 23 (2005): 785.

42. Carman, "Is GM Food Safe to Eat?" 82–93.

43. FLRAG of the PHAA of behalf of the PHAA, "Comments to ANZFA about Applications A372, A375, A378 and A379."

44. Gurian-Sherman, "Holes in the Biotech Safety Net, FDA Policy Does Not Assure the Safety of Genetically Engineered Foods."

45. E. Ann Clark, "Food Safety of GM Crops in Canada: toxicity and allergenicity," GE Alert, 2000.

46. European Communities submission to World Trade Organization dispute panel, 28 January 2005.

47. FLRAG, "Comments to ANZFA about Applications A346, A362 and A363," http://www.iher.org.au/

48. FLRAG, "Comments to ANZFA about Applications A372, A375, A378 and A379."

49. Clark, "Food Safety of GM Crops in Canada: toxicity and allergenicity."

50. Freese, "Genetically Engineered Crop Health Impacts Evaluation: A Critique of U.S. Regulation of Genetically Engineered Crops and Corporate Testing Practices, with a Case Study of *Bt* Corn."

51. Gurian-Sherman, "Holes in the Biotech Safety Net, FDA Policy Does Not Assure the Safety of Genetically Engineered Foods."

52. Clark, "Food Safety of GM Crops in Canada: toxicity and allergenicity."

53. Arpad Pusztai, "Why the Mon 863 Study Should Have Been Rejected," press backgrounder, June 22, 2005.

54. M. Cretenet, J. Goven, J. A. Heinemann, B. Moore, and C. Rodriguez-Beltran, "Submission on the DAR for Application A549 Food Derived from High-Lysine Corn LY038: to permit the use in food of high-lysine corn, 2006, www.inbi.canterbury.ac.nz

55. Friends of the Earth Europe, "Throwing Caution to the Wind."

56. FDA Note, "FDA Consultation Note on Monsanto's MON809 and MON810 *Bt* Corn Events," September 18, 1996. See Memo for BNF No. 34 at http://www.cfsan.fda.gov/~lrd/biocon.html

57. Freese and Schubert, "Safety Testing and Regulation of Genetically Engineered Foods."

58. Gurian-Sherman, "Holes in the Biotech Safety Net, FDA Policy Does Not Assure the Safety of Genetically Engineered Foods."

59. Cretenet, et al, "Submission on the DAR for Application A549 Food Derived from High-Lysine Corn LY038."

60. FLRAG, "Comments to ANZFA about Applications A346, A362 and A363."

61. Mae-Wan Ho, "Exposed: More shoddy science in GM maize approval," Science in Society 22 (Summer 2004).

62. Cretenet, et al, "Submission on the DAR for Application A549 Food Derived from High-Lysine Corn LY038."

63. Gurian-Sherman, "Holes in the Biotech Safety Net, FDA Policy Does Not Assure the Safety of Genetically Engineered Foods."

64. William Freese, "The StarLink Affair, Submission by Friends of the Earth to the FIFRA Scientific Advisory Panel considering Assessment of Additional Scientific Information Concerning StarLink Corn," July 17–19, 2001.

65. Freese, "Genetically Engineered Crop Health Impacts Evaluation: A Critique of U.S. Regulation of Genetically Engineered Crops and Corporate Testing Practices, with a Case Study of *Bt* Corn."

66. Jeffrey M. Smith, "Are You Critical of Genetically Engineered Foods? Watch Out." November 2004.

67. Jack Heinemann, letter to Hon. Kim Chance MLC, Centre for Integrated Research in Biosafety, July 31, 2006.

68. Mike Zelina, et al., "The Health Effects of Genetically Engineered Crops on San Luis Obispo County," A Citizen Response to the SLO Health Commission GMO Task Force Report, 2006.

69. Freese, "Genetically Engineered Crop Health Impacts Evaluation: A Critique of U.S. Regulation of Genetically Engineered Crops and Corporate Testing Practices, with a Case Study of *Bt* Corn."

70. Friends of the Earth Europe, "Throwing Caution to the Wind."

71. USDA-Office of Inspector General report, "APHIS controls over issuance of genetically engineered organism release permits," Washington, DC, December, 2005, http://www.usda.gov/oig/webdocs/50601-08-TE.pdf

PART 3: INDUSTRY STUDIES ARE NOT COMPETENT

1. "No-one will insure GM crops," FARM Press Release, October 7, 2003.

2. Christopher Preston, "Peer Reviewed Publications on the Safety of GM Foods: Results of a search of the PubMed database for publications on feeding studies for GM crops," AgBioWorld, December 2004, http://www.agbioworld.org/biotech-info/articles/biotech-art/peer-reviewed-pubs.html; Note: Preston claimed in his paper that 42 studies existed, but his list showed only 41

3. Preston, "Peer Reviewed Publications on the Safety of GM Foods."

4. Senior Lecturer in Weed Management, Univ. Of Adelaide. Comments re: Christopher Preston, 'Peer Reviewed Publications on the Safety of GM Foods. Results of a search of the PubMed database for publications on feeding studies for GM crops'; Unpublished mimeo. [Mounted at AgBioWorld.org],.

5. Jose L Domingo, "Health Risks of GM Foods: Many Opinions but Few Data," *Science* 288, June 9, 2000.

6. Ian F. Pryme and Rolf Lembcke, "In Vivo Studies on Possible Health Consequences of Genetically Modified Food and Feed—with Particular Regard to Ingredients Consisting of Genetically Modified Plan Materials," *Nutrition and Health* 17 (2003): 1–8.

7. A. Pusztai and S. Bardocz, "GMO in animal nutrition: potential benefits and risks," Chapter 17, *Biology of Nutrition in Growing Animals*, R. Mosenthin, J. Zentek and T. Zebrowska (Eds.) (Elsevier, October 2005)

8. Terje Traavik and Jack Heinemann, *Genetic Engineering and Omitted Health Research: Still No Answers to Ageing Questions,*

TWN Biotechnology & Biosafety Series 7, 2007

9.   William Freese, "Genetically Engineered Crop Health Impacts Evaluation: A Critique of U.S. Regulation of Genetically Engineered Crops and Corporate Testing Practices, with a Case Study of *Bt* Corn," Friends of the Earth U.S., http://www.foe.org/camps/comm/safefood/gefood/index.html

10. Freese, "Genetically Engineered Crop Health Impacts Evaluation: A Critique of U.S. Regulation of Genetically Engineered Crops and Corporate Testing Practices, with a Case Study of *Bt* Corn."

11. Sue Kedgley, testimony before the Royal Commission of Inquiry on Genetic Modification, January 29, 2001, as part of the Safe Food Campaign.

12. Michael Kuser, "Tests reveal presence of GM tomatoes in Turkey," *Turkish Daily News*, 26 May 2005, http://www.turkishdailynews.com.tr/article.php?enewsid=14143

13. John Ross, "The Sad Saga of Ignacio Chapela," *Anderson Valley Advertiser*, February 18, 2004.

14. Rex Dalton, "Superweed Study Falters as Seed Firms Deny Access to Transgene," *Nature* 419, no. 655 (Oct. 17, 2002).

15. Source: personal communication by report's author

16. Dalton, "Superweed study falters as seed firms deny access to transgene," 655.

17. "GM Science—Supported by a Tissue of Lies: Revealed: how the GM industry kills off "uncomfortable" research," Press release from GM Free Cymru, February 20, 2006, http://www.gmfreecymru.org/news/Press_Notice21February2006.htm

18. Marc Lappé and Britt Bailey, "American Soybean Association Response," Center for Toxics and Ethics, June 25, 1999, http://www.cetos.org/articles/asaresponse.html

19. Tom Knudson and Edie Lau, "Seeds of Doubt: Globe-trotting genes, welcome or not, modified strains pop up in crops near and far," *Sacramento Bee*, June 7, 2004.

20. Traavik and Heinemann, *Genetic Engineering and Omitted Health Research.*

21. Editorial, "Less Spin, More Science," *Sunday Independent* (London), May 23, 1999.

22. Jeffrey M. Smith, "GM Peas," *Ecologist*, March 2006; and Jeffrey M. Smith, "Science or Nonsense? Jeffrey Smith responds to Hans Lombard," *Noseweekonline*, January 2006.

23. V. E. Prescott, et al, "Transgenic Expression of Bean r-Amylase Inhibitor in Peas Results in Altered Structure and Immunogenicity," *J. Agric. Food Chem.* 2005: 53.

24. Steve Dube, "Ban These GM Foods Now," *Western Mail*, Dec 6, 2005, http://icwales.icnetwork.co.uk/farming/farming/tm_objectid=16451552&method=full&siteid=50082&headline=-ban-these-gm-foods-now--name_page.html

25. "GM crop failure shows rules force," CSIRO, November 19, 2005, http://www.theage.com.au/news/National/GM-crop-failure-shows-rules-force-CSIRO/2005/11/19/1132017013629.html

26. T. J. Higgins, personal communication, 2005.

27. G.E. Seralini, personal communication, 2005.

28. Smith, "GM Peas."

29. J. Lexchin, L. A. Bero, B. Djulbegovic, and O. Clark, "Pharmaceutical industry sponsorship and research outcome and quality: systematic review," *BMJ* 326 (2003):1167–1176.

30. Mark Friedberg, et al, "Evaluation of Conflict of Interest in Economic Analyses of New Drugs Used in Oncology," *JAMA* 282 (1999):1453–1457.

31. Freese, "Genetically Engineered Crop Health Impacts Evaluation: A Critique of U.S. Regulation of Genetically Engineered Crops and Corporate Testing Practices, with a Case Study of *Bt* Corn."

32. S. R. Padgette, N. B.Taylor, D. L. Nida, M. R. Bailey, J. MacDonald, L. R. Holden, R. L. Fuchs, "The composition of glyphosate-tolerant soybean seeds is equivalent to that of conventional soybeans," *J. Nutr.* 126 (1996):702–716.

33. Jeffrey M. Smith, *Seeds of Deception* (Fairfield, IA: Yes! Books, 2003).

34. Doug Gurian-Sherman, "Holes in the Biotech Safety Net, FDA Policy Does Not Assure the Safety of Genetically Engineered Foods," Center for Science in the Public Interest, http://www.cspinet.org/new/pdf/fda_report_final.pdf

35. Pryme and Lembcke, "In Vivo Studies on Possible Health Consequences of Genetically Modified Food and Feed," 1–8.

36. Gurian-Sherman, "Holes in the Biotech Safety Net, FDA Policy Does Not Assure the Safety of Genetically Engineered Foods."

37. FLRAG, "Comments to ANZFA about Applications A346, A362 and A363."

38. "Elements of Precaution: Recommendations for the Regulation of Food Biotechnology in Canada; An Expert Panel Report on the Future of Food Biotechnology prepared by The Royal Society of Canada at the request of Health Canada Canadian Food Inspection Agency and Environment Canada" The Royal Society of Canada, January 2001.

39. FIFRA Scientific Advisory Panel (SAP), Open Meeting, July 17, 2001.

40. Smith, *Seeds of Deception* (Fairfield, IA: Yes! Books, 2003).

41. Gurian-Sherman, "Holes in the Biotech Safety Net, FDA Policy Does Not Assure the Safety of Genetically Engineered Foods."

42. Friends of the Earth Europe, "Throwing Caution to the Wind: A review of the European Food Safety Authority and its work on genetically modified foods and crops," November 2004.

43. E. Ann Clark, "Food Safety of GM Crops in Canada: toxicity and allergenicity," *GE Alert*, 2000.

44. Food Legislation and Regulation Advisory Group (FLRAG) of the Public Health Association of Australia (PHAA) on behalf of the PHAA, "Comments to ANZFA about Applications A372, A375, A378 and A379," http://www.iher.org.au/

45. Smith, "GM Peas."

46. S. Blickling et al., "Structure of dihydrodipicolinate synthase of Nicotiana sylvestris reveals novel quaternary structure," *J. Mol. Biol.* 274 (1997): 608–621.

47. M. Cretenet, J. Goven, J. A. Heinemann, B. Moore, and C. Rodriguez-Beltran, "Submission on the DAR for Application A549 Food Derived from High-Lysine Corn LY038: to permit the use in food of high-lysine corn, 2006, www.inbi.canterbury.ac.nz

48. Mae-Wan Ho, "Exposed: More shoddy science in GM maize approval," *Science in Society* 22 (Summer 2004).

49. Judy Carman, "The Problem with the Safety of Round-Up Ready Soybeans," from Diverse Women for Diversity, 8th August 1999, http://members.iinet.net.au/~rabbit/notjcsoy.htm

50. Judy Carman, "Is GM Food Safe to Eat?" in R. Hindmarsh, G. Lawrence, eds., Recoding Nature Critical Perspectives on Genetic Engineering (Sydney: UNSW Press, 2004): 82–93.

51. FLRAG, "Comments to ANZFA about Applications A372, A375, A378 and A379."

52. Ho, "Exposed: More shoddy science in GM maize approval," *Science in Society* 22 (Summer 2004).

53. Carman, "Is GM Food Safe to Eat?" 82-93.

54. FLRAG, "Comments to ANZFA about Applications A346, A362 and A363."

55. Freese, "Genetically Engineered Crop Health Impacts Evaluation: A Critique of U.S. Regulation of Genetically Engineered Crops and Corporate Testing Practices, with a Case Study of *Bt* Corn."

56. E.C. Scientific Steering Committee. "Risk assessment in a rapidly evolving field: The case of genetically modified plants (GMP)," Scientific Opinion of the Scientific Steering Committee, European Commission, Health & Consumer Protection Directorate-General, October 26–27, 2000.

57. "Genetically Modified Pest-Protected Plants: Science and Regulation," Committee on Genetically Modified Pest-Protected Plants, National Research Council, National Academy of Sciences (2000): 65, http://books.nap.edu/catalog/9795.html; for similar recommendations, and examples of immunologic differences between nearly identical proteins, see "The StarLink Affair," Friends of the Earth, July 2001, sections 9.2 to 9.4, at www.foe.org/safefood/starlink.pdf

58. "Mammalian Toxicity Assessment Guidelines for Protein Plant Pesticides," EPA's Scientific Advisory Panel, SAP Report No. 2000-03B, (Sept. 28, 2000): 14, http://www.epa.gov/scipoly/sap/2000/june/finbtmamtox.pdf

59. William Freese, "A Critique of the EPA's Decision to Reregister *Bt* Crops and an Examination of the Potential Allergenicity of *Bt* Proteins," adapted from comments of Friends of the Earth to the EPA, Dec. 9, 2001, http://www.foe.org/safefood/comments.pdf

60. William Freese and David Schubert, "Safety Testing and Regulation of Genetically Engineered Foods," *Biotechnology and Genetic Engineering Reviews* 21 (November 2004).

61. Freese, "Genetically Engineered Crop Health Impacts Evaluation: A Critique of U.S. Regulation of Genetically Engineered Crops and Corporate Testing Practices, with a Case Study of *Bt* Corn."

62. B. Küster, T. N. Krogh, E. Mørtz, and D. J. Harvey, "Glycosylation analysis of gelseparated proteins," *Proteomics* 1 (2001): 350–361.

63. SAP MT, "Mammalian Toxicity Assessment Guidelines for Protein Plant Pesticides," FIFRA Scientific Advisory Panel, SAP Report No. 2000-03B: 23, http://www.epa.gov/scipoly/sap/2000/june/finbtmamtox.pdf

64. David Schubert, "A different perspective on GM food," *Nature Biotechnology* 20(2002): 969.

65. Freese and Schubert, "Safety Testing and Regulation of Genetically Engineered Foods."

66. Pryme and Lembcke, "In Vivo Studies on Possible Health Consequences of Genetically Modified Food and Feed," 1–8.

67. Cretenet, et al, "Submission on the DAR for Application A549 Food Derived from High-Lysine Corn LY038.

68. B. G. Hammond, J. L. Vicini, G. F. Hartnell, M. W. Naylor, C. D. Knight, E. H. Robinson, R. L. Fuchs, and S. R. Padgette, "The feeding value of soybeans fed to rats, chickens, catfish, and dairy cattle is not altered by genetic incorporation of glyphosate tolerance," *J. Nutr.* 126 (1996): 717–727.

69. A. Pusztai, SOAFED flexible fund project RO818 (a government funded project, coordinated by Dr Arpad Pusztai, involving three Scottish research institutes and described in detail in a recent Danish report (Lembcke 2000)). Audit report of data produced at the Rowett Research Institute (RRI) (21st, August 1998). Copies of the reports were circulated to a number of well-known international scientists prior to the announcement of the memorandum (signed by 23 scientists) in defense of Dr. Pusztai and his team at the RRI. The reports were made public on the Internet site of the RRI under the address http://www.rri.sari.ac.uk/. In a later revision of the site these were withdrawn. This review is based on the circulated copies; and A. Pusztai, "Can science give us the tools for recognizing possible health risks of GM food?" *Nutr. Health* 16(2002): 73–84; and A. Pusztai, G. Grant, S. Bardocz, R. Alonso, M. J. Chrispeels, H. E. Schroeder, L. M. Tabe, and T. J. V. Higgins, "Expression of the insecticidal bean-anylase inhibitor transgene has minimal detrimental effect on the

nutritional value of peas fed to rats at 30% of the diet," *J. Nutr.* 129(1999): 1567–1603.

70. Pryme and Lembcke, "In Vivo Studies on Possible Health Consequences of Genetically Modified Food and Feed," 1–8.
71. Pusztai and Bardocz, "GMO in animal nutrition: potential benefits and risks."
72. Pryme and Lembcke, "In Vivo Studies on Possible Health Consequences of Genetically Modified Food and Feed," 1–8.
73. Hammond, et al, "The feeding value of soybeans fed to rats, chickens, catfish and dairy cattle is not altered by genetic incorporation of glyphosate tolerance," 717–727.
74. Pusztai and Bardocz, "GMO in animal nutrition: potential benefits and risks."
75. Jeffrey M. Smith, "Genetically Modified Corn Study Reveals Health Damage and Cover-up," *Ecologist*, October 2005.
76. Ho, "Exposed: More shoddy science in GM maize approval."
77. Cretenet, et al, "Submission on the DAR for Application A549 Food Derived from High-Lysine Corn LY038."
78. Smith, "Genetically Modified Corn Study Reveals Health Damage and Cover-up."
79. H. P. J. M. Noteborn, M.E. Bienenmann-Ploum, J. H. J. van den Berg, G. M. Alink, L. Zolla, A. Reynerts, M. Pensa, and H. A. Kuiper, "Safety assessment of the *Bacillus thuringiensis* insecticidal Crystal Protein CRY1A(b) expressed in transgenic tomatoes," in *Genetically modified foods. Safety issues,* K. H. Engel, G. R. Takeola and R. Teranishi, eds. (Washington, DC: ACS Symposium Series 605), 134–147.
80. W. Hashimoto, K. Momma, H. J. Yoon, S. Ozawa, Y. Ohkawa, T. Ishige, M. Kito, S. Utsumi, and K. Murata, "Safety assessment of transgenic potatoes with soybean glycinin by feeding studies in rats," *Biosci. Biotechnol. Biochem.* 63(1999): 1942–1946.
81. Pryme and Lembcke, "In Vivo Studies on Possible Health Consequences of Genetically Modified Food and Feed." 1–8.
82. R. Teshima, H. Akiyama, H. Okunuki, J. I. Sakushima, Y. Goda, H. Onodera, J.I. Sawada, and M. Toyoda, "Effect of GM and non-GM soybeans on the immune system of BN rats and B10a mice," *J. Food Hyg. Soc. Japan* 41(2000):188–193.
83. K. J. Kramer, T. D. Morgan, J. E. Throne, F. E. Dowell, M. Bailey, J. A. Howard, "Transgenic avidin maize is resistant to storage insect pests," *Nat. Biotechnol.* 18: 670–674.
84. R. Teshima, T. Watanabe, H. Okunuki, K. Isuzugawa, H. Akiyama, H. Onodera, T. Imai, M. Toyoda, J. Sawada, "Effect of subchronic feeding of genetically modified corn (CBH351) on immune system in BN rats and B10A mice," *J. Food Hyg. Soc. Jpn.* 43(2002): 273–279.
85. Teshima et al., "Effect of GM and Non-GM soybeans on the immune system of BN rats and B10A mice," 188–193.
86. Pusztai and Bardocz, "GMO in animal nutrition: potential benefits and risks."
87. P. Gruber, W. M. Becker, and T. Hofmann, "Influence of the Maillard Reaction on the Allergenicity of rAra h 2, a Recombinant Major Allergen from Peanut Arachis hypogaea, Its Major Epitopes, and Peanut Agglutinin," *J. Agric. Food Chem.* 53(2005): 2289–2296.
88. Cretenet, et al, "Submission on the DAR for Application A549 Food Derived from High-Lysine Corn LY038."
89. Arpad Pusztai, "Can science give us the tools for recognizing possible health risks for GM food?" *Nutrition and Health*, 16 (2002): 73–84.
90. Carman, "The Problem with the Safety of Round-Up Ready Soybeans."
91. Pryme and Lembcke, "In Vivo Studies on Possible Health Consequences of Genetically Modified Food and Feed," 1–8.
92. Susan Bardocz and Arpad Pusztai, "The Pusztais' guide to GMOs and regulation," PowerPoint presentation.
93. Pusztai and Bardocz, "GMO in animal nutrition: potential benefits and risks."
94. Smith, *Seeds of Deception.*
95. Smith, "Genetically Modified Corn Study Reveals Health Damage and Cover-up."
96. Bardocz and Pusztai, "The Pusztais' guide to GMOs and regulation."
97. Smith, "Genetically Modified Corn Study Reveals Health Damage and Cover-up."
98. FLRAG, "Comments to ANZFA about Applications A346, A362 and A363."
99. Pusztai and Bardocz, "GMO in animal nutrition: potential benefits and risks."
100. Ibid.
101. Gilles-Eric Seralini, "Genome Fluidity and Health Risks for GMOs," *Epigenetics, Transgenic Plants & Risk Assessment, Proceedings of the Conference, December 1st 2005* (Frankfurtam Main, Germany: Literaturhaus, 2005).
102. Smith, "Genetically Modified Corn Study Reveals Health Damage and Cover-up."
103. V. L. Maggi, and S. R. Sims, "Evaluation of the Dietary Effects of Purified *B.t.k.* Endotoxin Proteins on Honey Bee Adults," California Agricultural Research, Inc., 1994, unpublished study submitted to the EPA by Monsanto, EPA MRID No. 434392-03; and A. Hilbeck, and M. S. Meier, "Critique of Monsanto's Environmental Safety Assessment for Cry3Bb Bt Corn," *Ecostrat GmbH.,* 2002, submitted to EPA on behalf of the Union of Concerned Scientists, www.ucsusa.org/publication.cfm?publicationID=480
104. US EPA, "Biopesticides Registration Action Document (BRAD)—*Bacillus thuringiensis* Plant-Incorporated Protectants: Environmental Assessment," EPA BRAD (2001a) (October 15, 2001): IIC34, http://www.epa.gov/pesticides/biopesticides/pips/bt_brad2/3-ecological.pdf; and M. Mendelsohn, J. Kough, Z. Vaituzis, and K. Matthews, "Are Bt Crops Safe?" *Nature*

Biotechnology 21, no 9(2003): 1003–1009 (see pg. 1009, Table 6).

105. Hilbeck and Meier, "Critique of Monsanto's Environmental Safety Assessment for Cry3Bb *Bt* Corn."

106. Freese and Schubert, "Safety Testing and Regulation of Genetically Engineered Foods."

107. Steve Kestin and Toby Knowles, Department of Clinical Veterinary Science, University of Bristol, testimony on behalf of Friends of the Earth, before the Chardon LL Hearings of the Advisory Committee on Releases to the Environment, November 2000.

108. Carman, "The Problem with the Safety of Round-Up Ready Soybeans."

109. Seralini, "Genome Fluidity and Health Risks for GMOs."

110. FLRAG, "Comments to ANZFA about Applications A346, A362 and A363."

111. Ibid.

112. Arpad Pusztai, "Genetically Modified Foods: Are They a Risk to Human/Animal Health?" June 2001 Action Bioscience http://www.actionbioscience.org/biotech/pusztai.html

113. "Science or Nonsense?" Jeffrey Smith responds to Hans Lombard, *Noseweekonline*, January 2006.

114. Arpad Pusztai, "Why the Mon 863 Study Should Have Been Rejected," press backgrounder, June 22, 2005.

115. Smith, "Genetically Modified Corn Study Reveals Health Damage and Cover-up."

116. "Draft risk analysis report, Application A382, Food produced from insect protected potato line BT-06," Australia New Zealand Food Authority, Canberra, 2000.

117. GE Foods and Human Health Safety Assessments (fuller citation needed)

118. Pusztai and Bardocz, "GMO in animal nutrition: potential benefits and risks."

119. Pryme and Lembcke, "In Vivo Studies on Possible Health Consequences of Genetically Modified Food and Feed," 1–8.

120. Clark, "Food Safety of GM Crops in Canada: toxicity and allergenicity."

121. Pusztai and Bardocz, "GMO in animal nutrition: potential benefits and risks."

122. Ho, "Exposed: More shoddy science in GM maize approval."

123. Pusztai, "Why the Mon 863 Study Should Have Been Rejected."

124. Smith, "Genetically Modified Corn Study Reveals Health Damage and Cover-up."

125. William Freese, "Organic, not Genetically Engineered," Comments of Friends of the Earth before the FIFRA Scientific Advisory Panel (SAP), Open Meeting on *Bt* Crop Re-Registrations, October 20, 2000.

126. Gurian-Sherman, "Holes in the Biotech Safety Net, FDA Policy Does Not Assure the Safety of Genetically Engineered Foods."

127. W. K. Novak, and A. G. Haslberger, "Substantial equivalence of antinutrients and inherent plant toxicants in genetically modified foods," *Food Chem. Toxicol.* 38(2000):473–483.

128. Marc Lappé and Britt Bailey, "ASA Response," June 25, 1999, http://cetos.org/articles/asaresponse.html

129. "Rammed Down Our Throats," *Noseweek magazine*, September 2005.

130. G. Le Gall, I. J. Colquhoun, A. L. Davis, G. J. Collins, M. E.Verhoeyen, "Metabolite profiling of tomato (lycopersicon esculentum) using 1H NMR spectroscopy as a tool to detect potential unintended effects following genetic modification," *J. Agric. Food Chem.* 51(2003): 2447–2456.

131. Pusztai and Bardocz, "GMO in animal nutrition: potential benefits and risks."

132. Ho, "Exposed: More shoddy science in GM maize approval."

133. Jack Heinemann et al, "Submission on Application A549 Food Derived from High Lysine Corn LY038: to permit the use in food of high lysine corn," Submitted to Food Standards Australia/New Zealand (FSANZ) by New Zealand Institute of Gene Ecology, January 22, 2005.

134. Bardocz and Pusztai, "The Pusztais' guide to GMOs and regulation."

135. Jeffrey M. Smith, "GM Peas," Ecologist, March 2006.

136. Gurian-Sherman, "Holes in the Biotech Safety Net, FDA Policy Does Not Assure the Safety of Genetically Engineered Foods."

137. Susan Bardocz and Arpad Pusztai, "The Pusztais' guide to GMOs and regulation," PowerPoint presentation.

138. Cretenet, et al, "Submission on the DAR for Application A549 Food Derived from High-Lysine Corn LY038."

139. FLRAG, "Comments to ANZFA about Applications A372, A375, A378 and A379."

141. FLRAG, "Comments to ANZFA about Applications A346, A362 and A363."

142. FLRAG, "Comments to ANZFA about Applications A372, A375, A378 and A379."

143. "Consensus Document on Compositional Considerations for New Varieties of Maize (*Zea Mays*): Key Food and Feed Nutrients, Anti-Nutrients and Secondary Plant Metabolites," OECD found at http://www.oecd.org/document/9/0,2340,en_2649_34385_1812041_1_1_1_1,00.html; access date: 2 May 2006.

144. Format for applying to amend the Australia/New Zealand Food Standards Code, Food Produced Using Gene Technology, updated June 2005, http://www.foodstandards.gov.au/_srcfiles/Application%20Format%20-%20GM%20June%2005.doc; access date: May 29, 2006.

145. Ibid.

146. Cretenet, et al, "Submission on the DAR for Application A549 Food Derived from High-Lysine Corn LY038."
147. CAC/GL 44-2003 (p. 2 paragraph 4); as cited in M. Cretenet, et al, "Submission on the DAR for Application A549 Food Derived from High-Lysine Corn LY038."
148. Cretenet, et al, "Submission on the DAR for Application A549 Food Derived from High-Lysine Corn LY038."
149. Format for applying to amend the Australia/New Zealand Food Standards Code.
150. Cretenet, et al. "Submission on the DAR for Application A549 Food Derived from High-Lysine Corn LY038."
151. FLRAG, "Comments to ANZFA about Applications A346, A362 and A363."
152. Gurian-Sherman, "Holes in the Biotech Safety Net, FDA Policy Does Not Assure the Safety of Genetically Engineered Foods."
153. R. S.Sidhu, B. G. Hammond, R. L. Fuchs, J. N. Mutz, L. R. Holden, B. George, T. Olson, "Glyphosate-tolerant corn: the composition and feeding value of grain from glyphosate tolerant corn is equivalent to that of conventional corn (*Zea mays* L.)," *J. Agric. Food Chem.* 48(2000): 2305–2312.
154. Padgette, et al, "The composition of glyphosate-tolerant soybean seeds is equivalent to that of conventional soybeans," 702–716.
155. Pusztai and Bardocz, "GMO in animal nutrition: potential benefits and risks."
156. Ibid., table 2.
157. Ibid.
158. Bardocz and Pusztai, "The Pusztais' guide to GMOs and regulation."
159. FLRAG, "Comments to ANZFA about Applications A346, A362 and A363."
160. T. L. Reynolds, M. A. Nemeth, K. C. Glenn, W. P. Ridley, and J. D. Astwood, "Natural Variability of Metabolites in Maize Grain: Differences Due to Genetic Background," *J. Agric. Food Chem.* 53(2005): 10061–10067.
161. Cretenet, et al, "Submission on the DAR for Application A549 Food Derived from High-Lysine Corn LY038."
162. Bardocz and Pusztai, "The Pusztais' guide to GMOs and regulation."
163. William Freese, "The StarLink Affair, Submission by Friends of the Earth to the FIFRA Scientific Advisory Panel considering Assessment of Additional Scientific Information Concerning StarLink Corn," July 17–19, 2001.
164. SAP III, "A Set of Scientific Issues Being Considered by the Environmental Protection Agency Regarding: Assessment of Scientific Information Concerning StarLink Corn," FIFRA Scientific Advisory Panel, SAP Report No. 2000-06 (December 1, 2000):15.
165. "Statement of Policy: Foods Derived from New Plant Varieties," Food and Drug Administration, Docket No. 92N-0139.
166. Rick Weiss, "Biotech Food Raises a Crop of Questions," *Washington Post*, August 15, 1999: A1.
167. Carl B. Johnson, Memo on the "draft statement of policy 12/12/91," January 8, 1992.
168. EPA Scientific Advisory Panel, "*Bt* Plant-Pesticides Risk and Benefits Assessments," March 12, 2001: 76, http://www.epa.gov/scipoly/sap/2000/october/octoberfinal.pdf
169. Weiss, "Biotech Food Raises a Crop of Questions."
170. D. D. Metcalfe, J. D. Astwood, R. Townsend, H. A. Sampson, S. L. Taylor, and R. L. Fuchs, "Assessment of the Allergenic Potential of Foods Derived from Genetically Engineered Crop Plants," *Critical Reviews in Food Science and Nutrition* 36(S)(1996): S165–186; and FAO-WHO, "Evaluation of Allergenicity of Genetically Modified Foods, Report of a Joint FAO/WHO Expert Consultation on Allergenicity of Foods Derived from Biotechnology," Jan. 22–25, 2001, http://www.fao.org/es/ESN/food/pdf/allergygm.pdf
171. Freese and Schubert, "Safety Testing and Regulation of Genetically Engineered Foods."
172. A. Pusztai and S. Bardocz, "GMO in animal nutrition: potential benefits and risks," Chapter 17, Biology of Nutrition in Growing Animals," R. Mosenthin, J. Zentek and T. Zebrowska (Eds.) (Elsevier, October 2005)
173. T. J. Fu, "Digestion Stability as a Criterion for Protein Allergenicity Assessment," *Ann. NY. Acad. Sci.* 964(2002): 99–110; and references within this article.
174. Cretenet, et al, "Submission on the DAR for Application A549 Food Derived from High-Lysine Corn LY038."
175. R. I. Vazquez Padron, L. Moreno Fierros, L. Neri Bazan, G. A. De la Riva, R. Lopez Revilla, "Intragastric and intraperitoneal administration of Cry1Ac protoxin from *Bacillus thuringiensis* induces systemic and mucosal antibody responses in mice," *Life Sci.* 64(1999): 1897–1912; and R. I. Vazquez Padron, J. Gonzalez Cabrera, C. Garcia Tovar, L. Neri Bazan, R. Lopez Revilla, M. Hernandez, L. Morena Fierros, G. A. De la Riva, "Cry1Ac protoxin from *Bacillus thuringiensis* sp. *kurstaki* HD73 binds to surface proteins in the mouse small intestine," *Biochem. Biophys. Res. Commun.* 271(2000): 54–58.
176. Pusztai and Bardocz, "GMO in animal nutrition: potential benefits and risks."
177. European Communities submission to World Trade Organization dispute panel, 28 January 2005.
178. Bardocz and Pusztai, "The Pusztais' guide to GMOs and regulation."
179. Gurian-Sherman, "Holes in the Biotech Safety Net, FDA Policy Does Not Assure the Safety of Genetically Engineered Foods."

180. Gruber, et al, "Influence of the Maillard Reaction on the Allergenicity of rAra h 2, a Recombinant Major Allergen from Peanut Arachis hypogaea, Its Major Epitopes, and Peanut Agglutinin," 2289–2296.

181. Cretenet, et al, "Submission on the DAR for Application A549 Food Derived from High-Lysine Corn LY038."

182. Ibid.

183. Fu, "Digestion Stability as a Criterion for Protein Allergenicity Assessment," 99–110.

184. J.D. Astwood, J.N. Leach and R.L. Fuch, "Stability of food allergens to digestion in vitro," *Nature Biotech.* 14(1996):1269–1273.

185. Fu, "Digestion stability as a criterion for protein allergenicity assessment," 99-110; and T. J. Fu, U. R. Abbott, C. Hatzos, "Digestibility of food allergens and nonallergenic proteins in simulated gastric fluid and simulated intestinal fluid – a comparative study," *J. Agric. Food Chem.* 50(2002):7154–7160.

186. Gurian-Sherman, "Holes in the Biotech Safety Net, FDA Policy Does Not Assure the Safety of Genetically Engineered Foods."

187. J. E. Ream, "Assessment of the *In vitro* Digestive Fate of *Bacillus thuringiensis* subsp. *kurstaki* HD-1 Protein," unpublished study submitted to the EPA by Monsanto, EPA MRID No. 434392-01 (1994).

188. H. Noteborn, "Assessment of the Stability to Digestion and Bioavailability of the LYS Mutant Cry9C Protein from *Bacillus thuringiensis serovar tolworthi*," submitted to the EPA by AgrEvo, EPA MRID No. 447343-05, 1998, (Cry1Ab was also tested for purposes of comparison); Noteborn, et al, "Safety assessment of the *Bacillus thuringiensis* insecticidal crystal protein CRYIA(b) expressed in transgenic tomatoes," 134–47.

189. Freese, "Genetically Engineered Crop Health Impacts Evaluation: A Critique of U.S. Regulation of Genetically Engineered Crops and Corporate Testing Practices, with a Case Study of *Bt* Corn."

190. Ream, "Assessment of the *In vitro* Digestive Fate of *Bacillus thuringiensis* subsp. *kurstaki* HD-1 Protein."

191. FAO-WHO, "Evaluation of Allergenicity of Genetically Modified Foods,"

192. Cretenet, et al, "Submission on the DAR for Application A549 Food Derived from High-Lysine Corn LY038.

193. Fu, "Digestion Stability as a Criterion for Protein Allergenicity Assessment," 99–110, Table 1.

194. Gurian-Sherman, "Holes in the Biotech Safety Net, FDA Policy Does Not Assure the Safety of Genetically Engineered Foods."

195. Metcalfe, et al., "Assessment of the allergenic potential of foods derived from genetically engineered crop plants," S165-S186; and R. L. Fuchs, and J. D. Astwood, "Allergenicity assessment of foods derived from genetically modified plants," *Food Technol.* 50, no 2(1996): 83–88.

196. Gurian-Sherman, "Holes in the Biotech Safety Net, FDA Policy Does Not Assure the Safety of Genetically Engineered Foods."

197. "Evaluation of Allergenicity of Genetically Modified Foods," Report of a Joint FAO/WHO Expert Consultation on Allergenicity of Foods Derived from Biotechnology, January 22-25, 2001, Rome, Italy, http://www.who.int/foodsafety/publications/biotech/en/ec_jan2001.pdf. Access date 15 May 2006.

198. Bardocz and Pusztai, "The Pusztais' guide to GMOs and regulation."

199. Ibid.

200. (MSL-18182 p. 16)

201. G. A. Kleter, and A. A. Peijnenburg, "Screening of transgenic proteins expressed in transgenic food crops for the presence of short amino acid sequences identical to potential IgE -binding linear epitopes of allergens," *BMC Struct. Biol.* 2(2002): 8.

202. Cretenet, et al, "Submission on the DAR for Application A549 Food Derived from High-Lysine Corn LY038.

203. US EPA, "Biopesticides Registration Action Document (BRAD)—Bacillus thuringiensis Plant-Incorporated Protectants: Product Characterization & Human Health Assessment."

204. S. Gendel, "The use of amino acid sequence alignments to assess potential allergenicity of proteins used in genetically modified foods," *Advances in Food and Nutrition Research* 42(1998): 45–62.

205. SAP MT, "Mammalian Toxicity Assessment Guidelines for Protein Plant Pesticides."

206. US EPA, "Biopesticides Registration Action Document (BRAD)—*Bacillus thuringiensis* Plant-Incorporated Protectants: Product Characterization & Human Health Assessment."

207. Noteborn, "Assessment of the Stability to Digestion and Bioavailability of the LYS Mutant Cry9C Protein from Bacillus thuringiensis serovar tolworthi"; Noteborn, et al, "Safety assessment of the *Bacillus thuringiensis* insecticidal crystal protein CRYIA(b) expressed in transgenic tomatoes," 134–47.

208. Noteborn, "Assessment of the Stability to Digestion and Bioavailability of the LYS Mutant Cry9C Protein from Bacillus thuringiensis serovar tolworthi." (Cry1Ab was also tested for purposes of comparison)

209. Freese and Schubert, "Safety Testing and Regulation of Genetically Engineered Foods."

210. Ibid.

211. Freese, "Genetically Engineered Crop Health Impacts Evaluation: A Critique of U.S. Regulation of Genetically Engineered Crops and Corporate Testing Practices, with a Case Study of *Bt* Corn."

212. Nagui H. Fares, Adel K. El-Sayed, "Fine Structural Changes in the Ileum of Mice Fed on -Endotoxin- Treated Potatoes and Transgenic Potatoes," *Natural Toxins* 6, no. 6 (1998): 219–233.

213. National Research Council, *Genetically Modified Pest-Protected Plants: Science and Regulation.* Washington, DC: National Academy Press, 2000).

214. Bardocz and Pusztai, "The Pusztais' guide to GMOs and regulation."

215. SAP *Bt* Plant-Pesticides, "*Bt* Plant-Pesticides Risk and Benefit Assessments," FIFRA Scientific Advisory Panel Report No. 2000-07(March 12, 2001): 76, http://www.epa.gov/scipoly/sap/2000/october/octoberfinal.pdf

216. Luca Bucchini, Ph.D. and Lynn R. Goldman, M.D., MPH, "A Snapshot of Federal Research on Food Allergy: Implications for Genetically Modified Food," a report commissioned by the Pew Initiative on Food and Biotechnology, June 2002.

217. Gurian-Sherman, "Holes in the Biotech Safety Net, FDA Policy Does Not Assure the Safety of Genetically Engineered Foods."

218. "Assessment of Additional Scientific Information Concerning StarLink Corn," FIFRA Scientific Advisory Panel Report No. 2001-09, July 2001.

219. Masaharu Kawata, "Dr. M. Kawata: Questions CDC and EPA testing of Starlink and allergies," *Renu Namjoshi*, June 28, 2001.

220. Smith, *Seeds of Deception.*

221. Robert Cohen, "Milk, the Deadly Poison," (Englewood Cliffs, New Jersey: Argus Publishing, 1998).

222. Judith C. Juskevich and C. Greg Guyer, "Bovine Growth Hormone: Human Food Safety Evaluation," *Science* 249(1990): 875–884.

223. Samuel Epstein and Pete Hardin, "Confidential Monsanto Research Files Dispute Many bGH Safety Claims," *The Milkweed,* January 1990

224. Text adapted from Jeffrey M. Smith, "Got Hormones—The Controversial Milk Drug that Refuses to Die," *Spilling the Beans,* Dec. 1, 2004.

225. Pat Howard and Arne Hansen, "Why genetic engineering is dangerous," Common Ground (Canada), August 2006, www.commonground.ca/iss/0608181/cg181_GMOs.shtml

226. Health Canada, "Novel Food Decisions," www.hc-sc.gc.ca/fn-an/gmf-agm/appro/index_e.html

227. Robert Mann, "GM-eggplant challenged in Supreme Court of India," Press Release, August 7, 2006. http://www.scoop.co.nz/stories/WO0608/S00085

228. The government (here DEFRA and ACRE) as well as the company in charge of the product (now Bayer Crop Science, formerly known as Aventis) explained in February 2002 in writing that the promoter regulating the *pat* gene (35S CaMV) was plant-specific and would thus not result in gene expression in the unlikely event of HGT. Thus no experiments with bacteria containing the transgene were required." U.K. Department of the Environment, Food and Rural Affairs & Advisory Committee on Releases into the Environment (ACRE) February 2002: *"In the unlikely event that the T25 maize pat gene is transferred to a soil bacterium then it would not be expressed This is because it is linked to the cauliflower mosaic virus promoter that expresses genes in plants - not bacteria."*

   AVENTIS CropScience—written submission to ACRE T25 Maize Hearing, 20 February 2002: *"The cauliflower mosaic promoter, associated with the pat gene is only active in plants, not in bacteria, thus even if horizontal gene transfer did take place, the PAT protein would not be expressed in the soil bacteria without the presence of a suitable promoter."* As cited in Ricarda A Steinbrecher and Jonathan R Latham, "Horizontal gene transfer from GM crops to unrelated organisms," *Econexus* technical paper

229. Barbara Keeler, "News Column," *Whole Life Times,* August 2000.

230. Susan Benson, Mark Arax, and Rachel Burstein, "Growing Concern: As biotech crops come to market, neither scientists—who take industry money—nor federal regulators are adequately protecting consumers and farmers," *Mother Jones,* January/February 1997, http://www.motherjones.com/mother_jones/JF97/biotech_jump2.html

231. Charles Yanofsky, personal correspondence (email) with William Crist, February 21, 2001.

232. "Scientists Warn of GM Crops Link to Meningitis," *Daily Mail,* April 26, 1999.

233. Mae-Wan Ho, "GM Ban Long Overdue, Dozens Ill & Five Deaths in the Philippines," ISIS Press Release, June 02, 2006.

234. Bardocz and Pusztai, "The Pusztais' guide to GMOs and regulation."

235. Ibid.

236. Ibid.

237. "The Committee considered the risk of genetic transfer to the human consumer or the gut micro-organisms of novel genes present in the GM maize through consumption of products made from the processed grain. It concluded that since processing would destroy any DNA present, the risk of genetic transfer from processed products could be discounted." Executive Summary, Advisory Committee on Novel Foods and Processes, Report on Processed Products from Genetically Modified Insect Resistant Maize.

238. Mae-Wan Ho, "Unstable Transgenic Lines Illegal," Institute for Science in Society, Press Release, March 12, 2003, http://www.i-sis.org.uk/UTLI.php

239. Food Standards Agency, UK, "GM food," http://www.eatwell.gov.uk/healthissues/factsbehindissues/gmfood/

240. Gruber, et al, "Influence of the Maillard Reaction on the Allergenicity of rAra h 2, a Recombinant Major Allergen from Peanut Arachis hypogaea, Its Major Epitopes, and Peanut Agglutinin," 2289–2296.

241. Cretenet, et al, "Submission on the DAR for Application A549 Food Derived from High-Lysine Corn LY038."

242. Smith, "GM Peas."

243. Heinemann et al, "Submission on Application A549 Food Derived from High Lysine Corn LY038."

244. Andreas Rang et al, "Detection of RNA variants transcribed from the transgene in Roundup Ready soybean," *Eur Food Res Technol* 220(2005):438–443.

245. Jonathan R Latham, PhD and Ricarda A Steinbrecher, PhD, "Horizontal gene transfer of viral inserts from GM plants to Viruses, GM Science Review Meeting of the Royal Society of Edinburgh on "GM Gene Flow: Scale and Consequences for Agriculture and the Environment" 27 January 2003—amended February 2004.

246. B. W. Falk and G. Bruening, "Will transgenic crops generate new viruses and new diseases," *Science* 263(1994): 1395–1396; "Environmental Assessment and finding of no significant impact for ZW-20 squash," USDA Docket No. 92-127-4; J. Hammond et al, "Epidemiological risks from mixed virus infections and transgenic plants expressing viral genes," *Adv. Virus Res.* 54(1999): 189–314.

247. H. Barker, "Specificity of effect of sap-transmissible viruses in increasing the accumulation of luteoviruses in co-infected cells," *Ann. Appl. Biol.* 115(1989): 71–78; and J. R. Latham et al, "Induction of plant cell division by beet curly top virus gene C4," *Plant J.* 11(1997): 1273–1283.

248. K.O. Simon, J. J. Cardamone, Jr., P. A. Whitaker-Dowling, J. S. Youngner, and C. C. Widnell, "Cellular mechanisms in the superinfection exclusion of vesicular stomatitis virus," *Virology* 177 (1990): 375–9.

249. Falk and Bruening, "Will transgenic crops generate new viruses and new diseases," 1395-1396; USDA, "Environmental Assessment and finding of no significant impact for ZW-20 squash"; and T. Rubio, M. Borja, H. B. Scholthof, A. O. Jackson, "Recombination with host transgenes and effects on virus evolution: An overview and opinion," *MPMI* 12(1999): 87–92.

250. M. Schwartz et al, "A positive strand RNA virus replication complex parallels form and function of retrovirus capsids," *Mol. Cell* 9(2002): 505–514.

251. M. Tepfer, "Risk assessment of virus-resistant transgenic plants," *Ann. Rev. Phytopathol* 40(2002): 467.

252. K. Kasschau and J. C. Carrington, "A counterdefensive strategy of plant viruses: suppression of post transcriptional gene silencingm" *Cell* 95(1998): 461–470; and Tepfer, "Risk assessment of virus-resistant transgenic plants," 467.

253. Falk and Bruening, "Will transgenic crops generate new viruses and new diseases," 1395-1396; AIBS 1995, Beltsville, Maryland; R. Aaziz, M. Tepfer, "Recombination in RNA viruses and in virus-resistant transgenic plants," *J Gen Virol* 80(June 1999): 1339–1346, Part 6; T. Rubio et al, "Recombination with host transgenes and effects on virus evolution: An overview and opinion," *MPMI* 12(1999): 87–92; and J. Hammond et al, "Epidemiological risks from mixed virus infections and transgenic plants expressing viral genes," *Adv. Virus Res.* 54 (1999): 189–314.

254. Falk and Bruening, "Will transgenic crops generate new viruses and new diseases," 1395-1396; Hammond et al, "Epidemiological risks from mixed virus infections and transgenic plants expressing viral genes," 189–314; Rubio et al, "Recombination with host transgenes and effects on virus evolution: An overview and opinion," 87–92.

255. For example R. Briddon et al, "Analysis of the nucleotide sequence of the treehopper-transmitted geminivirus, Tomato pseudo-curly top virus, suggests a recombinant origin," *Virology* 219(1996): 387–394; Zhou et al, "Evidence that the DNA-A of a geminivirus associated with severe cassava mosaic virus disease in Uganda has arisen by interspecific recombination," *J. Gen Virol.* 78(1997): 2101–2111; F. Moonan et al, "Sugarcane yellow leaf luteovirus: An emerging virus that has evloved by recombination between luteoviral and poleroviral ancestors, *Virology* 269(2000): 156–171.

256. Anderson et al, "Characterisation of a cauliflower mosaic virus isolate that is more severe and accumulates to higher concentrations than either of the strains from which it was derived, *MPMI* 5(1992): 48–54; S. Ding et al, "An interspecific hybrid RNA virus is significantly more virulent than either parental virus, *PNAS* 93(1996): 7470–7474; B. Fernandez-Cuartero et al, "Increase in the relative fitness of a plant virus RNA associated with its recombinant nature," *Virology* 203(1994): 373–377.

257. USDA, "Environmental Assessment and finding of no significant impact for ZW-20 squash."

258. O. Voinnet et al, "Suppression of gene silencing: a general strategy used by diverse DNA and RNA viruses of plants," *Proc. Natl. Acad. Sci. USA* 96(1999): 14147–52.

259. Falk and Bruening, "Will transgenic crops generate new viruses and new diseases," 1395–1396; Rubio et al, "Recombination with host transgenes and effects on virus evolution: An overview and opinion," 87–92.

PART 4: FLAWS IN THE ARGUMENTS USED TO JUSTIFY GM CROPS

1. Dan Sullivan, "Is Monsanto's patented Roundup Ready gene responsible for a flattening of U.S. soybean yields that has cost farmers an estimated \$1.28 billion?," Presentation at 2004 Midwest Soybean Conference explores the numbers...and the

potential causes behind them, September 28, 2004, http://www.newfarm.org/features/0904/soybeans/index_print.shtml

2. J. Fernandez-Cornejo and W. D. McBride, "Adoption of Bioengineered Crops," ERS Agricultural Economic Report No. AER810, May 2002, http://www.ers.usda.gov/publications/aer810/

3. C. M. Benbrook, "Troubled Times Amid Commercial Success for Roundup Ready Soybeans: Glyphosate Efficacy is Slipping and Unstable Transgene Expression Erodes Plant Defenses and Yields," Technical Paper No. 4, Northwest Science and Environmental Policy Center, Sandpoint Idaho, May 2001, http://www.biotech-info.net/troubledtimesfinal-exsum.pdf

4. M. A. Martinez-Ghersa, C. A. Worster, and S. R. Radosevich, "Concerns a weed scientist might have about herbicide-tolerant crops: a revisitation," *Weed Technol.* 17 (2003):202–210.

5. R. Eliason, and L. Jones, "Stagnating National Bean Yields," Midwest Soybean Conference, Des Moines, Iowa, 7 Aug 2004.

6. Benbrook, "Troubled Times Amid Commercial Success for Roundup Ready Soybeans."

7. Martinez-Ghersa, et. al, "Concerns a weed scientist might have about herbicide-tolerant crops: a revisitation," 202-210.

8. E. Ann Clark, "Has Ag Biotech Lived Up to Its Promise? (and what should the scientific community do about it?)," Presented at the 2004 Helen Battle Lecture, University of Western Ontario, November 25, 2004.

9. Abdul Qayum and Kiran Sakkhari, "Did *Bt* Cotton Save Farmers in Warangal? A season long impact study of *Bt* Cotton— Kharif 2002 in Warangal District of Andhra Pradesh," AP Coalition in Defence of Diversity & Deccan Development Society, Hyderabad, 2003.

10. "Marketing of *Bt* Cotton in India—Aggressive, Unscrupulous and False…," http://www.grain.org/research_files/Marketing_in_India.pdf

11. Peter Rosset, "Why Genetically Engineered Food Won't Conquer Hunger," *New York Times*, op-ed page, September 1, 1999.

12. Qayum and Sakkhari, "Did *Bt* Cotton Save Farmers in Warangal? A season long impact study of *Bt* Cotton - Kharif 2002 in Warangal District of Andhra Pradesh."

13. Ibid.

14. H. Jhamtani, "*Bt* cotton in Indonesia: A case for liability," Konphalindo. Paper presented at the Third World Network side event Liability and Redress: Lessons from Real Life during the First Meeting of the Parties to the Cartagena Protocol on Biosafety, 26 February 2004, Kuala Lumpur.

15. "Angry Andhra uproots Monsanto," *Financial Express*, June 04, 2005 http://www.financialexpress.com/fe_full_story.php?content_id=92868

16. NewKerala.com, November 14, 2005.

17. Gargi Parsai, "*Bt* cotton seeds fail to germinate," *The Hindu*, Nov 10, 2005.

18. J. Pretty and R. E. Hine, "Rural poverty, food security and sustainable agriculture: findings from research investigating 207 sustainable agriculture projects," DFID-University of Essex "Reducing Poverty through Sustainable Agriculture" Conference, St James's Palace, London, January 2001.

19. Fred Pearce, "An Ordinary Miracle," *New Scientist* 169, no. 2276 (February 3, 2001).

20. Ibid.

21. Talent Ngandwe, "'Conservation agriculture' boosts yields and incomes," SciDev.Net, January 25, 2006.

22. Pearce, "An Ordinary Miracle."

23. Miguel A. Altieri, *Why Are Transgenic Crops Incompatible With Sustainable Agriculture In The Third World?* (Berkeley: University of California, 2003).

24. Frances Moore Lappé, Joseph Collins, and Peter Rosset, *World Hunger: Twelve Myths* (New York: Grove Press, 1998), 8–9.

25. "Agriculture: Towards 2015/30," Food and Agriculture Organization of the United Nations, July 24, 2000.

26. Altieri, *Why Are Transgenic Crops Incompatible With Sustainable Agriculture In The Third World?*

27. Devinder Sharma, "The Great Trade Robbery: World Hunger and the Myths of Industrial Agriculture," in Brian Tokar, ed., *Gene Traders: Biotechnology, World Trade and the Globalization of Hunger* (Burlington, VT: Toward Freedom, 2004), 94, 98.

28. "No evidence that GM will help solve world hunger," ActionAid, UK, May 28, 2003, http://www.gene.ch/genet/2003/Jun/msg00004.html

29. "GM—The Facts (LEAFLET)," a leaflet published by the Soil Association, January, 2003, http://www.foresight-preconception.org.uk/booklet_gmfacts.htm

30. Dr Adrian C. Dubock, of Zeneca Plant Science (now Syngenta), at a conference on "Sustainable Agriculture in the New Millennium" in Brussels, May 28–31, 2000.

31. Greenpeace demands false biotech advertising be removed from TV, Letter, February 9, 2001.

32. "GE rice is fool's gold," Greenpeace, http://archive.greenpeace.org/~geneng/highlights/food/goldenrice.htm; *Note*, developers have since produced a golden rice variety with more beta carotene, but still not enough to meet recommended daily requirements for Vitamin A.

33. Benedikt Haerlin, "Opinion piece about Golden Rice," http://archive.greenpeace.org/~geneng/highlights/food/benny.htm

34. David Schubert, "A Different Perspective on GM Food," *Nature Biotechnology* 20, no. 10(October 2002): 969.

35. "Grains of Delusion," Jointly published by BIOTHAI (Thailand), CEDAC (Cambodia), DRCSC (India), GRAIN, MASIPAG (Philippines), PAN-Indonesia and UBINIG (Bangladesh), February 2001, www.grain.org/publications/delusion-en.cfm

36. Michael Pollan, "The Great Yellow Hype," *New York Times*, March 4, 2001, section 6, page 15.

37. Vitamin Angel Alliance, http://www.vitaminangelalliance.com/vitamina.html

38. Greenpeace demands false biotech advertising be removed from TV, Letter, February 9, 2001.

39. "Grains of Delusion."

40. Pollan, "The Great Yellow Hype."

41. Vandana Shiva, "Genetically Engineered 'Vitamin A Rice': A Blind Approach to Blindness Prevention," in *Redesigning Life? The Worldwide Challenge to Genetic Engineering*, Brian Tokar, ed. (London: Zed Books, 2001).

42. Devinder Sharma, "The Great Trade Robbery: World Hunger and the Myths of Industrial Agriculture."

CONCLUSION

1. NSW National Parks and Wildlife Service, "Rabbits—fact sheet," http://www.nationalparks.nsw.gov.au/npws.nsf/Content/rabbit_factsheet

2. "Environmental damage by wild rabbits: eating the heart out of the country," Australia and New Zealand Rabbit Calicivirus Disease Program, http://www.csiro.au/communication/rabbits/qa2.htm

3. European Communities submission to World Trade Organization dispute panel, 28 January 2005.

4. Nicholas Wade, "Scientists Say They've Found a Code Beyond Genetics in DNA," *New York Times*, July 25, 2006. http://www.nytimes.com/2006/07/25/science/25dna.html

5. Jack Heinemann et al, "Submission on Application A549 Food Derived from High Lysine Corn LY038: to permit the use in food of high lysine corn," Submitted to Food Standards Australia/New Zealand (FSANZ) by New Zealand Institute of Gene Ecology, January 22, 2005.

6. Professor Richard Lacey, microbiologist, medical doctor, and professor of Food Safety at Leeds University, personal communication.

7. Hugh Warwick and Gundala Meziani, "Seeds of Doubt," UK Soil Association, September 2002.

8. "Genetically modified foods, who knows how safe they are?" CBC News and Current Affairs, September 25, 2006.

9. Mike Zelina, et al., The Health Effects of Genetically Engineered Crops on San Luis Obispo County," A Citizen Response to the SLO Health Commission GMO Task Force Report, 2006.

10. Ziauddin Sardar, "Loss of Innocence: Genetically Modified Food," *New Statesman* (UK) 129, no. 4425, (February 26, 1999) 47

11. Abi Berger, "Hot potato," *Student BMJ, Medicine and the media* (April 1999), http://www.studentbmj.com/back_issues/0499/data/0499mm1.htm

12. *Public Sentiment About Genetically Modified Food* (2006 update). The Pew Initiative on Food and Biotechnology, December 2006, http://pewagbiotech.org/polls/

13. See for example, *GM Nation? The findings of the public debate*, http://www.gmnation.org.uk/ut_09/ut_9_6.htm#summary

14. Bruce Mohl, "2 dairies to end use of artificial hormones," *Boston Globe*, September 25, 2006.

15. Andrew Pollack, "Which Cows Do You Trust," *New York Times*, October 7th, 2006.

16. Email from Starbucks to consumers who had complained about rbGH, December 2006.

17. Carey Gillam, "Biotech dairy debate spills across U.S. markets," *Reuters*, Jan 18 2007.

18. *Public Sentiment About Genetically Modified Food* (2006 update). The Pew Initiative on Food and Biotechnology, December 2006, http://pewagbiotech.org/polls/

19. "Hot New Consumer and Retail Trends," The Natural Marketing Institute, Presented at Expo West, March 24, 2006.

20. "Caring for Life: Genetics, Agriculture, and Human Life," Discussion-document by the Working Group on Genetic Engineering of the Justice, Peace and Creation Team, Geneva, June 2005 http://www.wcc-coe.org/wcc/what/jpc/geneticengineering.pdf

21. "Some Past Escapes," side bar from "Out of Bounds," *Nature*, 10 January 2007, www.nature.com/news/2007/070108/box/445132a_BX1.html

22. "Communication Programmes for Europabio," Prepared by Burston Marsteller, Government and Public Affairs, January 1997.

23. Guy Cook, *Genetically Modified Language* (London and New York: Routledge, 2004).

24. "Transformation-induced Mutations in Transgenic Plants: Analysis and Biosafety Implications," *Biotechnology and Genetic Engineering Reviews* 23 (December 2006): 209–237.

APPENDIX

1. "Summary of All GRAS Notices," CFSAN/Office of Food Additive Safety, FDA, Accessed January 2007, http://www.cfsan.fda.gov/~rdb/opa-gras.html
2. M. Wolf, "World's Top Sweetener is Made with GM Bacteria," *The Independent*, June 6, 1999 www.wnho.net/gmbacteria.htm
3. Woodrow Monte, "Aspartame: Methanol And the Public Health", *Journal of Applied Nutrition*, Volume 36, Number 1, 1984. www.dorway.com/monte84.html
4. Ralph G. Walton, et al., "Adverse Reactions to Aspartame: Double-Blind Challenge in Patients from a Vulnerable Population," *Biol. Psychiatry* v.34 pp.13-17 1993
5. Woodrow Monte, "Aspartame: Methanol And the Public Health", *Journal of Applied Nutrition*, Volume 36, Number 1, 1984. www.dorway.com/monte84.html
6. Personal communication from Jeffrey Bada to H. J. Roberts. Bada is Professor of Chemistry at the University of California and researcher at the Amino Acid Dating Laboratory of the Scripps Institution of Oceanography.
7. Russell L. Blaylock, Excitotoxins: The Taste That Kills, Health Press, Sante Fe, NM, 1997
8. Russell L. Blaylock, Excitotoxins: The Taste That Kills, Health Press, Sante Fe, NM, 1997
9. Morando Soffritti, et al., Aspartame induces lymphomas and leukaemias in rats, Eur. J. Oncol., vol. 10, n. 2, pp. 107-116, 2005
10. Mike Adams, Interview with Dr. Russell Blaylock on devastating health effects of MSG, aspartame and excitotoxins, NewsTarget.com September 27 2006, http://www.newstarget.com/020550.html

Notes to Human Health Assessment Table (page 228)

(1)   "The Cry1Ab protein was digested at a similar, if slightly faster, rate than the E. coli-derived Cry9C protein in simulated gastric fluid." (Aventis CropScience 2000, "Cry9C Protein: The Digestibility of the Cry9C Protein by Simulated Gastric and Intestinal Fluids," study submitted to the EPA by Aventis CropScience, p. 17). In another study, Noteborn[1] found that it took two hours to achieve > 90% degradation of Cry1Ab(5) in SGF (165 µg/ml SGF, pH = 2.0) Noteborn, p. 21, Annex 1 – Table 1, p. 31.

(2)   "Studying the Cry1Ab5 protein a relatively significant thermostability was observed which was comparable to that of the Lys mutant Cry9C protein." Noteborn.[2]

(3)   "…the initial alignment between Cry1A(b) and vitellogenin located subsequences in which 9 to 11 amino acids were identical (82% similarity). Realignment indicated that these regions contained stretches of 11 biochemically similar and 12 evolutionarily similar amino acids (100% similarity over 11 or 12 amino acids)." "For example, the similarity between Cry1A(b) and vitellogenin might be sufficient to warrant additional evaluation."[3] The EPA apparently did not consider this study in its reassessment of Cry1Ab corn. The Agency states merely that companies did not submit structural comparisons: "Amino acid homology comparisons for Cry1Ab, Cry1Ac and Cry3A against the database of known allergenic and toxic proteins were not submitted."[4]

(4)   Monsanto conducted this study under conditions that proved extremely favorable to rapid digestion of the Cry1Ab/Ac hybrid protein: pH = 1.2, 2 µg test protein / ml SGF. Experts now recommend testing with much higher concentrations of test protein at a milder (at least pH = 2.0).

(5)   "Inactive" here means "unable to kill insects" in bioassays, which provide little or no information about degradation of the protein into amino acids and small peptides, which is what should have been measured (e.g. by HPLC or SDS-PAGE)

(6)   "Cry1A(c) has the same sequence as Cry1A(b) in the region involved, and therefore produced the same alignments, but this was not considered an independent alignment because the proteins are closely related."[5]

(7)   EPA fails to cite the pH value of SGF. If test conducted at pH = 1.2, it should be repeated at pH = 2.0. See note (4).

(8)   Many experts recommend a more stringent test than one based on 8 contiguous amino acids.

(9)   "No heat stability studies were available for Cry3A."[6]

(10)   "First, the initial alignment between Cry3A and β-lactoglobulin located subsequences in which 7 of 10 amino acids matched exactly. Realignment with both the evolutionary and biochemical matrices indicated that the intercalary amino acids were similar, meaning that the alignment was 100% similar over 10 amino acids."[7] The EPA apparently did not consider this study in its reassessment of Bt crops, stating merely that "additional amino acid sequence homology" data are needed to "complete product database" for Cry3A NewLeaf potatoes.[8]

---

1. Noteborn, "Assessment of the Stability to Digestion and Bioavailability of the LYS Mutant Cry9C Protein from *Bacillus thuringiensis serovar tolworthi*."

2. Ibid.

3. Steven M. Gendel, "The use of amino acid sequence alignments to assess potential allergenicity of proteins used in genetically modified foods," *Adv. in Food and Nutrition Research* 42(1998): 58–60.

4. US EPA, "Biopesticides Registration Action Document: Revised Risks and Benefits Sections—*Bacillus thuringiensis* Plant-Pesticides."

5. Gendel, "The use of amino acid sequence alignments to assess potential allergenicity of proteins used in genetically modified foods," 58–60.

6. US EPA, "Biopesticides Registration Action Document: Revised Risks and Benefits Sections—*Bacillus thuringiensis* Plant-Pesticides."

7. Gendel, "The use of amino acid sequence alignments to assess potential allergenicity of proteins used in genetically modified foods," 58–60.

8. US EPA "Biopesticides Registration Action Document: Revised Risks and Benefits Sections—*Bacillus thuringiensis* Plant-Pesticides."

Additional sources on *Bt*-toxin

Terje Traavik and Jack Heinemann include this excellent set of *Bt*-related citations in their *Genetic Engineering and Omitted Health Research: Still No Answers to Ageing Questions*, published by Third World Network in 2007.

Human and monkey cells exposed to *Bt*-toxins from the extra- or intra-cellular environment are killed or functionally disabled (Taybali and Seligy, 2000). Human cell exposure assays of Bacillus thuringiensis commercial insecticides: Production of Bacillus cereus-like cytolytic effects from outgrowth of spores. Environ Health Perspect online, 18 August 2000; Tsuda et al. (2003). Cytotoxic activity of Bacillus thuringiensis Cry proteins on mammalian cells transferred with cadherine-like Cry receptor gene of Bombyx mori (silkworm). Biochem J 369: 697–703;

Namba et al. (2003). The cytotoxicity of Bacillus thuringiensis subsp. coreanensis A 1519 strain against the human leukemic T cell. Biochimica et Biophysica Acta 1622: 29-35). Influenza A infections in mice were changed from silent to lethal encounters by co-exposing the animals to *Bt*-toxin (Hernandez et al. (2000). Super-infection by Bacillus thuringiensis H34 or 3a3b can lead to death in mice infected with the influenza A virus. FEMS Immunology and Med Microbiol 209: 177-181). Farmworkers exposed to *Bt* spores developed IgG and IgE antibodies to *Bt*-toxin (Cry1Ab) (Taylor et al. (2001). Will genetically modified foods be allergenic? Journal of Allergy and Clinical Immunology, May 2001, 765-771). The *Bt*-toxin Cry1Ac was found to have very strong direct and indirect immunological effects in rodents (Vazquez et al. (2000). Characterization of the mucosal and systemic immune response induced by Cry1Ac protein from Bacillus thuringiensis HD 73 in mice. Brazilian Journal of Medical and Biological Research 33: 147–155;

Moreno-Fierros et al. (2000). Intranasal, rectal and intraperitoneal immunization with protoxin Cry1Ac from Bacillus thuringiensis induces compartmentalized serum, intestinal, vaginal and pulmonary immune response in Balb/c mice. Microbes and Infection 2: 885–890; Moreno-Fierros et al. (2002). Slight influence of the estrous cycle stage on the mucosal and systemic specific antibody response induced after vaginal and intraperitoneal immunization with protoxin CryA1c from Bacillus thuringiensis in mice. ELSEVIER Life Sciences 71: 26672680).

Earthworms exposed to *Bt*-toxin Cry1Ab experience weight loss (Zwahlen et al. (2003). Effects of transgenic *Bt* corn litter on the earthworm Lumbricus terrestris. Molecular Ecology 12: 1077–1086). Cattle fed the *Bt* 176 maize variety demonstrated undegraded Cry1Ab through the whole alimentary tract, and the intact toxin was shed in faeces (Einspanier et al. (2004). Tracing residual recombinant feed molecules during digestion and rumen bacterial diversity in cattle fed transgene maize. Eur Food Res Technol 218: 269-273). Cry1Ab is much more resistant to degradation under field soil conditions than earlier assumed (Zwahlen et al. (2003). Degradation of the Cry1Ab protein within transgenic Bacillus thuringiensis corn tissue in the field. Mol Ecol 12: 765–775). Potentially IgE-binding epitopes have been identified in two *Bt*-toxins (Kleter and Peijnenburg (2002). Screening of transgenic proteins expressed in transgenic food crops for the presence of short amino acid sequences identical to potential IgE-binding linear epitopes of allergens. BMC Structural Biology 2:8), and it should be added that many IgE-binding epitopes are conformationally not linearly determined. Finally, it is a matter of concern that *Bt*-toxins have lectin characteristics (Akao et al. (2001). Specificity of lectin activity of Bacillus thuringiensis parasporal inclusion proteins. J Basic Microbiol. 41(1): 3-6). Lectins are notorious for finding receptors on mammalian cells. This may lead to internalization and intracellular effects of the toxins. Occupational exposure to novel proteins, and potential allergic sensitization, has had little study, but could be of public health significance. An amazing number of foods have been proven to evoke allergic reactions by inhalation (Bernstein et al. (2003). Clinical and laboratory investigation of allergy to genetically modified foods. Genetically Modified Foods, Mini-Monograph, Volume 111, No. 8, June 2003). In this connection the findings of serum IgG/IgE antibodies to B. thuringiensis spore extracts (Bernstein et al. (1999). Immune responses in farm workers after exposure to Bacillus thuringiensis pesticides. Environmental Health Perspectives 107(7): 575-582), in exposed farm workers should be given further attention. Inhalant exposure to *Bt*-toxin containing GMP materials may take place through pollen in rural settlements and also through dust in workplaces where foods are handled or processed.

INDEX

ARM. *See* antibiotic resistant marker
(ARM) genes
Arthur Anderson Consulting Group,
249
aspartame, 260
assumptions. *See* safety-related
assumptions
Australia, 4, 10
Australia New Zealand Food Authority
(ANZFA), 8, 101, 183, 184, 185,
203
Aventis, *See* Bayer CropScience
Azevedo, Kirk, Monsanto and, 1, 5–6

B

Bacillus thuringiensis (Bt), 94, 95
bacteria, 7, 117, 127, 129. *See also* gut
bacteria
antibiotic-resistant, 133
CaMV and, 135
identification of transgenic, 131
oral, 139
soil, pesticide from, 94, 95
bacterial infection method, 13
bacterium method, gene insertion, 9
Banerji, Debashish, 31
banning, 57, 133, 190
Bt 176 corn approval and, 133, 190
Bt 176 corn, Spain's, 133
peas, PR use of, 197–98
rbGH, approval and, 157
Bardocz, Susan, 71, 87, 133, 134, 194,
208, 212, 216, 220, 223, 224, 235
barnase, 100, 101
Barrett's esophagus, 23
barstar, 101
base pairs, 13
extra, 65
bases, 13
Bayer CropScience, 7, 55, 99, 115, 129,
145, 149
barnase contradiction of, 101
lawsuits of, 251
Baylor College of Medicine, 37
BBC, 138
Belgian Biosafety Advisory Council, 115
Benbrook, Charles, 240
beta-carotene, 243–44
Big Biotech, 195
biochemistry
evolution/study of, 87
human/rat similarity of, 49
Bioscience Resource Project, 106, 140
biotech companies, 7, 13, 248–49. *See
also* advocates; industry studies

circular logic of, 249
data ignored by, 153
debate avoidance by, 252
FDA and, 177–78
GM food tests of, 115
independent studies thwarted/
influenced by, 189, 194–97
public relations and, 180
regulation pressure of, 176–78,
194–95, 230
safety regulated by, 2–3, 176–78
science v., 176–78
self-regulating nature of, 198
strategies of, 252–53
study secrecy of, 199, 200
biotechnology, 13. *See also* advocates
(GM); arguments; safety-related
assumptions
application of, 122
power of, 179
irreversibility of, 238
recombinant DNA, 13, 141
*Biotechnology and Genetic Engineering
Reviews,* 10, 165, 177, 222
blood sugar, 27
blood test, StarLink protein, 229–30
BollGard Cotton, 228
Boston Globe, 250
bovine growth hormone. *See*
recombinant bovine growth
hormone
Boyles, John, 51
Brazil nut, 90, 91
breast cancer, 157
breathing
food processing dust, 138, 139
GM crop pollen, 34–35, 235
bribery, 157, 176, 230
Brunner, Eric, 167
Bt (Bacillus thuringiensis), 94, 95, 231
Bt 176 corn, 38–39, 115
ARM genes in, 133
banning/approval of, 133, 190
Bt corn, 26–27, 37, 54–55, 93, 115, 117,
125, 133
animals avoiding, 58, 59
Bt toxin consumed in, 97, 137
pollen, 34–35, 235
test data on, by company, 228
test methodology for, 216, 227, 228
Bt cotton, 30, 31, 32–33, 241
farmer suicides and, 241
Bt crops, 29, 93, 94, 95
Bt spray v., 96, 97
Bt gene transfer, 136, 137
Bt protein, 43, 91, 93, 95, 97, 99

Bt spray, 95, 231
Bt crop v., toxicity of, 96, 97
Bt-toxin, 4, 6, 26, 28–29, 33, 94, 95, 119,
136, 137, 151, 169–71, 266
allergic reactions to, 4, 26, 94, 95, 137
digestion and, 28–29, 223
immune response to, 97, 136, 169–70
spray v. crops, 96, 97
test methodology for, 205
Buiatti, Marcello, 116, 183
Burroughs, Richard, 230

C

CAC. *See* Codex Alimentarius
Commission
cadaverine, 103, 187
Calgene, 25, 59, 232
Campaign for Healthier Eating, 250
CaMV. *See* cauliflower mosaic virus
Canada. *See also* Royal Society of
Canada
cross-pollination in, 121
regulators/regulations in, 180, 184,
185, 199, 230, 231–32
studies submitted in, 212
cancer, 29, 83, 105, 147
IGF-1 in milk and, 157
canola, 232
contamination/recall of, 251
percentage of GM, 257
canola oil, 52–53, 86, 101, 185, 201, 217
carbohydrate problems, potatoes and, 86
Carman, Judy, 3, 10–11, 27, 28, 131, 183,
201–2, 203, 211, 217
case studies, IRT collecting, 256
cauliflower mosaic virus (CaMV),
promoter, 8, 14, 71, 74, 75, 129,
131, 135, 137
CDC. *See* Centers for Disease Control
cDHDPS, soil bacteria comparison to,
201, 205–6
cell growth, *22,* 22–23, 28–29
cells
damaged, 28–29
human, death of, 79
liver, 41
metabolism and, 41
pancreatic, 43
testicular, 44–45, 147
Center for the Biology of Natural
Systems, 116
Center for Veterinary Medicine (CVM),
151
Centers for Disease Control (CDC), 61
Centre for Integrated Research on

About the Author

International best-selling author Jeffrey M. Smith is a leading spokesperson on the health dangers of genetically modified organisms (GMOs). His globally respected research and magnetic communication style captured public attention in 2003 with his first book on the serious yet unknown side effects of genetically engineered foods, *Seeds of Deception*. *Seeds* became the world's best selling book on the health risks of GMOs and is credited with motivating changes in consumer buying habits to safer, non-GMO foods. In *Genetic Roulette*, Mr. Smith reveals insider documents about GMO safety trials that are sure to evoke strong emotions in the reader. *Genetic Roulette* shows how the world's most powerful Ag biotech companies bluff and mislead critics, Congress and the FDA about food safety research for the products Americans buy everyday.

Mr. Smith has counseled world leaders from every continent, influenced the first state laws regulating GMOs, and is now uniting leaders for The Campaign for Healthier Eating in America, a revolutionary industry and consumer movement to remove all GMOs from the natural food industry. A popular keynote speaker, he has lectured in 25 countries and has been quoted by government leaders and hundreds of media outlets across the globe including, *The New York Times*, *Washington Post*, BBC World Service, *Nature*, *The Independent*, *Daily Telegraph*, *New Scientist*, *The Times* (London), Associated Press, Reuters News Service, and *Genetic Engineering News*.

Mr. Smith directs the Campaign for Healthier Eating in America from the Institute for Responsible Technology, where he is executive director. He is also the producer of the docu-video series, *The GMO Trilogy* and writes an internationally syndicated monthly column, *Spilling the Beans*.

The Institute for Responsible Technology, www.responsibletechnology.org, nonprofit organization dedicated to public education, works on major public initiatives with scientists and concerned citizens from around the world to shine a spotlight on the dangers of GMOs. Prior to founding the Institute, Mr. Smith was the vice president of marketing communications for a GMO detection laboratory and a consultant to leading industry groups and organizations. Mr. Smith has written extensively on the GMO issue for more than a decade. He lives with his wife in Iowa, surrounded by genetically modified soybeans and corn.

More products by Jeffrey M. Smith

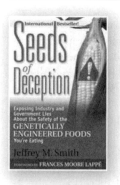

Seeds of Deception: Exposing Industry and Government Lies about the Safety of the Genetically Engineered Foods You're Eating

By Jeffrey M. Smith

Seeds of Deception is the world's best-selling and #1 rated book on GM foods. It reads like a thriller. Hard-to-put-down stories expose how industry manipulation and political collusion—not sound science—allowed dangerous genetically engineered food into our diet. Scientists were offered bribes or threatened. Evidence was stolen. Data was omitted or distorted. Government employees who complained were harassed, stripped of responsibilities, or fired. FDA officials withheld information from Congress after a genetically modified supplement killed nearly a hundred people and disabled thousands. $17.95 for 1. $12.50 ea. for 6 or more. $270 for a case of 27.

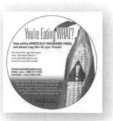

You're Eating WHAT? Stop eating genetically engineered foods and please copy this for your friends.

Jeffrey Smith presents a one hour talk on this popular audio CD.
At www.seedsofdeception.com, you can listen, download it onto a CD or iPod, or purchase copies for only $1.20.

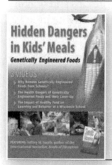

Hidden Dangers in Kids' Meals: Genetically Engineered Foods, DVD

By Jeffrey M. Smith

Shocking research results, inadequate regulations, and warnings from eminent scientists explain why GM foods are dangerous and should be removed from kids' meals. The dramatic story of how student behavior in a Wisconsin school was transformed with a healthy diet provides added motivation to make a change. $14.95

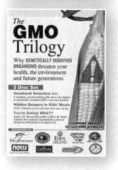

The GMO Trilogy

Combines *Hidden Dangers in Kids' Meals* and *You're Eating WHAT?* (described above), with *Unnatural Selection*, a stunning, award-winning film that reveals several harsh consequences of genetic engineering worldwide: A failed GM cotton crop prompts farmer suicides in India. GM pigs are born with ghastly mutations in the United States. Windborne GM canola threatens farms in Canada, forcing one farmer to the Supreme Court. A company breeds giant GM salmon, despite its threat to natural fish populations. Alarming findings convince a scientist that GMOs may lead to a catastrophe. And corporations deceive the public, while trying to patent and control the food supply. It features Vandana Shiva, Andrew Kimbrell, Percy Schmeiser, and others.

By Bertram Verhaag and Gabriele Kröber. $19.95

Order online at www.seedsofdeception.com or call 1.888.717.7000 (orders only), Fax: 1.888.FAX (329).7000